Essentials *of* Rehabilitation Research

A *Statistical Guide to* Clinical Practice

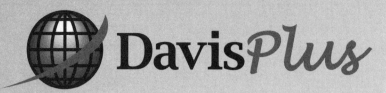

Davis*Plus*

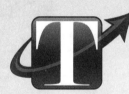

Online Resource Center

Davis*Plus* is your online source for a wealth of learning resources and teaching tools, as well as electronic and mobile versions of our products.

Visit **davisplus.fadavis.com**

STUDENTS

Unlimited FREE access.
Sign up today to see what's available for your title.

INSTRUCTORS

Upon Adoption.
Password-protected library of title-specific, online course content.

Taber's online resources are now available across many of the **DavisPlus** resource pages.

Look for this icon **T** to find Taber's resources!

Explore more online resources from F.A.Davis

DAVIS'S DRUG GUIDE ONLINE

www.DrugGuide.com

The complete Davis's Drug Guide for Nurses® database with over 1,100 monographs on the web.

Taber's Online

www.Tabers.com

The power of Taber's® Cyclopedic Medical Dictionary on the web. Find more than 60,000 terms, 1,000 images, and more.

DAVIS'S Laboratory and Diagnostic Tests with Nursing Implications

www.LabDxTest.com

The complete database for Davis's Comprehensive Handbook of Laboratory and Diagnostic Tests with Nursing Implications online. Access hundreds of detailed monographs.

powered by
unbound
MEDICINE

www.FADavis.com

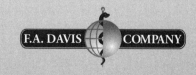

F.A. DAVIS COMPANY

Essentials *of* Rehabilitation Research

A *Statistical Guide to* Clinical Practice

Dr. Richard Di Fabio, PhD, PT

Professor
Fesler-Lampert Chair in Aging Studies (2002–2003)
Department of Physical Medicine & Rehabilitation
University of Minnesota
Minneapolis, MN

F.A. Davis Company • Philadelphia

F. A. Davis Company
1915 Arch Street
Philadelphia, PA 19103
www.fadavis.com

Copyright © 2013 by F. A. Davis Company

All rights reserved. This product is protected by copyright. No part of it may be reproduced, stored in a retrieval system, or transmitted in any form or by any means, electronic, mechanical, photocopying, recording, or otherwise, without written permission from the publisher.

Printed in the United States of America

Last digit indicates print number: 10 9 8 7 6 5 4 3 2 1

Acquisitions Editor: Melissa Duffield
Manager of Content Development: George W. Lang
Developmental Editor: Stephanie Kelly
Manager of Art and Design: Carolyn O'Brien

As new scientific information becomes available through basic and clinical research, recommended treatments and drug therapies undergo changes. The author(s) and publisher have done everything possible to make this book accurate, up to date, and in accord with accepted standards at the time of publication. The author(s), editors, and publisher are not responsible for errors or omissions or for consequences from application of the book, and make no warranty, expressed or implied, in regard to the contents of the book. Any practice described in this book should be applied by the reader in accordance with professional standards of care used in regard to the unique circumstances that may apply in each situation. The reader is advised always to check product information (package inserts) for changes and new information regarding dose and contraindications before administering any drug. Caution is especially urged when using new or infrequently ordered drugs.

Library of Congress Cataloging-in-Publication Data

Di Fabio, Richard P.
  Essentials of rehabilitation research : a statistical guide to clinical practice / Richard Di Fabio.
     p. ; cm.
  Includes bibliographical references and index.
  ISBN 978-0-8036-2564-8 (pbk. : alk. paper)
  I. Title.
  [DNLM: 1. Disabled Persons—rehabilitation. 2. Health Services Research—methods. 3. Rehabilitation—methods. 4. Research Design. 5. Statistics as Topic—methods. WB 320]
  LC-classification not assigned
  617'.03072—dc23

                                                                    2011025987

Authorization to photocopy items for internal or personal use, or the internal or personal use of specific clients, is granted by F. A. Davis Company for users registered with the Copyright Clearance Center (CCC) Transactional Reporting Service, provided that the fee of $.25 per copy is paid directly to CCC, 222 Rosewood Drive, Danvers, MA 01923. For those organizations that have been granted a photocopy license by CCC, a separate system of payment has been arranged. The fee code for users of the Transactional Reporting Service is: 8036-2564-8/ + $.25.

To my wife, Betsy and my daughters, Danielle and Diana
who will forever be the source of my inspiration
and
to my students, whose inquisitive nature and
dedication to scholarship made this text a reality

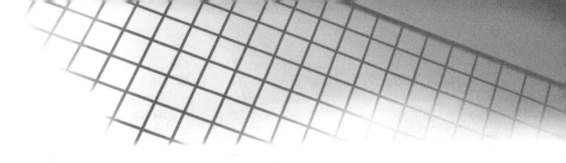

Foreword

In 1975 Dr. John Basmajian wrote an article titled, "Research or Retrench: The Rehabilitation Fields Challenged."[1] In this article, Dr. Basmajian argued that the rehabilitation specialties, particularly occupational and physical therapy, were at a crossroads in their professional development. He observed that the members of the disciplines could actively pursue professional status by encouraging research and scholarly activity or, alternatively, they could continue on their 1975 course and become what Dr. Basmajian called "respected technologies."[1] The rehabilitation fields responded to the challenge and have made dramatic progress in creating a research knowledge base and developing the discipline of rehabilitation science.

The challenge identified by Dr. Basmajian 37 years ago was to build research capacity and generate a knowledge base for the professional practice of rehabilitation to be based on scientific evidence. Earlier, many of the rehabilitation specialties were "debtor professions," borrowing the research evidence to support their clinical practice from other disciplines.[1] Accomplishing this goal also established rehabilitation practitioners as true professionals, responsible for developing the research necessary to guide and refine clinical practice.

In 2012, we face a new challenge, which is to ensure our research results are clinically relevant and useful. How do we translate our scientific knowledge and findings into treatments that improve the lives of persons with disability and chronic disease?

One of the most important research-related advances has been the development of evidence-based practice. The concept of evidence-based practice was introduced in the early 1990s, and, while not a research method, it has had a pervasive and profound influence on how we interpret and use clinical research.[2]

Broadly defined, evidence-based practice is the process of systematically locating, appraising, and using research findings as the basis for making clinical decisions. Evidence-based practice involves asking questions, finding and evaluating relevant data, and integrating that information into and interpreting it in the context of everyday practice. The goal of evidence-based practice is to use research information to help make decisions about treatment options for individual patients or clients. This goal is reflected in the most widely cited definition of evidence-based practice, developed by Sackett and colleagues, who state that it is the "conscientious, explicit and judicious use of evidence in making decisions about the care of individual patients. The practice of evidence-based medicine [practice] means integrating individual clinical expertise with the best available external clinical evidence from systematic research."[2] The focus is on intervention decisions for individual patients; in contrast, the goal of traditional research is to answer scientific questions and test theoretically derived hypotheses.

Excellent resources exist in the field of rehabilitation that describe evidence-based practice and clinical research. For example, *Evidence-Based Rehabilitation: A Guide to Practice,* edited by Law and MacDermid,[3] provides valuable information for rehabilitation professionals. *Foundations of Clinical Research: Applications to Practice,* by Portney and Watkins,[4] contains excellent information on designs, measurement issues, data analysis procedures, and ethical considerations in conducting clinical research. Each text includes a brief description of the complementary area (evidence-based practice/clinical research). For example, Portney and Watkins include a three-page description of evidence-based practice, including the definition presented above, but the actual methodology is not integrated in the remainder of the text.

Essentials of Rehabilitation Research: A Statistical Guide to Clinical Practice by Dr. Di Fabio is important because it is the first book in rehabilitation to blend and integrate evidence-based practice and clinical research. Other authors have hinted at this integration. For example, Law refers to the potential collaboration of evidence-based practice and clinical research as one the "greatest forgotten strengths of evidence-based practice."[3] She goes on to note that "Not only does evidence-based practice enable the use of the current best evidence in treatment, it can also be used to direct research advances. This conception of evidence-based practice closely links applied practice with research aspects of health care. Evidence-based practice is a force for integration, bringing these two often separate domains together and aiming to further streamline the process of generating new clinical knowledge.[3(p.7)]

In this book, Dr. Di Fabio has begun the process of integration, with a focus on the quantitative aspects for clinical research. This is an excellent place to begin as the quantitative aspects of clinical research are frequently the most difficult to interpret and translate in the clinical decision-making process at the core of evidence-based practice.

This book has a number of unique and useful features, including demonstration data sets patterned after real rehabilitation research questions, problem-solving exercises accompanied by video tutorials that guide the learner through relevant statistical procedures, and assistance with interpretation of output from statistical software. One of the most useful features of the text is the organization and focus of the chapters. Instead of the traditional chapters on sample or research design, Dr. Di Fabio has used an approach consistent with the philosophy of evidence-based practice that emphasizes clinical relevance. Following the introductory chapters, in which Dr. Di Fabio describes how to use the book, how clinical practice can be viewed as clinical research, and how contingency tables can be applied to clinical practice, Chapter 3, titled, "Diagnostic and Clinical Assessment Accuracy," provides a clear explanation of methods involved in quantifying patient progress and classifying persons into risk or diagnostic categories. The description begins with methods associated with basic 2×2 tables and continues to receiver operating characteristic (ROC) curves and likelihood ratios. Chapter 4 focuses on "Assessing Meaningful Clinical Change" and includes descriptions of change scores, clinically meaningful change, and minimal detectable change, among others. Continuing with the focus on clinical relevance, Chapter 5 addresses the responsiveness of clinical assessments and introduces the minimum important difference proportion and the reliable change proportion.

Other indices of responsiveness include the effect size for responsiveness, the standardized response mean, and Guyatt's responsiveness index. All these measures of change and responsiveness are regularly used in evidence-based practice reports. They have been described and illustrated in journal articles, but *Essentials of Rehabilitation Research* is the first text to aggregate and explain these concepts and indexes in one source with examples relevant to rehabilitation practitioners and investigators.

Chapters 6 through 9 follow the pattern of addressing topics relevant to the quantitative application of evidence-based practice, including clinical prediction rules, patient profiles, methods of identifying persons most likely to respond to treatment, and ways to examine associations among clinical variables. Chapter 10, "Assessment of Outcome Over Time," addresses specific methods that can be used in clinical outcome assessments that enhance documentation of patient progress. The key aspects of evaluating clinical practice guidelines are covered in Chapter 11. A series of practice exercises from the rehabilitation literature with illustrations and exercises relevant to the various topics, issues, and indexes described in chapters 2 through 11 can be found in Appendix A. Each study exercise includes a demonstration data set that allows the learner a chance to practice the approaches and methods presented in earlier chapters. Appendix C provides solutions to the exercises from previous chapters, and Appendix B contains a number of useful statistical tables.

In Joseph Campbell's book, titled *The Hero with a Thousand Faces,* which examines the role of myth and legend in modern culture, the author makes the observation that we can have only those adventures in life that we are ready for.[5] Some 30 years ago, we were ready for the adventure of establishing rehabilitation science and creating a body of knowledge to support clinical practice. In the current age of consumer-based health care and evidence-based accountability, we face a new challenge as important and difficult as the one identified by Dr. Basmajian in 1975. Our challenge is to translate the research knowledge we have generated into clinical practice that improves the lives of individual patients and persons with disabilities. With the support of Dr. Di Fabio, we are ready to begin this adventure.

—KENNETH J. OTTENBACHER, PhD, OTR
Russell Shearn Moody Distinguished Chair
Professor and Director, Division of Rehabilitation Sciences
Associate Director, Sealy Center on Aging
University of Texas Medical Branch
Galveston, Texas

References

1. Basmajian JV. Research or retrench: the rehabilitation fields challenged. Phys Ther 1975; 55:607-610.
2. Sackett DL, Straus S, Richardson S, et al. Evidence-Based Medicine: How to Practice and Teach EBM, 2nd ed. Edinburgh, UK: Churchill Livingstone; 2000.
3. Law MC, MacDermid J. Evidence-Based Rehabilitation: A Guide to Practice, 2nd ed. Thorofare, NJ: Slack; 2008.
4. Portney LG, Watkins MP. Foundations of clinical research: applications to practice. Upper Saddle River, NJ: Prentice Hall; 2000.
5. Campbell J. The Hero with a Thousand Faces, 2nd ed. Princeton University Press; 1968.

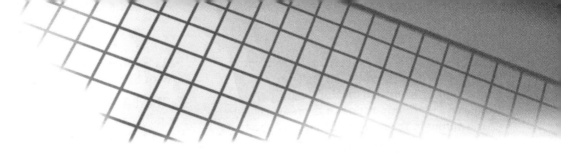

Preface

How to Use This Book

This book is based on the premise that clinical practice requires (1) a fundamental understanding of clinical research that has the potential to augment the care of patients in rehabilitation settings and (2) active practitioner involvement to analyze clinical information as well as the assessment methods used to measure patient progress.

The text is intended for advanced students and practitioners seeking clinically relevant statistical tools to enhance their practice in the fields of:

- Physical therapy
- Occupational therapy
- Rehabilitation medicine

The book is designed as an interactive primer that highlights carefully selected statistical methodologies that are important to clinicians seeking to integrate essential statistical methodologies into their practice. The book is a guide to the interpretation of commonly used statistics in a specific context, providing information to clinicians that has the potential to enhance the quality of care. It is *not* a comprehensive treatment of statistics that have a primary role in research.

Individuals reading this text can expect to learn about the implementation of simple data analyses in local clinical environments in order to evaluate outcomes of care systematically. Also, clinicians will immediately find a guide to understanding and/or initiating diagnostic validity assessments, implementing or developing prognostic prediction models, and piloting the first phases of developing new clinical prediction rules. The reader will also become familiar with methods of selecting assessment tools that are responsive to patient change while reducing the burden on both the patient and the health-care professional.

Fixed Chapter Sequence: Knowledge Is Cumulative

Each chapter builds on the information presented in the previous chapter. It is recommended that the reader progress through the book in sequence. This design facilitates "concept building" and allows the reader to appreciate the similarities and differences of related statistical methodologies that have clinical importance for a variety of applications.

In each chapter the reader will find:

- An overview of the link between clinical practice and the statistical procedures that enhance clinical practice
- Hypothetical data sets that allow the reader to perform analyses that are patterned after common types of rehabilitation research
- Problem-solving exercises that guide the reader through clinically relevant statistical analyses
- "Calculators" (in selected chapters), created using Excel spreadsheets, so the reader can check manual calculations of simple biostatistics, verify statistics during a literature review, and reduce reliance on more cumbersome statistical software. The calculators have not been validated externally and are presented in this text for the convenience of the reader.[1]

---

[1]No liability is implied or intended in the use of statistical programs or spreadsheet calculators herein (the "programs"). You should attempt to verify the accuracy of results using validated software programs that are not included with this text. There is no warranty for the spreadsheet calculators, and the copyright holders and other parties provide the calculators "as is" without warranty of any kind, either expressed or implied, including but not limited to the implied warranties of merchantability and fitness for a particular application. The entire risk as to the quality and performance of the program is with you. Should the programs prove defective, you assume the cost and all necessary servicing, repair, or correction.

- Video tutorials (in selected chapters) that show the step-by-step procedures to generate and interpret output from statistical software
- Guidance with interpretation of the results of statistical output in the context of clinical applications

Hypothetical Data Sets

This primer uses data sets with imaginary data. The variables included in each data set reflect commonly used clinical variables that are reported in studies cited throughout this text. The data are scaled to be realistic, but values entered into these practice data sets are not real. Throughout the primer, the terms "demonstration data set" or "hypothetical replication study" are used to denote hypothetical data. While it is possible in some cases to derive data from tables published in actual articles, it is not feasible to verify data accuracy independently. Therefore, the reader should view "derived" data as hypothetical data with results from imaginary patients. These demonstration data sets have no link to any real study and should be used only in the context of promoting *understanding* of statistical methodology.

Statistical Software as a Primer Companion

Many calculations demonstrated in this text can be performed simply in a Microsoft Excel spreadsheet. In fact, nearly all the examples in Chapters 2 to 6 can be implemented exclusively in an Excel spreadsheet. For the best results, however, it is recommended that the reader also use a statistical software program to analyze more complex clinical questions using the demonstration data sets as each chapter is reviewed. The essential concepts presented in this primer are learned most effectively by interpreting relevant statistical outputs from statistical software.

A bound-in disk included with this text holds the demonstration data sets and step-by-step video tutorials using Excel, SPSS version 18, and NCSS 2007 statistical software. Other statistical software programs will generate similar outputs. It is up to the reader to select and purchase a statistical software program separately from this book.

Practice data sets are presented in three forms in the online component of the text:

- As Excel spreadsheets that can be imported into most statistical programs
- As NCSS data sets that are immediately usable with NCSS software[2]

[2]Users who wish to use statistical software other than NCSS can also download the trial version of NCSS and export the practice data sets to the preferred program file type (File→Export→choose file type).

- As SPSS data sets that are immediately usable with SPSS and PSPP software

The disk menu is organized so that data sets corresponding to each chapter and software program can be accessed easily.

Suggestions for Obtaining Statistical Software

Free Statistical Software

At this writing, a compiled version of a program called PSPP is an open source program that provides output very similar to that of SPSS. The free PSPP software can be obtained at PSPP Statistical Software (free)[3] (www.gnu.org/software/pspp/get.html). Select the software version under MS Windows for PC users or Mac OS X for Apple users.

Examples in the tutorial videos that illustrate SPSS procedures will provide the fundamental information needed to analyze data in PSPP. Also, the demonstration data sets for SPSS are directly compatible with PSPP software. Users should note that PSPP provides most, but not all, statistical analyses discussed in this text.

Trial Versions of Commercial Software and Software Purchase

Trial downloads of NCSS and SPSS are available free of charge for use during a short-term trial period, but special *student and group pricing requested by course instructors* make the software very accessible for a longer term, particularly for use in the classroom setting. Contact Microsoft, NCSS, or SPSS directly to determine the best method of acquiring the software:

Microsoft Excel (copyright Microsoft Corporation)

- To download a trial version: http://office.microsoft.com/en-us/excel/microsoft-excel-2010-FX101825647.aspx
- Support: http://technet.microsoft.com/en-us/office/default.aspx

NCSS Statistical Software

- To download a trial version: www.ncss.com
- To contact by phone: 801-546-0554
- To email: sales@ncss.com

[3]Copyright © 1996, 1997, 1998, 1999, 2000, 2001, 2002, 2003, 2004, 2005, 2006, 2007 Free Software Foundation, Inc., 51 Franklin St - Suite 330, Boston, MA 02110, USA - Verbatim copying and distribution of this entire article are permitted worldwide, without royalty, in any medium.

IBM SPSS Statistics (also called PASW Statistics)

- To download a trial version: www.spss.com/statistics/
- To contact by phone: 1-312-651-3000
- To email: sales@spss.com

Opening Demonstration Data Sets

Once statistical software is installed on your computer, insert the disk that comes with this book into your computer's drive (Note: the software is not compatible with Apple computers, but Apple software such as Parallels can be used as a gateway for installation of most PC-compatible software). Open the statistical program (Excel, NCSS, SPSS, or PSPP) by clicking on the corresponding desktop icon. Then navigate to the demonstration data set of interest.

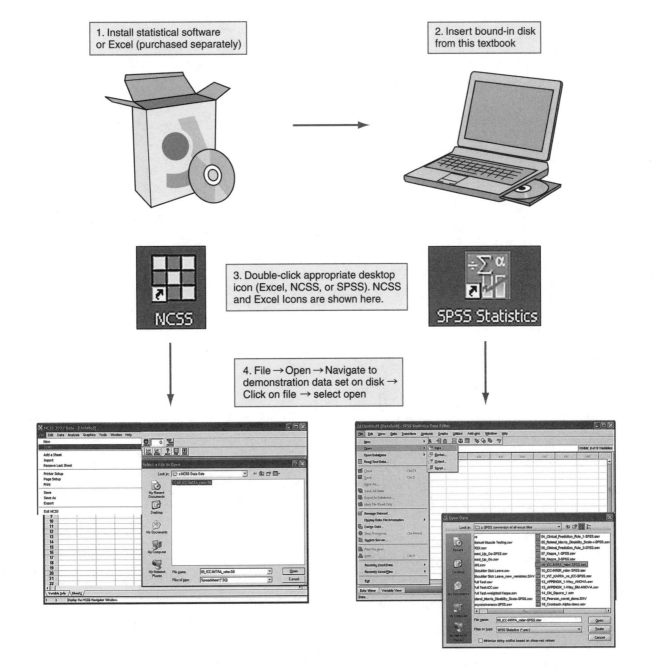

1. Install statistical software or Excel (purchased separately)

2. Insert bound-in disk from this textbook

3. Double-click appropriate desktop icon (Excel, NCSS, or SPSS). NCSS and Excel Icons are shown here.

NCSS

SPSS Statistics

4. File → Open → Navigate to demonstration data set on disk → Click on file → select open

Updates to Statistical Software

Commercially available statistical software packages undergo frequent revision. The video tutorials in the bound-in disk that accompany this text are based on the most current version of each software program available at the time of publication. Keep in mind that software updates may alter the basic steps for using Excel, NCSS, or SPSS.

A Note About Appendixes

Several chapters have an appendix that covers technical statistical details and provides exercises to enable a deeper understanding of statistical methodology. These appendixes address basic concepts that are the foundation for clinically applied statistics presented in the body of the text. Although review of appendixes could be considered optional, this content is highly recommended, especially for readers who are uninitiated in the field of biostatistics.

About the Author

Richard P. Di Fabio, PT, PhD is Professor in the Department of Physical Medicine and Rehabilitation at the University of Minnesota. He has served on the editorial board of the American Physical Therapy Association's Physical Therapy Journal and was Editor-in-Chief of the *Journal of Orthopaedic and Sports Physical Therapy*. His research in rehabilitation and motor dysfunction has been funded by the National Institute on Aging as well as the National Institute for Disability and Rehabilitation Research. Dr. Di Fabio has an extensive record of peer-reviewed publications and holds the distinguished Golden Pen Award for outstanding scientific writing. He has also received the Rose Award for excellence in research and the Fesler-Lampert Chair in Aging Studies. In addition he served as the Director of Physical Therapy Rehabilitation services at the University of Wisconsin Hospitals and Clinics. Dr. Di Fabio has worked closely with rehabilitation professionals, including occupational and physical therapists as well as physicians, nurses, and speech therapists specializing in rehabilitation medicine. His experiences as a clinician, academic faculty, and health-care administrator give him a unique perspective for developing new approaches to teaching outcome assessment and methods for integrating evidence into clinical practice.

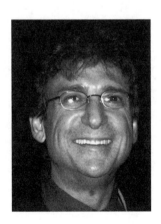

In loving memory of Dr. Rick Di Fabio (1952-December 2011), whose passionate love for learning and clinical research inspired this book. May he live on through his words and the knowledge he has passed down to his students and family. The profound lessons he has taught us will forever impact our lives.

Consultant

STEVEN P. GULKUS, PhD
Associate Professor
Arcadia University
Education Department
Glenside, Pennsylvania

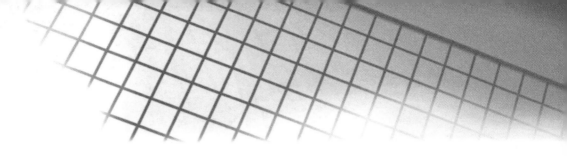

Reviewers

CHRISTINE BERG, PhD, OTR/L
Instructor
Washington University
Program in Occupational Therapy
St. Louis, Missouri

M. J. BLASCHAK, PT, PhD
Associate Professor and Program Coordinator
Northern Illinois University
College of Health & Human Sciences
School of Allied Health & Communicative Disorders
Physical Therapy Program
DeKalb, Illinois

LORI BORDENAVE, PT, DPT, MEd
Assistant Chair and Associate Professor
A.T. Still University
Arizona School of Health Sciences
Physical Therapy Program
Mesa, Arizona

KIMBERLY K. CLEARY, PT, PhD
Associate Professor
Eastern Washington University
College of Science, Health & Engineering
Department of Physical Therapy
Spokane, Washington

KEVIN K. CHUI, PT, PhD, GCS
Assistant Professor
Sacred Heart University
College of Education & Health Professions
Department of Physical Therapy
Fairfield, Connecticut

CLIFTON F. FRILOT, PhD, MBA
Assistant Professor
Louisiana State University Health Sciences Center
School of Allied Health Professions
Program in Physical Therapy
Shreveport, Louisiana

JOHN H. HOLLMAN, PT, PhD
Associate Professor of Physical Therapy
Mayo Clinic
Department of Physical Medicine and Rehabilitation
Rochester, Minnesota

BETH M. JONES, PT, DPT, MS, OCS
Assistant Professor
University of New Mexico Health Sciences Center
School of Medicine
Physical Therapy Program
Albuquerque, New Mexico

LISA KENYON, PT, MHS, PCS
Assistant Professor
Arkansas State University
College of Nursing and Health Professions
Department of Physical Therapy
State University, Arizona

JENNIFER MAI, PT, DPT, MHS, NCS
Assistant Professor
Clarke College
Department of Physical Therapy
Dubuque, Iowa

GUY SIMONEAU, PhD, PT
Professor
Marquette University
College of Health Sciences
Department of Physical Therapy
Milwaukee, Wisconsin

BARBARA S. SMITH, PhD, PT
Professor
Wichita State University
College of Health Professions
Department of Physical Therapy
Wichita, Kansas

LAURA K. VOGTLE, PhD, OTR/L, FAOTA
Professor & Director Post Professional Program
University of Alabama at Birmingham
School of Health Professions
Department of Occupational Therapy
Birmingham, Alabama

Acknowledgments

Thank you to the University of Minnesota for providing time and material support to complete this text. Also, to Diana Di Fabio for her expertise in photographing and arranging the cover image for this book.

Contents

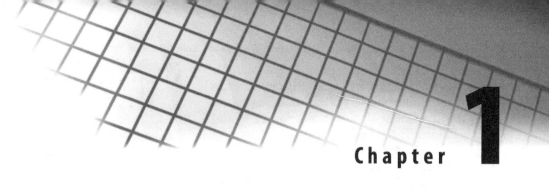

Chapter **1**

Clinical Practice *Is* Clinical Research

Introduction

Developing a clinical practice based on evidence in any health profession requires an understanding of treatment concepts and the manner in which those treatments are tested and evaluated in published clinical studies. Law and MacDermid view evidence-based practice (EBP) as a force for integration of applied research and clinical practice.[1] A central barrier to the integration of practice and research is a prevailing notion that these domains are separate entities.[2] Recently, however, the idea that clinical practice *requires* elements of clinical research redefines the traditional role of the practitioner.

Evidence supporting the theme that "clinical *practice is clinical research*" is emerging from national health professions organizations. Practice and accreditation standards for medical residency programs in the field of Physical Medicine and Rehabilitation[3] as well as the fields of Occupational[4] and Physical Therapy[5] have linked patient care with the process of developing and participating in patient-centered clinical research to enhance clinical outcomes.

Residency programs in Physical Medicine, governed by the Accreditation Council for Graduate Medical Education (ACGME), require that: "The curriculum must advance residents' knowledge of the basic principles of research, including how research is conducted, evaluated, explained to patients, and applied to patient care" (Standard IV B1).

The Accreditation Council for Occupational Therapy Education (ACOTE)[4] mandates that educational programs must prepare students to: "Organize, collect, and analyze data in a systematic manner for evaluation of practice outcomes, report evaluation results and modify practice as needed to improve outcomes" (Standard B.5.26).

Also, the ACOTE requires that students: "Demonstrate the ability to design ongoing processes for quality improvement (e.g., outcome studies analysis) and develop program changes as needed to ensure quality of services and to direct administrative changes" (Standard B.7.8).

From the *Guide to Physical Therapist Practice:* "The physical therapist engages in outcomes data collection and analysis—that is, the systematic review of outcomes of care in relation to selected variables (e.g., age, sex, diagnosis, interventions performed)—and develops statistical reports for internal or external use."[5(p.S40)]

Additional support for the concept that clinical practice involves aspects of clinical research comes from the American Physical Therapy Association's clinical outcome assessment tool, developed to enable practicing clinicians to audit the efficacy of their care and establish performance standards to satisfy third-party payors.[6]

While accreditation agencies for professional schools of rehabilitation and national rehabilitation associations promote clinical research as part of clinical practice,[3-5,7] the practitioner has little guidance for systematically analyzing clinical information collected during routine clinical care.

Patient Assessments: Potential to Enhance Care Through Statistical Analyses[a]

Information gathered during the course of routine clinical practice is valuable for guiding ongoing changes in

[a]In any research project, the person(s) conducting the research must secure permission from the appropriate institutional review board before initiating the project. This includes data collection through the use of retrospective chart review.

1

the assessment and treatment of patients. For example, the assessment of patients in clinical environments has promoted the evaluation of diagnostic or screening tools,[8,9] the assessment of patient prognosis,[10-13] and protocols to identify responders versus nonresponders to rehabilitation interventions.[14-16]

There are calls for increasing clinical research in clinical practice settings because a broad representation of both the patient populations and clinical environments that serve patients might improve the foundations of EBP.[17] Chen and Worrall[17] warn, however, that practitioners who wish to seek a higher level of practice that includes the integration of clinical research with practice should be aware of a "conflict of commitment." The conflict of commitment arises when clinical research is not viewed as an integrated component of clinical practice: "A [health care provider] seeks to advance this patient's best interests (medical and otherwise) and improve this patient's well-being. Clinical research aims to improve the well-being of future individuals. Although improvement in the medical condition of research participants is hoped for, it is a secondary effect ('side effect') and is not the primary intention of research."[17(p.134)]

The conflict of commitment can be avoided by ongoing reevaluation of best practices that are acceptable in view of current standards of care. In other words, the systematic evaluation of assessments and interventions *is* the process of providing care that is thought to improve the patient's well-being. There are many aspects of routine rehabilitation practice that could be enhanced through the application of statistical analyses to guide care (Table 1-1).

Role of the Clinician to Validate Surrogate Outcomes

As the gap between clinical practice and clinical research narrows, practitioners will find an important role in validating surrogate outcomes. DiCenso et al.[18] describe surrogate outcomes as "an intermediate outcome used as a substitute for an end point that directly measures how a patient feels, functions, or survives."[p.224]

Examples of surrogate outcomes in a rehabilitation context include interventions to improve:

- Protective stepping with the assumption that modifying the number of steps will decrease falls.[19]
- Posture because it is a presumed cause of shoulder impairment.[20]
- Hand range of motion with the assumption that better movement range will improve overall hand function.[21]

When evaluating surrogate outcomes in the literature, it will be critical to determine the validity of

Table 1-1	Aspects of Clinical Practice Enhanced by Statistical Analyses Performed by the Clinician.	
Aspect of Routine Clinical Practice	**Corresponding Chapter in This Text**
Determining diagnostic validity	3
Describing meaningful clinical change	4
Measuring assessment responsiveness	5
Determining consensus among clinicians in patient assessment	6
Establishing relationships among clinical variables	7
Prediction of prognosis and outcome	8
Identifying "Responders" to treatment	9
Measuring change in patient outcome over time	10
Evaluating and applying clinical practice guidelines	11

these intermediate outcomes. DiCenso et al.[18] ask the clinician to determine if there is a strong association between the surrogate outcome (e.g., hand motion) and the target outcome (e.g., hand function). Consistent, strong associations between the surrogate and target outcomes will be an important step toward validating research that uses surrogate outcomes in the assessment of rehabilitation efficacy.

Guidance for the Clinician Seeking Statistical Tools to Enhance Practice: Learn EBP by Doing

In order to meet practice and accreditation standards, there is a need to prepare clinicians to analyze clinical data and answer clinical questions directly relevant to patient care. When teaching EBP, "integration means applying the steps [of analysis] to real and current clinical problems."[22] This model of teaching EBP is based on the concept of "learn by doing."

Producing and interpreting statistical output is a new approach to EBP that can be transferred directly to clinical practice. This approach differs from traditional approaches to teaching applied statistics because the student and clinician are working with data sets that can be used as templates in the classroom or local clinic for real clinical research (Fig. 1-1).

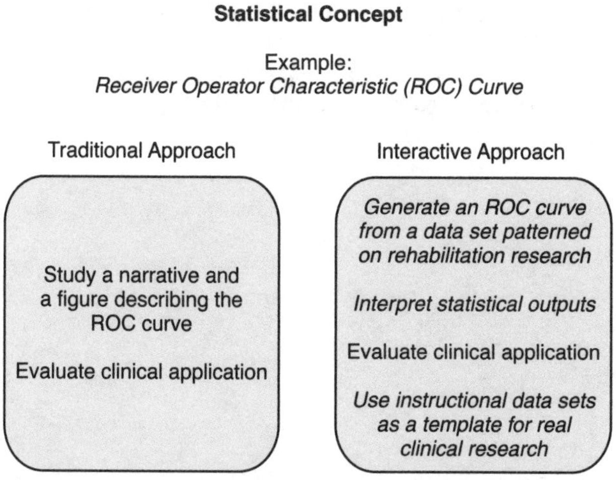

Statistical Concept

Example:
Receiver Operator Characteristic (ROC) Curve

Traditional Approach

Study a narrative and
a figure describing the
ROC curve

Evaluate clinical application

Interactive Approach

*Generate an ROC curve
from a data set patterned
on rehabilitation research*

Interpret statistical outputs

Evaluate clinical application

*Use instructional data sets
as a template for real
clinical research*

Figure 1-1 Comparison of traditional and interactive methods of teaching (and learning) applied statistics to support EBP. The receiver operator characteristic curve is used as an example of the statistical concept of interest.

SUMMARY

A critical component of clinical practice is clinical research. That is, clinical practice requires elements of research. National organizations representing the health-care professions not only encourage but in some cases mandate and promote the integration of clinical research with practice as a part of entry-level education. Prime examples of practice-research integration are the systematic evaluation of the quality of clinical assessment tools and outcomes of care in local clinics. Statistical analysis is needed to answer many clinical questions and serves as an important methodology supporting routine clinical care and the implementation of EBP. A "learn by doing" approach can help students and rehabilitation practitioners consolidate research and practice aspects into the role of rehabilitation practitioner.

REFERENCES

1. Law MC, MacDermid J. Evidence-based Rehabilitation: A Guide to Practice, 2nd ed. Thorofare, NJ: Slack, 2008.
2. Segal NA, Wilson Garvan C, Basford JR. Factors influencing involvement in research and career choice: A survey of graduating physical medicine and rehabilitation residents. Arch Phys Med Rehabil 2006; 87:1442–1446.
3. ACGME Program Requirements for Graduate Medical Education in Physical Medicine and Rehabilitation, www.acgme.org/acWebsite/RRC_340/340_prIndex.asp, 2007.
4. Accreditation Council for Occupational Therapy Education. The American Occupational Therapy Association Inc. Standards and interpretive guidelines, www.aota.org/Educate/Accredit/StandardsReview.aspx, 2008.
5. Guide to Physical Therapist Practice: Chapter 1: Who are physical therapists and what do they do? Phys Ther 2001; 81:S31–S121.
6. Guccione AA, Mielenz TJ, DeVellis R, et al. Development and testing of a self-report instrument to measure actions: Outpatient Physical Therapy Improvement in Movement Assessment Log (OPTIMAL). Phys Ther 2005; 85:515–530.
7. Commission on Accreditation in Physical Therapy Education (CAPTE). Evaluative criteria for accreditation of education programs for the preparation of physical therapists, 2007.
8. Bohannon RW. Manual muscle testing: Does it meet the standards of an adequate screening test? Clin Rehabilitation 2005; 19:662–667.
9. Schmitt J, Di Fabio RP. Reliable change and minimum important difference (MID) proportions facilitated group responsiveness comparisons using individual threshold criteria. J Clin Epidemiol 2004; 57:1008–1018.
10. Freeman JA, Hobart JC, Playford ED, et al. Evaluating neurorehabilitation: Lessons from routine data collection. J Neurol Neurosurg Psychiatry 2005; 76:723–728.
11. Kay ED, Deutsch A, Wuermser LA. Predicting walking at discharge from inpatient rehabilitation after a traumatic spinal cord injury. Arch Phys Med Rehabil 2007; 88:745–750.
12. Mazer BL, Korner-Bitensky NA, Sofer S. Predicting ability to drive after stroke. Arch Phys Med Rehabil 1998; 79:743–750.
13. Stineman MG, Ross RN, Granger CV, et al. Predicting the achievement of 6 grades of physical independence from data routinely collected at admission to rehabilitation. Arch Phys Med Rehabil 2003; 84:1647–1656.
14. Flynn T, Fritz J, Whitman J, et al. A clinical prediction rule for classifying patients with low back pain who demonstrate short-term improvement with spinal manipulation. Spine 2002; 27:2835–2843.
15. Kuijpers T, van der Windt DAWM, Boeke AJP, et al. Clinical prediction rules for the prognosis of shoulder pain in general practice. Pain 2006; 120:276–285.
16. Wainner RS, Fritz JM, Irrgang JJ, et al. Development of a clinical prediction rule for the diagnosis of carpal tunnel syndrome. Arch Phys Med Rehabil 2005; 86:609–618.
17. Chen DT, Worrall BB. Practice-based clinical research and ethical decision making—Part I: Deciding whether to incorporate practice-based research into your clinical practice. Semin Neurol 2006; 26: 131–139.
18. DiCenso A, Guyatt G. Evidence-Based Nursing: A Guide to Clinical Practice. St Louis, MO: Elsevier Mosby, 2005.
19. Hilliard MJ, Martinez KM, Janssen I, et al. Lateral balance factors predict future falls in community-living older adults. Arch Phys Med Rehabil 2008; 89:1708–1713.

20. Borstad JD. Resting position variables at the shoulder: evidence to support a posture-impairment association. Phys Ther 2006; 86:549–557.

21. Poole JL, Cordova KJ. Can hand assessments designed for persons with scleroderma be valid for persons with rheumatoid arthritis? J Rheumatology 2005; 33:2278.

22. Del Mar C, Glasziou P, Mayer D. Teaching evidence-based practice. BMJ 2004; 989–990.

Chapter 2

Clinical Practice Requires Contingency Tables

An Overview

Clinical Questions
Contingency tables help answer clinical questions like:
- Do clinical tests used for patient assessment accurately determine the patient's classification for diagnosis and treatment?
- How much change must a patient demonstrate to be *functionally meaningful*?
- Does my clinical assessment adequately identify changes in the patient's status when they occur?
- When different clinicians evaluate the same patient do they reach the same conclusion?
- Is treatment related to patient outcome?
- Are certain patient symptoms good predictors of diagnosis or prognosis?

Introduction

When reviewing the literature to support evidence-based practice, students and clinicians will see contingency tables that help answer questions like:

- Does the selected clinical test accurately guide determination of patient classification for subsequent intervention or the diagnosis? (diagnostic and assessment accuracy)
- How much change must a patient demonstrate to be *meaningful clinical change*?
- Does my clinical assessment identify changes in patients when they occur? (responsiveness)
- When therapists evaluate patients do they reach the same conclusion to guide patient care? (consensus)

- Is treatment related to patient outcome? (association)
- Are certain patient symptoms good predictors of diagnosis or prognosis?

What Is a Contingency Table?

A contingency table is a table of counts. The table is named by the number of rows and columns. For example a 2×2 contingency table has 2 rows and 2 columns, whereas a 3×2 contingency table has 3 rows and 2 columns. In this text, each cell for a 2×2 contingency table has a standardized label A through D **(Fig. 2-1)**. The demonstration in Figure 2-1 shows 5 patients counted for cell A, 11 patients for cell B, and so on.

How Does a Contingency Table Relate to Clinical Practice?

The content of a contingency table will determine which aspect of clinical practice is addressed. The clinical application of a 2×2 table is addressed in Chapters 3 through 8. Note from **Table 2-1** that the size of the contingency table remains the same, but the labels identifying the content of each cell in the table vary with the purpose of the table.

Diagnostic and Assessment Accuracy

For example, when diagnostic accuracy of a clinical test is addressed, does the test accurately classify the patient for treatment or accurately identify the diagnosis?

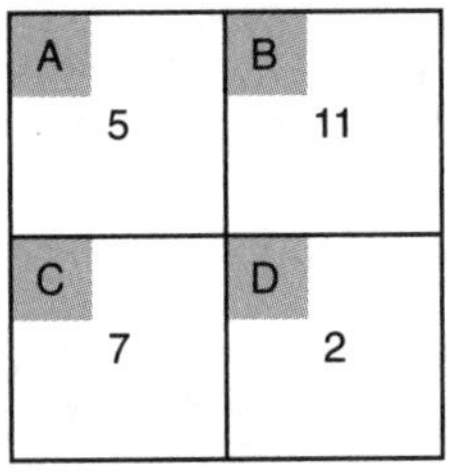

Figure 2-1 Cell labels for any 2×2 contingency table. Counts of observations or patients (whole numbers) are shown to demonstrate how counts are placed into the table.

Table 2-1, panel 1, labels of counts across the top of the table show the number of patients meeting the criterion standard for the presence of pathology. The side of the table shows the counts of patients for example who are also diagnosed with that pathology according to the test used in the clinic. When put together, each cell has unique information about the clinical assessment. Cell A shows the number of patients with true positive results for pathology (positive on both the criterion and the clinical test *for pathology*). Cell B shows the number of patients with false positive results (positive on the clinical test *for pathology*, but not the criterion standard). Cell C shows the number of patients with false negative results (negative on the clinical test *for pathology*, but positive on the criterion). Cell D shows the number of patients with true negative results (negative on both the criterion standard and the clinical test of interest; *the patient is deemed to be free of pathology and classified as unimpaired*).

An easy way to remember these relationships is to view the diagonal cells. The counts for cells A and D agree with the criterion standard *for pathology*, and

Table 2-1	**Overview of Contingency Table Format to Answer Different Clinical Questions.** Additional dotted cells and arrow in the reliability and association contingency tables indicate that some applications might require larger tables.

Panel	Clinical Question	Contingency Table Format
1	Diagnostic Accuracy	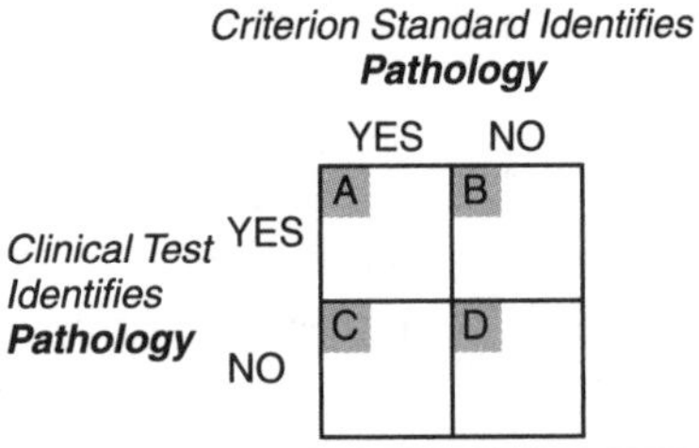
2	Meaningful Clinical Change	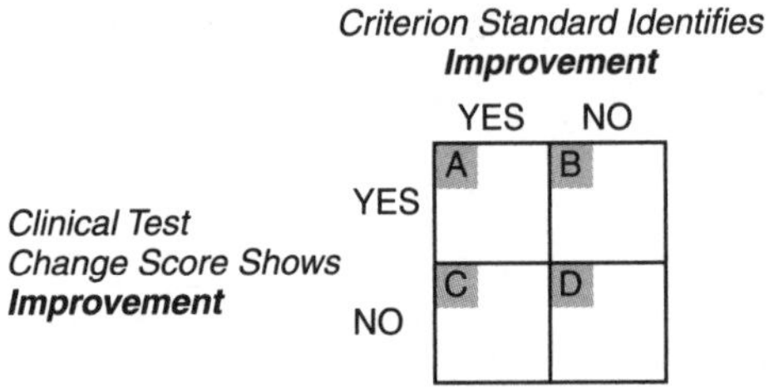
3	Responsiveness	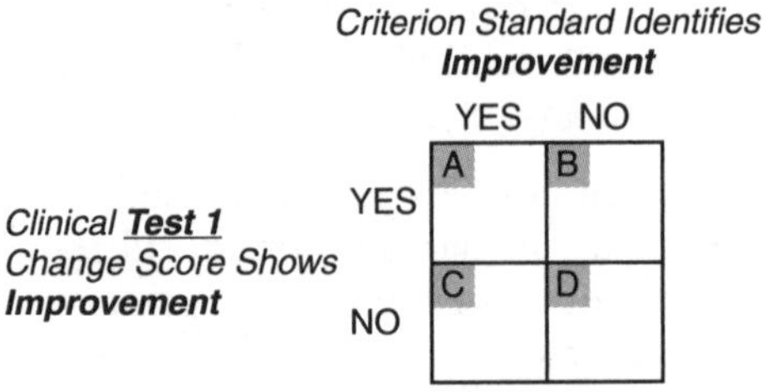 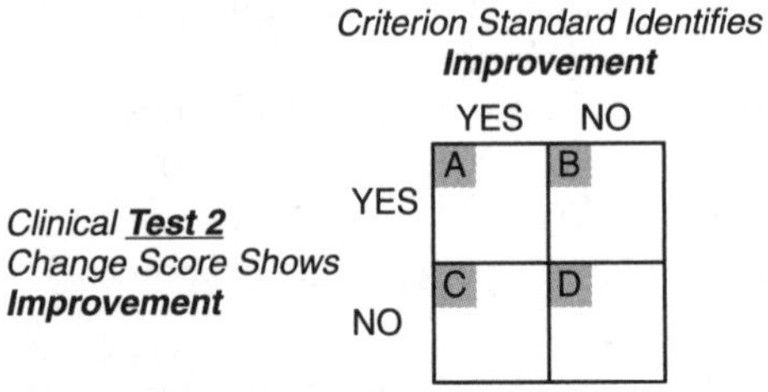

| Table 2-1 | **Overview of Contingency Table Format to Answer Different Clinical Questions.** Additional dotted cells and arrow in the reliability and association contingency tables indicate that some applications might require larger tables.—cont'd |

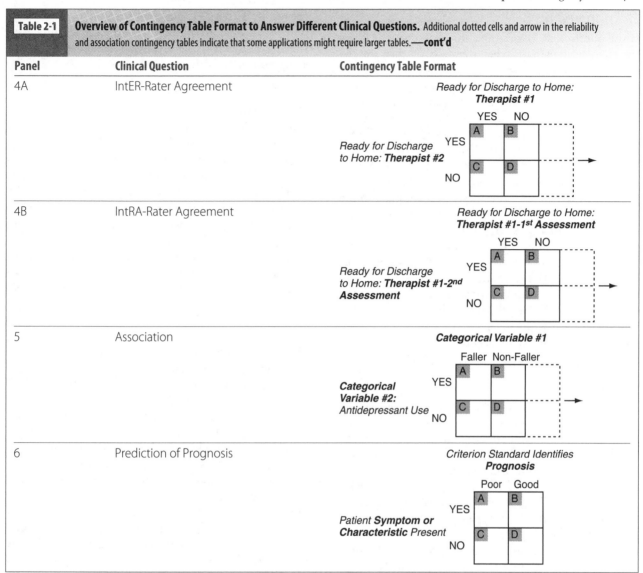

Panel	Clinical Question	Contingency Table Format
4A	IntER-Rater Agreement	
4B	IntRA-Rater Agreement	
5	Association	
6	Prediction of Prognosis	

cells B and C disagree with the criterion. More patient counts on the "agreement" diagonal relative to fewer counts on the "disagreement" diagonal give a preliminary indication that the test might be useful for identifying true results in the clinical setting (i.e., those who truly have a disorder and those who truly do not).

Meaningful Clinical Change

In order to answer different clinical questions, the content of the 2×2 contingency table changes. If the question relates to meaningful clinical change rather than diagnostic validity (**Table 2-1, panel 2;** also refer to Chapter 4), then the counts in each cell represent something different from a diagnostic validity table. In this case, the criterion standard shown across the top of the table indicates the number of patients who

were judged to improve, whereas the side of the table counts the number of patients that also have change scores on a selected clinical assessment tool (initial assessment minus follow-up assessment during the course of care) that are associated with improvement or worsening. Here, cell A shows the number of patients with true positive results for *improvement* (positive on both the criterion and the clinical test). Cell B shows the number of patients with false positive results (positive on the clinical test *for improvement* but not the criterion standard). Cell C shows the number of patients with false negative results (negative on the clinical test *for improvement*, but positive on the criterion). Cell D shows the number of patients with true negative results (negative on both the criterion standard and the clinical test of interest; *the patient is deemed worse or unchanged*).

Responsiveness

If the question is, "Does my clinical assessment identify changes in patients when they occur?" then the clinician is interested in selecting the clinical assessment tool that is most responsive. In this case, the analysis of responsiveness involves a contingency table for each assessment tool under consideration for use in the clinic. For example, when comparing two different assessment tools, the analysis of responsiveness will involve two contingency tables (**Table 2-1, panel 3**). Each contingency table uses the same criterion standard for measuring improvement and is applied to the same patient group. The responsiveness of clinical test #1 is then compared to the responsiveness of clinical test #2 (see Chapter 5 for statistical calculations and method details). In essence, the analysis of responsiveness compares the amount of meaningful clinical change for each tool under consideration for use in the clinic. In general, the tool that shows greater meaningful change has greater responsiveness, but several statistical indices may be needed to support this conclusion (Chapter 5).

Consensus

Using assessment tools in the clinic that yield consistent results gives practitioners confidence that the same patient, if evaluated by different therapists, would be functionally classified in a similar way (Chapter 6). The contingency table demonstration for interrater reliability (**Table 2-1, panel 4A, IntER-Rater**) has two clinicians evaluating the same patients to determine if it is appropriate to recommend discharge from the hospital to home. Notice that cells A and D show the number of patients where both raters agreed on the discharge plan, whereas cells B and C show the number of patients where raters disagreed (see Chapter 6). If the question is changed to "does a single therapist show agreement when rating a patient two times," then the contingency table is modified to place the same therapist on each side of the contingency table and then to count the agreements and disagreements on patient assessment for that particular clinician's rating the first and second time (**Table 2-1, panel 4B, IntRA-Rater**).

There are cases where the classification of patients exceeds two levels. For example, the patient might be rated as minimal, moderate, or maximum impairment. In this case, a 3×3 contingency table would be used (the expanded table indicated by the dotted cells and arrows in **Table 2-1, panels 4A** and **4B**). Regardless of the number of patient classifications, however, the contingency table is always balanced with the same number of rows and columns (i.e., 2×2, 3×3, or 4×4, etc.).

Association

The relationships between categorical variables (e.g., variables that are discrete and form distinct categories like gender and sex) are often used by practitioners to create an awareness of unique associations that might alter the care of the patient (Chapter 7). For example, if a therapist was aware that there was a strong association between fall status (falling vs. not falling) and antidepressant use (yes vs. no), action might be taken to reduce or modify the use of antidepressants (**Table 2-1, panel 5**). In this case, the contingency table does not need to be "balanced" and can take many forms (i.e., 3×2, 4×4, or 4×3).

Prediction of Prognosis

A common question asked by patients as they begin treatment is "What can I expect from the treatment you will give me?" The use of clinical prediction rules is one way to help practitioners answer that question. Clinical prediction rules rely on a statistical method that uses various forms of prediction methodology. Odds ratios derived from a 2×2 contingency table provide an index of risk (Chapter 8). In other words, if a patient has a particular symptom at the initial evaluation, what are the odds that patient will have a good outcome at the end of treatment? Contingency tables for predicting prognosis are unidimensional, meaning that usually only one symptom can be evaluated at any given time (**Table 2-1, panel 6**). In real-world clinical applications, a cluster of symptoms more accurately predicts the outcome of care. Advanced statistics that evaluate more than one predictor at a time are covered in Chapters 8 and 9.

SUMMARY

Contingency tables help practitioners answer a wide array of important clinical questions. The particular question addressed by a contingency table will determine the format of the table. In the chapters that follow, detailed statistical procedures derived from each type of contingency table are described so that practitioners can interpret and apply the results of table analyses.

PRACTICE

1. Name the labels across the top and along the side of contingency tables designed to answer the following clinical questions:

	Label Across Top	**Label Along Side**
a. IntER-Rater reliability		
b. Meaningful clinical change		
c. Responsiveness		
d. Association		
e. Prediction of Prognosis		
f. Diagnostic accuracy		

2. Match the contingency table with the clinical scenario:

CLINICAL SCENARIOS

a. A patient with Parkinson's disease enters a gait rehabilitation program. The goal is to determine the target change in gait speed (from initial evaluation to postrehabilitation assessment) needed to establish that the patient made progress that equates to a meaningful functional improvement in gait mobility.

b. Before implementing a new assessment tool that measures driving ability in people poststroke, the clinic supervisor wants to determine if the conclusion of "OK to drive" versus "not OK to drive" is consistent among therapists evaluating the patient.

c. A patient with a brain injury presents at initial evaluation with a low motor function score. The therapist's goal is to determine if low motor function at the initial assessment is a strong predictor of outcome at 6 months postinjury.

d. The burden on the patient enduring multiple patient assessments is a concern. The goal is to identify the single best clinical assessment of low back disability among two choices: Oswestry vs. Roland-Morris disability assessments.

e. A therapist who sees patients with shoulder dysfunction frequently uses the Neer test to evaluate each patient for impingement syndrome. After using the test for some time, the therapist finds that many patients who appear to have impingement by other clinical measures do not seem to have a positive Neer test. The literature is reviewed to determine if the Neer test, when used alone, provides an accurate diagnostic finding.

Chapter 3

Diagnostic and Clinical Assessment Accuracy

Clinical Question

Do the clinical tests used for patient assessment accurately determine the patient's classification for treatment or diagnosis?

What Is "Diagnosis" in Rehabilitation?

Diagnosis is both a reasoning process as well as a label.[1] The term *diagnosis* is "the name given to a collection of relevant signs and symptoms."[2(p.1703)] The process of diagnosis involves clinical reasoning that summarizes a patient's dysfunction and serves as a basis for planning subsequent interventions.[1,3]

Rehabilitation practice usually requires an evaluation to assess the patient's status followed by implementation of a care plan that is designed to treat the patient's problem. Some have termed the results of this initial assessment a "diagnosis" in physical[1] and occupational therapy.[3] The use of the term *diagnosis* by physical therapists is controversial,[1] but the literature has many examples of nonphysician authors using the term. For example, "diagnosis" has been attached to the classification of patients with high fall risk,[4] the patterns of movement dysfunction in people with stroke,[5] and the description of anatomical and biomechanical faults contributing to shoulder dysfunction.[6]

It should be recognized first and foremost that clinicians are limited to providing services that are consistent with the scope of their education and the laws regulating their practice.[2] *To practice in an effective manner, clinicians should use the best assessment tools available to accurately describe patient dysfunction or impairment within the scope of their practice.* To this end, the central focus of this chapter is to (1) help rehabilitation physicians and clinicians understand the literature addressing the diagnostic accuracy of patient assessment tools and (2) provide a foundation for those professionals to determine the accuracy of assessment tools currently used or intended for use in their respective clinical settings.

Accuracy of Clinical Assessments

Clinical assessment tools are used to quantify patient progress or to classify patients into risk or diagnostic categories.[7-9] The "target condition" is a certain type of dysfunction or pathology that needs to be confirmed before treatment decisions can be made. Patient function, cognitive status, and quality of life are measured by scores on various assessment tools. Some examples of common clinical assessments are illustrated in **Table 3-1.**

The value of an assessment tool is determined by its diagnostic or assessment accuracy (validity). Tools with good diagnostic validity accurately measure the presence or absence of disease or dysfunction.[a]

---

[a]The term *diagnosis* used throughout this text must be interpreted within the scope of practice allowed by the readers' qualifications.

Diagnosis by a physician will not be the same as "diagnosis" (e.g., patient classification for rehabilitation interventions or measurements of functional impairment) by physical and occupational therapists.

The use of the term *diagnosis* should **not** in any way be construed as a recommendation for readers to act outside of the scope of their legally defined practice.

Table 3-1	Selected Examples of Clinical Outcome Assessments			
Assessment	Domains of Clinical Measurement	Scale	Composite Score Range	As Composite Score ↑, Function:
Western Ontario McMaster Osteoarthritis Index (WOMAC)[10]	Pain, Stiffness, Physical Function	Continuous	0–2400 mm*	↓
Roland-Morris Disability Questionnaire[11]	Self-perceived low back disability	Continuous	0–24 points	↑
Timed Up & Go[9]	Mobility		6.4 s–49.6 s	↓
Modified Ashworth Scale[12]	Abnormal muscle tone	Ordinal	0–4++	↓
Manual Muscle Testing[13]	Strength	Ordinal	0–12	↑
Berg Balance Scale[14]	Balance and Mobility	Ordinal	0–56	↑

*Visual analog scale reported here, but other methods of scoring, including a Likert-type scale, are available.

++ Scale points range from 0 to 4 but include +/– gradations, which increase scale resolution.

Research Design to Determine the Diagnostic Validity

Most research designed to evaluate the diagnostic validity of clinical assessment tools shares these common characteristics:

- The use of a 2×2 contingency table (see Fig. 3-1 later in this chapter for an example);
- Identification of a criterion standard that serves as the reference to judge the presence or absence of pathology or dysfunction;
- Identification of a cut-point in the clinical assessment score that serves as the boundary between a positive test for dysfunction and a negative test.

Several statistics can be used to determine the diagnostic validity of any clinical assessment. These statistics are intended to assist the clinician to make a diagnosis, classify the patient for selected rehabilitation interventions, or to compare the accuracy of different clinical tests as part of a review of literature when the goal is to establish an evidence-based practice. The most commonly used measures of diagnostic validity are sensitivity, specificity, and positive or negative likelihood ratios.

Sensitivity

The ratio of the number of patients who have the target disorder (judged by agreement of the clinical test with the criterion standard in cell A) with the total count of patients who have positive findings (judged by the criterion standard) indicates the percentage of patients correctly identified *with* dysfunction when the clinical test is applied. Higher numbers indicate better

sensitivity. Referring to the cells in the 2×2 contingency table:

$$\text{Sensitivity} = A/A+C \qquad \textbf{eq 3-1}$$

Specificity

The ratio of the number of patients who **do not** have the target disorder (judged by agreement of the clinical test with the criterion standard in cell D) with the total count of patients who have negative findings (judged by the criterion standard) indicates the percentage of patients correctly identified *without* dysfunction when the clinical test is applied. Higher numbers indicate better specificity. Referring to the cells in the 2×2 contingency table:

$$\text{Specificity} = D/B+D \qquad \textbf{eq 3-2}$$

Likelihood Ratios

The likelihood ratios (LRs) are statistics used to determine the probability that the target condition is present. Positive LRs (+LRs) apply to situations where the clinical test is positive for pathology, whereas negative LRs (−LRs) illustrate the likelihood of pathology or impairment when the clinical test is negative. The magnitudes of LRs are judged descriptively (see Table 3-2 later in this chapter). A clinician interpreting LRs is seeking information about diagnostic certainty. In other words, what level of confidence should practitioners have when administering the clinical test?

Positive likelihood ratio (+LR): large +LRs indicate that the patient with a positive clinical test is very likely to have the target condition, whereas smaller +LRs reduce diagnostic certainty and cast doubt on the validity of the diagnosis. The +LR differs from sensitivity because the calculation of +LR has a "correction" for false positives (see the denominator of **equation 3-3**). Also, the +LR is used in conjunction with prevalence to determine how much the clinical test of interest adds to diagnostic certainty beyond the baseline occurrence of the target condition in the population (prevalence). The coupling of prevalence with the +LR to determine diagnostic certainty is discussed in more detail in the section on nomograms. Prevalence can be estimated from a contingency table using **equation 3-4**. In summary, *the +LR, conceptually, is the true positive rate corrected for the false positive rate.*

$$\text{+Likelihood Ratio= Sensitivity/}$$
$$\text{(1-Specificity)} \qquad \textbf{eq 3-3}$$
$$\text{Prevalence (estimated) =}$$
$$\text{A+C/(A+ B+C+D)} \qquad \textbf{eq 3-4}$$

Negative likelihood ratio (–LR): small negative LRs indicate that the patient with a negative clinical test is *not likely* to have the target condition. In contrast, larger –LRs reduce diagnostic certainty and cast doubt on the validity of the diagnosis.

Negative LRs differ from specificity because the focus is on false negative test results. The clinician interpreting –LRs is interested in the relative prominence of the false negative rate. Thus, *the –LR is essentially the false negative rate corrected for the true negative rate.* A low value of –LR is desired because this indicates that the true negative rate (the denominator of the ratio in **equation 3-5**) overpowers the false negative rate (shown in the numerator of equation 3-5). The coupling of prevalence with the –LR is also used to evaluate diagnostic certainty in a nomogram (discussed later).

$$\text{–Likelihood Ratio = (1 - Sensitivity)/}$$
$$\text{Specificity} \qquad \textbf{eq 3-5}$$

Interpretation of the Magnitude of LRs

Large +LR (>5) and small –LRs (≤0.20) are thought to improve diagnostic certainty in a meaningful way.[15] When either the positive or negative LR = 1, the clinical test does not yield any improvement in diagnostic certainty because results on the clinical test provide no additional certainty of diagnosis beyond the prevalence of the disorder.

Point Estimates and Confidence Intervals for Diagnostic Validity Statistics

Diagnostic validity statistics from a single study or a single contingency table are called *point estimates* because the accuracy of diagnosis is determined from a single measure derived from a limited sample.[b] Point estimates of diagnostic validity could bias the clinician's decision to use or not use the test of interest because single measures might be better or worse than what is actually true. The concept of confidence intervals (CIs) provides some protection against point estimate bias. If a study were repeated an infinite number of times with different patients sampled from the target population, a range of values for each diagnostic validity statistic would be expected across multiple study repetitions. This occurs because each replication study samples different patients from the "universe" of all patients with a defined "target" disorder. Also, there is measurement error associated with each independent replication of a diagnostic validity study that can alter the results with each replication. For these reasons, it is important to report the confidence intervals surrounding each point estimate of diagnostic validity. [16-18]

The CI can be thought of as an "error interval" and is expressed as an upper and lower limit (a range) surrounding the point estimate. For example, if sensitivity = 0.80 with a 95% CI of 0.60 to 0.90, the best guess of true sensitivity is 0.80, but the true value for sensitivity could be anywhere between 0.60 and 0.90. Thus, the 95% CI provides a range of reasonable values for the diagnostic validity statistic.[19] The point estimate including the CI in this example is written as "Sensitivity = 0.80 (0.60-0.90)."

This means that with many theoretical replications of the study with different samples of patients, the CIs calculated from those studies would hold the true value of the statistic 95% of the time.[20] If the range of the CI includes low values of sensitivity, specificity, +LRs, or high values for –LRs, then it is possible that the true value of the point estimate reflects poor diagnostic validity. For LRs, a CI that includes 1 nullifies the significance of a positive or negative LR, regardless of the size of the ratio. Hand calculation of the CI is beyond the scope of this text. Instead, the reader should use the Consensus Calculator on the disk at the back of this textbook. (refer to Video 3-1).

Clinicians need to decide which values to consider as a high priority. If misdiagnosis of the target condition is life-threatening, then it might be best to consider the lower limit of the CI as the true value of the diagnostic test.[19] In rehabilitation practice there are instances where assessment might require close scrutiny of the CI before making decisions (e.g., certifying the

---

[b]Point estimates can also be derived from a single contingency table that has data from multiple patients. Diagnostic validity statistics remain point estimates because not all patients in the target population are possible to include in a single study.

driving ability of a patient with stroke).[21] However, there are other areas of clinical practice where trial treatments are provided based on an initial classification of the patient. If the first attempt at therapy is not effective, then the therapist reviews the patient's symptom profile and may try an alternative treatment (see Flynn et al.[7] or Maluf et al.[21] for examples). In these cases the practitioner might decide to focus on the point estimate for diagnostic validity.

Demonstration of Diagnostic Validity Assessment

The vertebral artery test is sometimes used prior to manipulation or mobilization of the cervical spine to identify patients who might be injured by treatment.[23] The patient lies supine and the practitioner rotates and then extends the patient's neck. The practitioner is looking for signs of vertebral artery insufficiency (e.g., numbness, tingling in the arms, visual changes). Any sign of insufficiency is a positive test for impairment, whereas the patient with no vertebral artery signs has a negative test. The validity of the vertebral artery test as a screening tool for preventing injuries related to cervical manipulation has been discussed in the literature.[23,24] One way to test the diagnostic accuracy of this clinical test is to compare the results of the test to a criterion, or "gold," standard in a 2×2 contingency table. The use of ultrasound imaging to document findings of vertebral artery insufficiency has served as one criterion standard (see Richter and Reinking[23] for a review).

For this demonstration, 100 imaginary patients were evaluated using both the clinical test and ultrasound imaging as the criterion standard (Fig. 3-1). The clinicians performing the vertebral artery test in this hypothetical exercise were not aware of the results from the ultrasound imaging.

Diagnostic validity statistics were calculated from the hypothetical results shown in Figure 3-1 using the Diagnostic Validity Calculator on the bound-in disk. The results are summarized in **Table 3-2**. The 95% CIs surrounding the point estimates for the demonstration data were calculated by applying the formulas of Simel et al.[24] and Agresti and Coull.[25]

The data in the vertebral artery test demonstration with imaginary patients show that while *specificity* is high, sensitivity is very low. An initial impression from these hypothetical results is that the vertebral artery test might have reasonable utility as a tool that could rule out arterial occlusion (e.g., it labels 89% of non-impaired subjects as normal). However, sensitivity is unacceptably low. In addition, a positive vertebral artery test in this imaginary study makes only a tiny contribution to diagnostic certainty that an occlusion is present (+LR <2). A negative vertebral artery test also contributes only a "tiny" amount to diagnostic certainty (–LR >0.5 but <1.0).[15] The 95% CIs for both LRs contain 1, which means that this value could be the true LR and thus make no contribution to diagnostic certainty.

Calculating Diagnostic Certainty Using the Nomogram

When patients enter the clinic, the likelihood, before any diagnostic test is given, that they have a particular disorder is equal to the prevalence of that particular impairment. In other words, the odds in favor of the patient having the target condition before the initial assessment are related to the prevalence of the disorder. A review of literature can establish an estimate of prevalence, or prevalence can be estimated from a contingency table using **equation 3-4**. Another term for prevalence is "pretest probability." This simply means that before using a clinical test, the probability of the

Criterion Standard-Imaging reveals Vertebral Artery Compression

		Yes	No
Hypothetical Data	"Yes" --- Positive for Dysfunction	A 7 True Positive	B 6 False Positive
	Clinical Assessment: Vertebral Artery Test		
	"No" --- Negative for Dysfunction	C 38 False Negative	D 49 True Negative
		A+C=45	B+D=55

Figure 3-1 2×2 contingency table with hypothetical data for a clinical assessment tool that has a dichotomous outcome.

Table 3-2	95% CIs Surrounding the Point Estimates of Diagnostic Validity Statistics Derived From Figure 3-1. (See bound-in disk, Diagnostic Validity Calculator for calculations.)		
Point Estimate of Diagnostic Validity Statistic		**Lower 95% CI Limit**	**Upper 95% CI Limit**
Sensitivity	0.16	0.08	0.29
Specificity	0.89	0.78	0.95
+LR	1.43	0.52	3.94
–LR	0.95	0.81	1.11

Video Tutorial 3-1

P Calculator for Diagnostic Validity Statistics

Application:
• Illustration of how to use counts in a 2×2 contingency to calculate diagnostic validity statistics and corresponding confidence intervals.

Demonstration Data:
• Figure 3-1 but also applicable to other 2×2 diagnostic validity tables.

Steps:
1. Open disk and navigate to this chapter.
2. Select Video Tutorial 3-1: Calculator for Diagnostic Validity Statistics.
3. View how diagnostic validity statistics are automatically calculated.

Use of Calculator:
1. Navigate to the P Calculator.
2. Open this Excel spreadsheet and select the worksheet tab entitled "**95% Confidence Intervals.**"
3. Enter the frequency counts for cells A through D.
4. The 95% CIs are calculated automatically once the counts are entered.

---

correct diagnosis is no better than the prevalence of the disorder in the population.

If a condition has a prevalence of 45%, the chances of it being present are 45 out of every 100 people. In the demonstration data shown in Figure 3-1 for vertebral artery occlusion, the hypothetical prevalence is:

$$\text{Prevalence (estimated)} = \text{A+C/(A+ B+C+D)}$$
$$45/(7+6+38+39) = 0.45 = 45\%$$
eq 3-4

This means that a person entering the clinic with neck symptoms has a 45% chance of having vertebral artery occlusion before any assessment of function is initiated.

Once patient function is assessed using the clinical test, the question becomes: How much has diagnostic certainty improved through administration of the vertebral artery test? Diagnostic certainty, or "post-test probability," shows the amount of improvement in diagnostic accuracy after the test results are known.

Assuming the following information about the vertebral artery test:

• prevalence of 45% (pretest probability),
• +LR of 1.43 (see Table 3-2),
• −LR=0.95 (see Table 3-2).

The clinician can use a nomogram[27] to estimate post-test probability (**Fig. 3-2** and also Jaeschke et al.[15] and Deeks and Altman[16]). A straight line is drawn from the pretest probability, through the value of the

+LR to yield a post-test probability of approximately 50%. This means that the diagnostic certainty for identifying patients with vertebral artery occlusion improves a tiny amount (around 50%) after the vertebral artery test is applied. When the vertebral artery test is negative, the nomogram reveals that around 45% of patients would *actually have* occlusions (see Fig. 3-2). The magnitude of the +LR is too small and the −LR is too large to improve diagnostic accuracy in a meaningful way beyond prevalence.

In summary, the use of a nomogram provides a simple method to visualize the impact of prevalence (pretest probability) and the magnitude of LRs on diagnostic accuracy (post-test probability). The clinician must judge the usefulness of any diagnostic test by considering the point estimates of diagnostic validity statistics in conjunction with their respective CIs and post-test probabilities. The magnitude of post-test probabilities in the field of rehabilitation that is required to initiate a given treatment protocol depends upon risk versus benefit.[19] Higher-risk procedures should require higher post-test probabilities for +LR and lower post-test probabilities for −LRs compared to low-risk procedures.[19] After viewing the nomogram in Figure 3-2, the clinician should ask, "Do I believe it is justified to initiate a particular rehabilitation intervention knowing that a positive diagnostic test is only 50% accurate while approximately 45% of patients with negative tests have the target disorder?" Clinicians seeking a more precise method of calculating post-test probabilities should use the Post-test Probability calculator on the bound-in disk. The calculator is based on the formulas provided by Fritz et al.[27] Overall, if these data were real, the outcome would not support the use of vertebral artery testing in a clinical setting.[24]

Video Tutorial 3-2

P Calculator for Post-test Probability

Application:
• Illustration of how to calculate the precise post-test probability without the use of a nomogram.

Demonstration Data:
• Cell counts in Figure 3-1, but also applicable to any 2×2 diagnostic contingency table where cell counts are known.

Steps:
1. Open disk and navigate to this chapter.
2. Select Video Tutorial 3-2: Post-test Probability Calculator.
3. View how post-test probability is automatically calculated.

Continued

Use of Calculator:

1. Navigate to the P Calculator
2. Open this Excel spreadsheet and select the work sheet tab entitled "Post-test Probability Calculator."
3. Enter the frequency counts for cells A through D.
4. The post-test probability is calculated automatically once the counts are entered.
5. Compare results with nomogram or with hand calculations of the post-test probability.

Data Type and Cut-Point for Determining Patient Classification

When the diagnostic outcome measure is dichotomous (impaired versus nonimpaired), then the classification of patients in a 2×2 contingency table is not ambiguous (see Fig. 3-1). However, when the data type for the outcome assessment is continuous (i.e., a score on a scale from 0% to 100%, or walk time in seconds), then determination of the cut-point showing the boundary between impaired and nonimpaired requires an assessment of each score to determine which

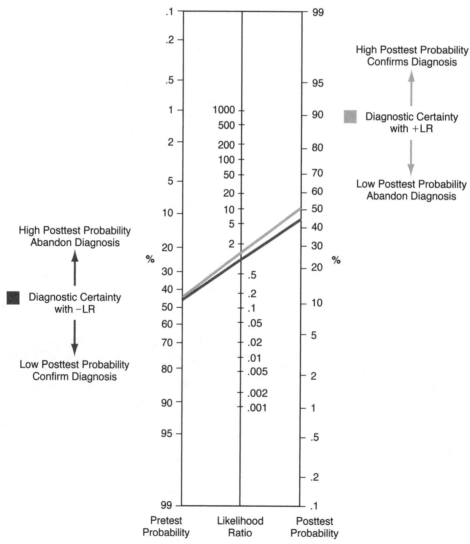

Figure 3-2 Fagan's nomogram[26] for the rapid calculation of post-test probability. The lines across the nomogram show the calculation of post-test probability of a vertebral artery test with a prevalence of 5% and a +LR = 4.24 and –LR = 0.98. (Reprinted and adapted with permission from Fagan TJ. Letter: *Nomogram for Bayes's theorem.* N Engl J Med 1975; 293:257. Copyright © 1975 Massachusetts Medical Society. All rights reserved.)

score serves as the best boundary that correctly classifies patients with and without the target condition. For example, the Timed Up & Go test (TUG)[28] is commonly used in clinical settings to evaluate the mobility status of older adults who live in the community. The test requires patients to stand from a chair, walk 10 feet, turn, walk back to the start point, and then sit down.[28] Longer TUG times are associated with reduced mobility. Time is a continuous outcome measure that requires a cut-point or boundary that creates a dichotomous classification (**Fig. 3-3**). *When the goal is to optimize both sensitivity and specificity, what is the method to identify the best cut-point (in seconds) on a continuous outcome measure like the TUG?*

Determining the Cut-Point for Diagnostic Validity Research

The cut-point selected as the threshold for establishing the presence or absence of dysfunction in the contingency table is a critical step that will influence the accuracy of outcome and hence the diagnostic validity of the tool. A cut-point too liberal may falsely classify subjects as dysfunctional, whereas a cut-point too conservative may miss identifying people with a disorder.

In the example illustrated in Figure 3-3, cell A indicates the number of true positive results (fallers who are classified with dysfunction on the TUG), cell B indicates false-positives (nonfallers who are classified with dysfunction on the TUG), cell C shows the count of false-negatives (fallers classified as having no impairment on the TUG), and cell D shows the number of true negatives (non-fallers classified as no dysfunction when the TUG assessment is applied).

Two methods could be employed to determine the optimal cut-point for the TUG: logistic regression[9] or the "receiver operating characteristic (ROC) curve analysis. The method used here to demonstrate the cut-point determination is the ROC analysis.[30] This analysis generates a contingency

table for every possible cut-point and plots a curve of true positives (sensitivity) versus false-positives (1-specificity) for each of these contingency tables. The goal is to find the optimal cut-point for use in a particular clinical setting.

Raw Data Set Up for Generating a ROC Curve

Using hypothetical TUG data for 30 imaginary patients, the organization of the data set for this exercise is shown in **Figure 3-4**. The criterion standard is fall history, and the clinical assessment is TUG measured in seconds.

Statistical software run on the demonstration data set (see Fig. 3-4) yields the output in **Table 3-3**. The procedures for generating the ROC outputs are outlined at the end of this chapter along with video tutorial 3-3 on the bound-in disk, entitled "ROC Analysis for Diagnostic Validiy."

Interpretation of ROC Curve Analysis on Hypothetical Data

There are several aspects of the ROC output that require interpretation by practitioners: the sensitivity and specificity associated with each cut-point and the selection of optimal cut-points in the ROC plot summary. The calculations for sensitivity and specificity are illustrated in **Figure 3-5**.

Subject_ID	Criterion_standard	TUG_seconds
1	faller	9
2	faller	23.6
3	faller	16.0
4	faller	14.9
5	faller	8
6	faller	12.4
7	faller	33.4
8	faller	16.1
9	faller	14.6
10	faller	11
11	faller	14.4
12	faller	16.6
13	faller	22.5
14	faller	30.5
15	faller	21.3
16	non-faller	7.6
17	non-faller	7.3
18	non-faller	8.3
19	non-faller	6.4
20	non-faller	9.8

Figure 3-4 Hypothetical data, set up to generate an ROC curve for identifying the best cut-point for the TUG test (see the data file "CH3-Timed Up & Go" with the NCSS or SPSS and PSPP freeware extension on the bound-in disk). Only a portion of the data set is shown.

Figure 3-3 2×2 contingency table for determining diagnostic validity of the Timed Up & Go Test for a cut-point to be determined.

| Table 3-3 | Data for Contingency Tables Shown at Multiple Cut-Points Generated From NCSS ROC Analysis of TUG Scores (in seconds). Cells A, B, C, and D are described in Figure 3-2. Optimal cut-point, sensitivity, 1-specificity (false-positive), and specificity are highlighted. Output here is from NCSS statistical software. See bound-in disk Video Tutorial 3-3 "ROC Analysis for Diagnostic Validity" for analogous output in SPSS or PSPP freeware. |

HYPOTHETICAL DATA

ROC Curve Outputs

TUG-seconds Cut-off Value	Count A	Count B	Count C	Count D	Sensitivity A/(A+C)	C/(A+C)	False+ B/(B+D)	Specificity D/(B+D)
6.39	15	15	0	0	1.00000	0.00000	1.00000	0.00000
6.75	15	14	0	1	1.00000	0.00000	0.93333	0.06667
7.33	15	13	0	2	1.00000	0.00000	0.86667	0.13333
7.60	15	12	0	3	1.00000	0.00000	0.80000	0.20000
8.00	15	11	0	4	1.00000	0.00000	0.73333	0.26667
8.01	14	11	1	4	0.93333	0.06667	0.73333	0.26667
8.26	14	10	1	5	0.93333	0.06667	0.66667	0.33333
8.27	14	9	1	6	0.93333	0.06667	0.60000	0.40000
8.59	14	8	1	7	0.93333	0.06667	0.53333	0.46667
8.63	14	7	1	8	0.93333	0.06667	0.46667	0.53333
8.71	14	6	1	9	0.93333	0.06667	0.40000	0.60000
9.00	14	5	1	10	0.93333	0.06667	0.33333	0.66667
9.17	13	5	2	10	0.86667	0.13333	0.33333	0.66667
9.77	13	4	2	11	0.86667	0.13333	0.26667	0.73333
11.00	13	3	2	12	0.86667	0.13333	0.20000	0.80000
11.17	12	3	3	12	0.80000	0.20000	0.20000	0.80000
12.38	12	2	3	13	0.80000	0.20000	0.13333	0.86667
14.35	11	2	4	13	0.73333	0.26667	0.13333	0.86667
14.60	10	2	5	13	0.66667	0.33333	0.13333	0.86667
14.93	9	2	6	13	0.60000	0.40000	0.13333	0.86667

Sensitivities and Specificities Linked to the ROC Analysis

All possible cut-points are generated to show sensitivity and specificity at each cut-point (see Table 3-3). *Note that each row shows the data for a different 2×2 contingency table.* For example, with N = 30, at a cut-point of 12.38 ~ 12 seconds (highlighted in Table 3-3), 12 of 15 fallers were correctly identified by the TUG (count in cell A) and 13 of 15 nonfallers were correctly identified by the test (count in cell D).

Selecting Optimal Cut-Points

There are two methods that clinicians can use to select optimal cut-points from a ROC curve analysis: a quantitative method or selecting points from the ROC curve.

- **Quantitative Method for Selecting Optimal Cut-Points.** When using the quantitative method, find the cut-point(s) with the highest number of correctly classified subjects (adding the cells A and D to yield the total of true positives and true

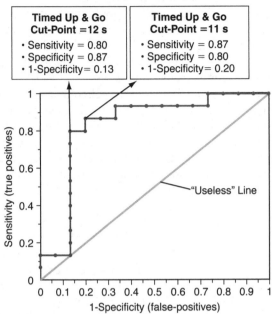

Figure 3-5 ROC plot within a box showing the distribution of true and false positives for all possible cut-points generated from the clinical assessment tool (the TUG). The hypothetical data points highlighted illustrate optimal cut-points based on the highest accuracy (tally of true positive and true negative results in the data set). Refer to video tutorial **3-3**: "ROC Analysis for Diagnostic Validity."

negatives).[30] The highest number of correctly classified subjects in the hypothetical data listing TUG scores is 25 (out of 30 subjects). This magnitude of true positives and true negatives by row is found at two cut-points (11 seconds and 12 seconds; see Table 3-3).

> *Optimal Cut-point Selection = Greatest (True Positives + True Negatives)*   **eq 3-6**

- **ROC Plot Inspection Method.** When using the ROC plot inspection method, statistical software produces the plot of true positives versus false-positive results at every possible cut-point (see Fig. 3-5). The plot occurs in a box with an area equal to 1 unit. The box has a diagonal line that splits the area into two equal parts, each part with an area of 0.50. This diagonal is called the "useless" line because points on or below this line represent cut-points that generate an equal number of true positives and false-positives or more false-positives than true positives (hence, useless in determining diagnosis).
- The ROC plot of the hypothetical TUG data set provides a visual illustration of the location of the

optimal cut-points for this demonstration (see Fig. 3-5). The cut-points in this example shape the curve toward the upper left corner and make the area under the ROC curve inside the box considerably larger than the area below the useless line. *The point(s) in the farthest upper left corner of the plot are the optimal cut-points because they have the highest sensitivity coupled with the lowest false positive rate.* The ROC plot confirms that two points in this hypothetical data set are candidates for the optimal cut-point (the same two points discovered by using the quantitative method).

- When more than one optimal cut-point is identified, the decision about which to use relies on clinical judgment and the introduction of the positive and negative likelihood ratios.[20] For the optimal cut-points shown in Figure 3-5, the +LR = 6 for the 12 s cut-point is larger than the +LR = 4.33 for the 11 s cut-point (also refer to Fig. 3-6). A +LR = 6 will result in a meaningful improvement in diagnostic confidence from baseline prevalence because it is >5. By contrast, a +LR = 4.33 will have only small effect on the power of the TUG to identify the target condition ("fallers") beyond prevalence. Thus, diagnostic accuracy of a positive test result will improve to a greater extent using the 12 s cut-point derived from the hypothetical TUG data.
- On the other hand, the −LR for the 12 s cut-point is larger (worse) than the 11 s cut-point **(Fig. 3-6)**. When using TUGs less than 12 s as a negative result on the clinical test, the negative LR = 0.23 will improve diagnostic accuracy only a "small" amount. However, TUGs less than 11 s (with a −LR = 0.17) will shift post-test probability lower than the 12 s cut-point, so there is "moderate" protection against false-negative results (refer to Table 3-2).

Video Tutorial 3-3

ROC Analysis for Diagnostic Validity Using Statistical Software

Application:
- Illustrates how to reproduce ROC numeric outputs for all possible cut-points (see Table 3-3). Illustrates how to reproduce ROC plot (see Fig. 3-5).

Demonstration Data:
- *Ch3-Timed Up & Go.**S0*** (for NCSS)
- *Ch3-Timed Up & Go.**Sav*** (for SPSS or PSPP freeware)

Steps:
1. Open disk and navigate to this chapter.

Continued

2. Select the Video Tutorial 3–3: ROC Analysis for Diagnostic Validity that is appropriate for the software you are using.
3. View how to run the analysis.

Use of Software:
1. Verify that you have either NCSS , SPSS, or PSPP freeware statistical software loaded on your computer.
2. Run the analysis illustrated in the video using the appropriate data set for the statistical software that you have installed.

Hypothetical TUG Diagnostic Validity Analysis

The summary of the ROC results so far are depicted in a nomogram (**Fig. 3-7**). It is easy to see that the optimal TUG cut-point of 12 s provides better diagnostic accuracy for positive TUG tests, whereas 11 s provides better diagnostic accuracy for negative TUG tests.

In the hypothetical data set holding TUG test results for each patient, the LR 95% confidence intervals for the *11 and 12 second cut-points* are illustrated in **Table 3-4.** Note that the number 1 does not appear in the interval for either the positive or negative LR for either cut-point. As noted previously, when 1 appears in the 95% CI, it means that a possible value for the LR conveys no change in diagnostic accuracy from that of the prevalence of the target patient group.

Gilbert et al.[19] note that "the choice of a particular cutoff value depends on how the test result will be used—to rule out disease, to rule in disease, or to screen the population (p. 407)." Both positive and negative likelihood ratios should be considered.[17] It would appear from the comparison of +LRs in Figure 3-5 that the 12 s cut-point is the best choice based on the +LR. However, clinical judgment might deem that higher sensitivity is needed for a screening test where misclassifying nonimpaired persons is not a large concern. In this case, using the 11 s cut-point will result in more nonfallers being misclassified as fallers on the TUG, but the benefit of identifying and treating a greater number of "true positives" (cell A; fallers) might offset the cost of including more "false-positives" (cell B; non-fallers) in the treatment program.

"SnNOut" and "SpPIn" Rules

Some authors recommend the use of the "SnNOut" and "SpPIn" rules to rule out disease or confirm a diagnosis.[20,31] The proposed logic is that "tests with high sensitivity have few false-negative results, and so high sensitivity effectively rules out the disorder ("SnNout"). Tests with high specificity are proposed to have the fewest false-positives and thus effectively confirm the diagnosis ("SpPIn")." The problem with this approach is that both sensitivity and specificity must be very high (on the order of 0.90) for "SnNOut" and "SpPIn" assumptions to be true.[32] Fritz and Wainner[27] point out that in the fields of rehabilitation it is rare to see clinical assessment tools with high levels of both sensitivity and specificity. The recommendation, therefore, is to include the LRs to guide judgments concerning the diagnostic validity of a selected cut-point.[32]

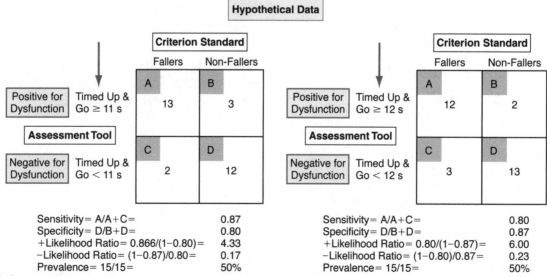

Figure 3-6 Comparison of contingency tables based on two different cut-points (highlighted by arrows) generated from a ROC analysis of hypothetical data on 30 imaginary patients.

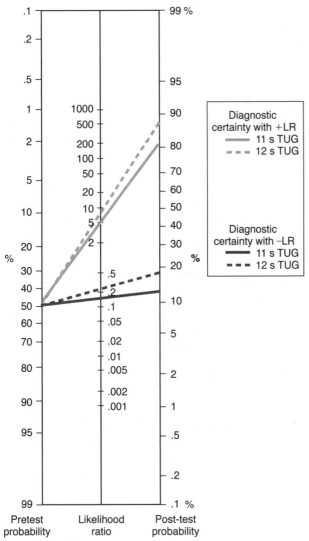

Hypothetical Timed Up & Go Diagnostic Validity Analysis

Diagnostic certainty with +LR
— 11 s TUG
--- 12 s TUG

Diagnostic certainty with −LR
— 11 s TUG
--- 12 s TUG

Pretest probability — Likelihood ratio — Post-test probability

Figure 3-7 Fagan's nomogram[26] applied to hypothetical TUG ROC analysis. (Reprinted and adapted with permission from Fagan TJ. Letter: *Nomogram for Bayes's theorem.* N Engl J Med 1975; 293:257. Copyright (c) 1975 Massachusetts Medical Society. All rights reserved.)

ROC Plot and Analysis Synopsis

The ROC analysis is used to dichotomize continuous clinical measures (examples in Table 3-1) so that an optimal cut-point for dysfunction can be identified. The cut-point fits the format of the 2×2 contingency tables used to determine the diagnostic validity of the clinical test. The best cut-points have the greatest number of true positives plus true negatives. When more than one optimal cut-point exists, the best point for ruling dysfunction "in" is usually the point with the largest +LR.[28] The cut-point with the smallest −LR is usually the best point for ruling dysfunction "out."[28]

Table 3-4	95% CIs for the 12-Second Cut-Point in the Hypothetical TUG Data Set (calculated by using the bound-in disk P calculator for this chapter; see the worksheet "95% Confidence Interval").		
Diagnostic Statistic		Lower Limit 95% Confidence Interval	Upper Limit 95% Confidence Interval
11 s TUG Cut-point:			
+ Likelihood Ratio = 4.33		1.54	12.16
− Likelihood Ratio = 0.17		0.04	0.62
12 s TUG Cut-point:			
+ Likelihood Ratio = 6.00		1.61	22.34
− Likelihood Ratio = 0.23		0.06	0.65

Clinical judgment is an important element in setting the optimal cut-point for a clinical test. When screening a population of subjects for dysfunction (fall risk in the demonstration example), the clinician must weigh the trade-off between maximizing sensitivity (with a loss of specificity) and "being swamped by patients labeled as having a positive result on a screening test who do not have the condition of interest."[20(p. 408)]

Positive and Negative Predictive Values

Positive and negative predictive values are additional statistics that have been evaluated as measures of diagnostic accuracy.[20,32-34] Predictive values show the absolute probability that a disorder is present (positive predictive value, "PPV") or absent (negative predictive value, "NPV"). Using 2×2 contingency table cell designations:

$$\text{Positive Predictive Value} = \frac{A}{A+B} \quad \textbf{eq 3-7}$$

$$\text{Negative Predictive Value} = \frac{D}{C+D} \quad \textbf{eq 3-8}$$

Positive predictive values (PPVs) are equal to post-test probability when the clinical test result is positive. Negative predictive values (NPVs) are equal to 1- post-test probability when the clinical test is negative.[32] For example, in Table 3-3, the PPV and NPV for a cut-point of 11 are:

$$\text{Positive Predictive Value} = \frac{A}{A+B} = \frac{13}{13+3} = 0.81$$

$$\text{Negative Predictive Value} = \frac{D}{C+D} = \frac{12}{2+12} = 0.86$$

The PPV in this example means that the TUG test is truly positive 13 times out of every 16 times it *appears* to be positive. Stated in a generic way, the PPV for a clinical test shows how many times the test identifies a true positive (cell A) out of every time it appears to be positive (cells A + B). The same logic applies to the NPV. The NPV for a clinical test shows how many times the test identifies a true negative (cell D) out of every time it appears to be negative (cells C + D).

The PPV and NPV (and by extension the post-test probability), however, have several limitations that restrict their use as diagnostic validity statistics. The PPV and NPV should only be used when clinicians are evaluating patients from a population where the prevalence is similar to that reported in respective studies of diagnostic validity.[20] In other words, the value of these statistics change according to the prevalence of the disorder (see **Fig. 3-8** and Fischer et al.[18] or Bogduk[32] for a demonstration of this effect). The example in Figure 3-8 uses hypothetical data to show how prevalence can influence PPV and NPV. In this example, the constants are: sensitivity = 0.75,

specificity = 0.95, and N = 100 patients. Note that the PPV increases and the NPV decreases as prevalence increases.

When prevalence of dysfunction is low, the number of nonimpaired clients will be relatively large, yielding a relatively large number of false positives (cell B), increasing the denominator of the ratio and thereby reducing the PPV (**eq. 3-7**). When prevalence of dysfunction is high, however, the number of nonimpaired clients will be relatively small, yielding a relatively small number of false positives (cell B), decreasing the denominator of the ratio and thereby increasing the PPV. Thus, predictive values not only change due to the test properties but also vary based on the prevalence of disease in the population.[18] By contrast, the LR is resistant to the influence of prevalence. For additional reading on this subject, refer to Fletcher and Fletcher.[34]

SUMMARY

Literature evaluating the diagnostic accuracy of a clinical test typically involves classifying patients in a contingency table. When the clinical test and the criterion standard yield dichotomous results (e.g., "impaired" vs. "nonimpaired"), diagnostic accuracy can be calculated directly from the 2×2 contingency table. However, when the clinical test yields a continuous result (e.g., walk time), a ROC curve provides a statistical method that dichotomizes continuous scores and facilitates selection of optimal cut-points for diagnostic validity statistics.

Several measures (and their associated CIs, where applicable) are important to consider when establishing the diagnostic validity of an assessment tool:

- Sensitivity
- Specificity
- Positive and negative LRs
- Prevalence
- Post-test probability (along with positive and negative predictive values)

The clinician must establish the priority for application of the clinical test (rule out, rule in, or screen a population[20]) so that the cut-points selected appropriately address the intended use of the tool.

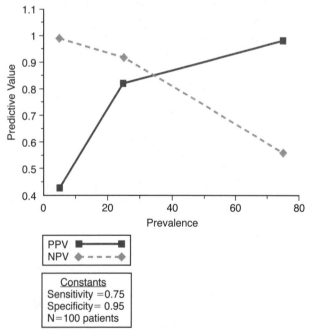

Figure 3-8 Demonstration of the effect of prevalence on PPV and NPV predictive values. See text for discussion.

PRACTICE

1. Determine the point estimates and 95% CIs for sensitivity, specificity, +LR, and –LR for each of the following contingency tables. (Note: The tables show hypothetical data representing a count of patients. Each cell is a count of patients with results from an unspecified criterion standard versus an unspecified clinical test outcome.)

Example X	
A	B
9	61
C	D
30	22

Example Y	
A	B
33	77
C	D
12	131

Example Z	
A	B
146	39
C	D
53	172

2. From question 1 above, which contingency table has:
   a. the least error for finding sensitivity?
   b. the least error for finding specificity?
   c. the greatest post-test probability for a positive impairment finding?
3. What is the pretest probability and the prevalence for the unspecified dysfunction in the contingency table in question 1, Example Y?
4. Given the data in Table 3-3, which point on the ROC curve below corresponds to a cut-point of 9 s on the TUG test?

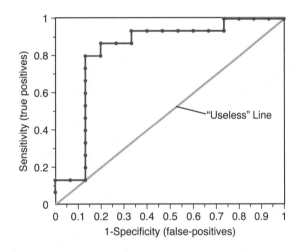

5. When sensitivity, specificity and the number of patients across diagnostic validity studies are held constant, what happens to the following statistics as prevalence increases?
   a. PPV
   b. NPV

REFERENCES

1. Norton BJ. Harnessing our collective professional power: diagnosis dialog. Phys Ther 2007; 87:635–638.
2. Sahrmann SA. Diagnosis by the physical therapist—a prerequisite for treatment. A special communication. Phys Ther 1988; 68:1703–1706.
3. Rogers JC, Holm MB. Occupational therapy diagnostic reasoning: a component of clinical reasoning. Am J Occup Ther 1991; 45:1045–1053.
4. Dibble LE, Christensen J, Ballard DJ, et al. Diagnosis of fall risk in Parkinson disease: an analysis of individual and collective clinical balance test interpretation. Phys Ther 2008; 88:323–332.

5. Scheets PL, Sahrmann SA, Norton BJ. Use of movement system diagnoses in the management of patients with neuromuscular conditions: a multiple-patient case report. Phys Ther 2007; 87:654–669.
6. Schmitt L, Snyder-Mackler L. Role of scapular stabilizers in etiology and treatment of impingement syndrome. J Orthop Sports Phys Ther 1999; 29:31–38.
7. Flynn T, Fritz J, Whitman J, et al. A clinical prediction rule for classifying patients with low back pain who demonstrate short-term improvement with spinal manipulation. Spine 2002; 27:2835–2843.
8. Razmjou H, Kramer JF, Yamada R. Intertester reliability of the McKenzie evaluation in assessing patients

with mechanical low-back pain. J Orthop Sports Phys Ther 2000; 30:368–389.

9. Shumway-Cook A, Brauer S, Woollacott M. Predicting the probability for falls in community-dwelling older adults using the Timed Up & Go Test. Phys Ther 2000; 80:896–903.

10. Deyle GD, Henderson NE, Matekel RL, et al. Effectiveness of manual physical therapy and exercise in osteoarthritis of the knee: a randomized, controlled trial. Ann of Intern Med 2000; 132:173–181.

11. Ostelo RWJG, deVet HCW, Knola DL, et al. 24-item Roland-Morris Disability Questionnaire was preferred out of six functional status questionnaires for post-lumbar disc surgery. J Clin Epidem 2004; 57:268–276.

12. Blackburn M, van Vliet P, Mockett SP. Reliability of measurements obtained with the Modified Ashworth Scale in the lower extremities of people with stroke. Phys Ther 2002; 82:25–34.

13. Bohannon RW. Manual muscle testing: does it meet the standards of an adequate screening test? Clin Rehabilitation 2005; 19:662–667.

14. Riddle DL, Stratford PW. Interpreting validity indexes for diagnostic tests: an Illustration using the Berg Balance test. Phys Ther 1999; 79:939–948.

15. Jaeschke R, Guyatt GH, Sackett DL. Users' guides to the medical literature, III: how to use an article about a diagnostic test, B: What are the results and will they help me in caring for my patients? JAMA 1994; 271:703–707.

16. Deeks JJ, Altman DG. Diagnostic tests 4: likelihood ratios. BMJ 2004; 329:168–169.

17. Dujardin B, Van den Ende J, Van Gompel A, et al. Likelihood ratios: a real improvement for clinical decision making? European J Clin Epi 1994; 10:29–36.

18. Fischer JE, Bachmann LM, Jaeschke R. A readers' guide to the interpretation of diagnostic test properties: clinical example of sepsis. Intensive Care Med 2003; 29:1043–1051.

19. Gilbert R, Logan S, Moyer VA, et al. Assessing diagnostic and screening tests: Part 1. Concepts. Western J Med 2001; 174:405–409.

20. Mazer BL, Korner-Bitensky NA, Sofer S. Predicting ability to drive after stroke. Arch Phys Med Rehabil 1998; 79:743–750.

21. Maluf KS, Sahrmann SA, Van Dillen LR. Use of a classification system to guide nonsurgical management of a patient with chronic low back pain. Phys Ther 2000; 80:1097–1111.

22. Di Fabio RP. Manipulation of the cervical spine: risks and benefits. Phys Ther 1999; 79:50–65.

23. Richter RR, Reinking MF. How does evidence on the diagnostic accuracy of the vertebral artery test influence teaching of the test in a professional physical therapist education program? Phys Ther 2005; 85:589–599.

24. Simel DL, Samsa GP, Matchar DB. Likelihood ratios with confidence: sample size estimation for diagnostic test studies. J Clin Epidemiol 1991; 44:763–770.

25. Agresti A, Coull B. Approximate is better than 'exact' for interval estimation of binomial proportions. American Statistician 1998; 52:119–126.

26. Fagan TJ. Letter: nomogram for Bayes's theorem. N Engl J Med 1975; 293:257.

27. Fritz JM, Wainner R. Examining diagnostic tests: an evidence-based perspective. Phys Ther 2001; 81:1546–1564.

28. Podsiadlo D, Richardson S. The timed "Up & Go": a test of basic functional mobility for frail elderly persons. J Am Geriatr Soc 1991; 39:142–148.

29. Zweig MH, Campbell G. Receiver-operating characteristic (ROC) plots: a fundamental evaluation tool in clinical medicine. Clin Chem 1993; 39:561–577.

30. Sackett DL, Haynes RB, Guyatt GH, et al. Clinical Epidemiology: A Basic Science for Clinical Medicine. Boston, MA: Little, Brown and Co., Inc., 1992.

31. Pewsner D, Battaglia M, Minder C, et al. Ruling a diagnosis in or out with "SpPIn" and "SnNOut": a note of caution. BMJ 2006; 329:209–213.

32. Bogduk N. Truth in musculoskeletal medicine: truth in diagnosis—validity. Australasian Muskeletal Medicine 1999; May:32–39.

33. Smith JE, Winkler RL, Fryback DG. The first positive: computing positive predictive value at the extremes. Ann Intern Med 2000; 132:804–809.

34. Fletcher RH, Fletcher SW. Clinical Epidemiology: The Essentials. Baltimore, MD: Lippincott Williams & Wilkins, 2005.

Chapter 4

Assessing Meaningful Clinical Change

Clinical Questions
- What is "clinically significant" change?
- How much improvement or worsening must a patient demonstrate to show functionally meaningful change?

The assessment of a patient before and then after a course of treatment allows the practitioner to determine if the patient's functional or cognitive status has changed. The question facing clinicians in rehabilitation practice is how much change in function represents meaningful change? Clinical assessment tools used in the fields of rehabilitation often "lack a clear external criterion (also referred to as an 'anchor' or 'global measure' of change) to help with the interpretation of scores."[1](p.740) For example, Haley and Fragala-Pinkham[1] pose the questions:

- "What can a person do differently if he or she is able to lift an additional 5 kg in knee extension?
- What does it mean to a person's involvement in sports if his or her energy expenditure index improves 0.5 beat per meter walked?
- What does it mean for the child to improve 5 to 10 points on the PEDI Functional Skills Mobility Scale?"[1](p.740)

Meaningful clinical change is defined differently, depending upon the perspective of interest.[2] From the patient's perspective, it is defined as the smallest difference in outcome pre- versus postrehabilitation where the patient still perceives the change as beneficial.[3] From the clinician's perspective, meaningful clinical change is the minimal difference in outcome across the time of intervention, "which would mandate, in the absence of troublesome side effects and excessive cost, a change in the patient's management."[3](p.408) Crosby et al. note that the clinician's perspective of meaningful clinical change may not always be in agreement with the patient's perspective.[2] It is recommended that both patient and clinician perspectives be considered when analyzing meaningful clinical change.[2]

Approaches to Identifying Meaningful Clinical Change

Clinicians seeking to identify a meaningful clinical change (MCC) threshold must rely on the literature to determine the optimal values of MCC for each clinical assessment selected. For example, the patient might be an elderly person who has suffered a hip fracture. What is the amount of improvement needed in gait speed to be functionally meaningful for the patient? This clinical question relates to the goal of therapy.

The literature review reveals a study by Palombaro et al.,[4] where the MCC for gait speed in elderly people recovering from a hip fracture was 0.10 m/s. Clinicians using this study to support their practice might reasonably establish a goal to improve gait speed by 0.10 m/s because this value is the amount of change identified from statistical procedures that assess MCC and then supported by a panel of clinical experts.[4] Thus, the MCC threshold reported in the literature helps clinicians establish treatment goals that are likely to represent change that will be helpful to the patient. Identifying the MCC threshold for any clinical assessment, therefore, requires a review of literature *prior to initiating patient assessment and treatment in the clinic.*

The purpose of this chapter is to help clinicians understand the literature addressing MCC and the underlying statistical procedures used to establish the MCC threshold. There are two approaches to identifying meaningful clinical change in the literature: the *anchor method* and the *distribution method*.[2,5] The terms associated with each method and commonly used synonyms are listed in **Table 4-1**.

Anchor Method

The anchor method uses an external criterion as the reference for distinguishing between patient improvement and worsening.[1] Examples of criterion standards derived from the anchor method include patient perception of change or the judgment of a panel of expert clinicians. These criterion standards are measures that, in theory, reflect overall "global" change in the patient's status from the beginning to the end of rehabilitation.[6] There is no uniformly accepted criterion standard to estimate true clinical change.[6]

A common, but problematic, procedure when using the anchor method is to simply ask the patient or caregiver if the subject improved over the course of rehabilitation.[1,6,7] In this scenario, change scores on the clinical assessment tool are compared with the patient's or therapist's perception of functional change over the course of treatment (**Fig. 4-1**). This type of rating is a retrospective rating of global change, because the therapist and patient must recall health status at the time of initial evaluation in order to compare that status with the postrehabilitation status.

The retrospective global rating is then presented as an external criterion to differentiate between patients who have improved or are worse (or unchanged) over the period of intervention. However, the use of retrospective global change ratings has been challenged because of recall bias.[9,10] The problem of recall bias exists with all retrospective global change criteria, including patient satisfaction ratings,[11-13] retrospective rating of change in overall pain or function,[14] or estimates of the degree of recovery from surgery.[15] In each case, recall to an earlier state is required to make judgments about change over time. The validity of retrospective ratings from the clinician perspective might be enhanced when clinicians receive training and practice their evaluations on case examples prior to rendering a judgment of patient change in longitudinal studies.[16] Nevertheless, authors continue to use retrospective global instruments as a criterion to define treatment success.[17,18]

Other "anchor" methods include consensus from expert panels,[4] a measure of the patient's ability to meet improvement criteria, and the use of prognostic rating scales completed by the clinician (see Wells et al.[19] for a review).

The Anchor Method and Contingency Tables

The "anchors" are the criterion standards for the MCC contingency tables. The criterion standard in the anchor method is dichotomized (meaning that the global change standard classifies patients as either improved or worse).[19] For example, the Expanded Disability Status Scale (EDSS) was used as a criterion standard to judge functional status in people with multiple sclerosis.[20] The EDDS is a standard measure of disease progression and degree of neurological impairment. Function is rated by the clinician in eight systems: pyramidal, cerebellar, brainstem, cerebral, bowel and bladder, sensory, visual, and "other." Scores are summed across the eight systems and vary from 0 (no neurological abnormality) to 10 (death from multiple sclerosis). A change of +1 point on the EDSS indicated global improvement of patients with multiple sclerosis, whereas a change of −1 point indicated deterioration of function.[20]

In some designs, the format of the anchor allows for separate analysis of MCC for improvement versus

Table 4-1	Terminology Used in the Literature to Describe MCC		
Term	**Abbreviation**	**Same As**	**Abbreviation**
Meaningful clinical change	MCC	• Clinically significant change	—
		• Clinical change threshold	—
Anchor method			
• Minimal clinically important difference	MCID	Minimal important difference	MID
Distribution method			
• Minimal detectable change	MDC	• Minimal detectable difference	MDD
		• Reliable change index	RCI
		• Smallest real difference	SRD
• Standard error of measure	SEM	—	—

1. How would you say this patient is today compared with the visit when he or she first completed the back questionnaire? (Circle your choice)			2. How important would you say this change is? (Circle your choice)		
__ No Change			__ No Change		
__ Worse			__ Worse		
__ Better			__ Better		
1	A tiny bit, almost the same	1	1	A tiny bit, almost the same	1
2	A little bit	2	2	A little bit	2
3	Somewhat	3	3	Somewhat	3
4	Moderately	4	4	Moderately	4
5	Quite a bit	5	5	Quite a bit	5
6	A great deal	6	6	A great deal	6
7	A very great deal	7	7	A very great deal	7

*The patient's version is identical to the clinician's version; however, the words "this patient is" are replaced by the words "you are."

Figure 4-1 Example of retrospective global change rating completed by both the therapist and the patient. Patient and therapist scores are averaged to provide an estimate of true change and then scores are dichotomized by arbitrary definition of improved versus worse so that the criterion standard will conform to a 2×2 contingency table. (Reprinted from Stratford PW, Binkley JM, Riddle DL. Health status measures: strategies and analytic methods for assessing change scores. Phys Ther 1996; 76:1109–1123[8] with permission of the American Physical Therapy Association. This material is copyrighted and any further reproduction or distribution requires written permission from APTA.)

decline. For example, Brach et al.[21] used self-report of walking difficulty as the global criterion standard when evaluating functional mobility of elderly people residing in the community. They analyzed MCC at initial and follow-up sessions. They first identified those who reported *no difficulty at baseline*. At follow-up, some people in this cohort developed difficulty (declining performance) and some continued to have no difficulty ("stable"). The criterion standard thus allowed for a comparison of those declining versus those who remained stable. The MCC produced from this anchor format measured a decline in performance.

Continuing with their analysis, they then identified those who *reported difficulty at baseline*. At follow-up, some people in this cohort reported improvement in walking ability while some continued to have difficulty ("stable" because walking was difficult at both initial and follow-up). This part of the analysis allowed for the calculation of an MCC reflecting improvement. Using the criterion standard in this way produced two MCCs on various gait parameters, one reflecting a threshold for improvement and one showing a threshold for decline. The anchor in this study was used in conjunction with a comparison of mean change scores for each category of the anchor. This variation of the anchor method did not use a contingency table. Refer to Brach et al.[21] for additional information.

If the clinical test matched to the criterion standard produces a continuous outcome measure, then an ROC analysis is needed to dichotomize the clinical assessment

change scores to enable selection of the optimal cut-point for meaningful clinical change. A demonstration of this method is shown later in this chapter.

The contingency table for establishing MCC has some similarities and some important differences compared to the contingency table used to determine the diagnostic accuracy (Chapter 3) of a clinical assessment tool (Fig. 4-2).

Similarities

- The contingency tables are always 2×2.
- Both types of contingency tables show counts of patients in each cell of the table.
- An optimal cut-point for clinical assessment tools that produce continuous outcomes are typically identified from a ROC curve analysis in both types of research.

Differences

- The presentation of the criterion standard in clinical change research is "reversed" from that in diagnostic validity (see Fig. 4-2). Note that the criterion standard for meaningful clinical change indicates "improvement" in the first column of the contingency table, whereas the criterion standard for diagnostic validity shows "dysfunction" in that column.
- The *meaningful clinical change score* on the clinical assessment tool is identified as the variable of interest (e.g., the change in function from initial assessment to post-treatment or follow-up) in

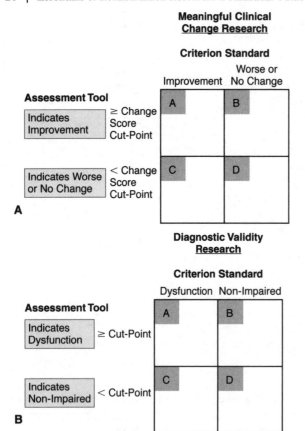

Figure 4-2 Comparison of the contingency table used to evaluate meaningful clinical change (A) versus the table used in diagnostic validity research (B). It is assumed that higher change scores for meaningful change tables indicate clinical improvement.

research on clinically meaningful change. *The scores are usually subtracted in a way that makes positive scores reflect improvement (but this is not always the case).* Thus, change scores exceeding or equal to the cut-point indicate *clinical improvement*, whereas change scores below the cut-point indicate *no change or worse* functional status following treatment. Diagnostic validity research does not use a *change score* for the clinical test of interest.

- The definitions of true and false-positive, as well as the respective true and false-negative cells in the contingency tables differ among clinical change versus diagnostic validity research (Table 4-2).

The calculation of sensitivity, specificity, and ± likelihood ratios is the same for clinical change and diagnostic validity, but the interpretation of these statistics differs depending upon the type of research that generated the contingency table (see Fig. 4-2 and Table 4-2).[22,23]

Sensitivity Compared

- In diagnostic validity, of all the people identified with dysfunction by the criterion standard, a proportion of that group is classified as having dysfunction by the clinical assessment tool. *This is sensitivity in the context of diagnostic validity.*
- For meaningful clinical change, of all the people identified who clinically improved by the criterion standard, a proportion of that group is classified as "improved" by the change score on the clinical assessment tool. *This is sensitivity in the context of meaningful clinical change.*

Specificity Compared

- In diagnostic validity, of all the people identified as non-impaired by the criterion standard, a proportion of that group is classified as nonimpaired by the clinical assessment tool. *This is specificity in the context of diagnostic validity.*
- For meaningful clinical change, of all the people identified who did not improve by the criterion standard, a proportion of that group is classified as "no improvement" by the change score on the clinical assessment tool. *This is specificity in the context of meaningful clinical change.*

+Likelihood Ratio Compared

- In *diagnostic validity, the +likelihood ratio* is the likelihood that a person identified as dysfunctional on the clinical assessment will actually have the target disorder.
- For *meaningful clinical change, the +likelihood ratio* is the likelihood that a person identified as "improved" by the change score on the clinical assessment will actually be classified as improved by the criterion standard.

–Likelihood Ratio Compared

- In *diagnostic validity, the –likelihood ratio* is the likelihood that a person with a negative clinical test has the target disorder.
- For *meaningful clinical change, the –likelihood ratio* is the likelihood that a person identified as "not improved" by the change score on the clinical assessment will actually be classified as improved by the criterion standard.

Direction of Scale Change in the Outcome Measure

When reviewing the literature, it is necessary to know the scale of the outcome measure and what a high versus low score indicates for the patient's outcome. For example, when measuring distance walked during a 6-minute walk test,[24] higher scores indicate better

Contingency Table Cell	Meaningful Clinical Change	Research	Diagnostic Validity	Research
	Table 4-2 Definitions of True and False Positives and Negatives in Meaningful Clinical Change Vs. Diagnostic Validity Research			
A	True positive for clinical improvement	Both the criterion standard and clinical change score indicate *improvement*	True positive for dysfunction	Both the criterion standard and clinical assessment indicate *dysfunction*
B	False positive for clinical improvement	The criterion standard indicates no improvement but the change score indicates improvement	False positive for dysfunction	The criterion standard indicates no impairment but the clinical assessment indicates dysfunction
C	False negative for clinical improvement	The criterion standard indicates improvement but the change score indicates no improvement	False-negative for dysfunction	The criterion standard indicates impairment but the clinical assessment indicates no dysfunction
D	True negative for clinical improvement	Both the criterion standard and clinical change score indicate *no improvement*	True negative for dysfunction	Both the criterion standard and clinical assessment indicate *no dysfunction*

performance. A change score for a patient who walked 300 m at initial evaluation (pretest) and 400 m following 2 weeks of rehabilitation would have a negative change score of

$$\text{Change Score} = \text{Pretest} - \text{Post-test}$$
$$= 300 - 400 \text{ meters}$$
$$= \textbf{-100 meters}$$

The negative change score in the case of a 6-minute walk test shows that the patient **improved** from baseline to discharge.

By comparison, the scale on the Roland-Morris disability questionnaire[25] is 0 to 24, with higher scores indicating more disability (this scale is discussed in more detail later in the chapter). In this example, a patient reporting a disability level of 10 at the initial evaluation and a score of 19 following rehabilitation would have a negative change score of

$$\text{Change Score} = \text{Pretest} - \text{Post-test}$$
$$= 10 - 19$$
$$= \textbf{-9}$$

In this case, however, a negative change score indicates that the patient's self-perceived disability **worsened** after treatment.

These scenarios highlight the fact that a negative (or positive) change score must be interpreted in light of the outcome variable scale. In one outcome measure, a negative change score indicates improvement,

while in another case, a negative change score indicates worsening status. Thus, when interpreting the results of meaningful change research, the author's order of subtracting baseline versus discharge scores must be considered so that the meaning of a positive or negative change score is correctly interpreted.

Demonstration of the Anchor Method

In order to demonstrate the analysis of meaningful clinical change, a hypothetical data set was constructed based on the Roland-Morris Disability Scale **(Fig. 4-3)**.[26] This scale is a widely used measure of self-perceived disability related to low back dysfunction.[25,27-29] Patients check the number of questions that pertain to their current status. The number of questions checked is the disability score (range from 0 = no disability to 24 = maximum disability). The data set holding hypothetical disability scores is shown in **Figure 4-4**. In this demonstration 88 imaginary patients have an initial evaluation and receive a rehabilitation intervention followed by a postrehabilitation assessment (follow-up).

For the anchor method of MCC analysis, the criterion standard in this demonstration is return to work. The clinical test of interest is the change score (baseline minus follow-up to make a positive change score equal improvement) on the Roland-Morris Disability Scale. The change score in this demonstration is considered a continuous variable (i.e., the variable has many values designating various levels of

---

Roland Morris Disability Questionnaire

When your back hurts, you may find it difficult to do some things you normally do. This list contains sentences that people have used to describe themselves when they have back pain. When you read them, you may find that some stand out because they describe you today. As you read the list, think of yourself today. When you read a sentence that describes you today, put a tick against it. If the sentence does not describe you, then leave the space blank and go on to the next one. Remember, only tick the sentence if you are sure it describes you today.

___ 1. I stay at home most of the time because of my back.
___ 2. I change position frequently to try and get my back comfortable.
___ 3. I walk more slowly than usual because of my back.
___ 4. Because of my back I am not doing any of the jobs that I usually do around the house.
___ 5. Because of my back, I use a handrail to get upstairs.
___ 6. Because of my back, I lie down to rest more often.
___ 7. Because of my back, I have to hold on to something to get out of an easy chair.
___ 8. Because of my back, I try to get other people to do things for me.
___ 9. I get dressed more slowly than usual because of my back.
___ 10. I only stand for short periods of time because of my back.
___ 11. Because of my back, I try not to bend or kneel down.
___ 12. I find it difficult to get out of a chair because of my back.
___ 13. My back is painful almost all the time.
___ 14. I find it difficult to turn over in bed because of my back.
___ 15. My appetite is not very good because of my back pain.
___ 16. I have trouble putting on my socks (or stockings) because of the pain in my back.
___ 17. I only walk short distances because of my back.
___ 18. I sleep less well on my back.
___ 19. Because of my back pain, I get dressed with help from someone else.
___ 20. I sit down for most of the day because of my back.
___ 21. I avoid heavy jobs around the house because of my back.
___ 22. Because of my back pain, I am more irritable and bad tempered with people than usual.
___ 23. Because of my back, I go upstairs more slowly than usual.
___ 24. I stay in bed most of the time because of my back.

The score is the total number of items checked—*i.e.,* from a minimum of 0 to a maximum of 24.

Figure 4-3 Roland-Morris Disability Scale. (Reprinted from Roland M, Fairbank J. The Roland-Morris Disability Questionnaire and the Oswestry Disability Questionnaire. Spine 2000; 25:3115–3124).[25]

Figure 4-4 Hypothetical data, set up to generate a ROC curve for analyzing meaningful clinical change. All imaginary patients were *not working* at the initial evaluation. Twenty-nine of 88 rows are shown. RM = Roland-Morris. Data from initial visit, follow-up postrehab, and the change score are illustrated. (See the data file "Ch4_Roland_Morris_Disability_Scale" for NCSS, SPSS, or PSPP on the bound-in disk.)

Subject	Return_to_Work	Initial_RM	RM_followup	RM_change
1	No	16	18	−2
2	No	18	18	0
3	Yes	20	3	17
4	Yes	20	17	18
5	No	2	18	−16
6	No	5	8	−3
7	No	20	22	−2
8	No	18	23	−5
9	No	21	21	0
10	Yes	23	16	7
11	No	20	21	−1
12	Yes	10	2	8
13	No	9	7	2
14	Yes	23	8	15
15	Yes	23	8	15
16	No	17	19	−2
17	No	11	15	−4
18	No	12	15	−3
19	No	8	10	−2
20	Yes	20	10	10
21	Yes	24	15	9
22	Yes	12	6	6
23	No	4	7	−3
24	Yes	23	12	11
25	No	23	23	0
26	Yes	23	13	10
27	No	21	17	4
28	Yes	21	11	10
29	Yes	10	2	8

function). Therefore, a ROC curve analysis is required to dichotomize the change scores. The ROC curve analysis yields the output shown in **Table 4-3** and **Figure 4-5**. The cut-point(s) with the highest number of correctly classified subjects (adding the cells A + D to yield the total of true positives and true negatives) will be the optimal cut-point for detecting meaningful clinical change.[28] That point on the ROC curve is the MCID. In other words, the minimal amount of change from the initial evaluation to follow-up that is considered clinically meaningful is the change score that identifies the truest results on the ROC curve.

The highest number of correctly classified subjects in this demonstration occurs at a Roland-Morris *change score* of 5, where 80 (out of 88 patients) are correctly classified (see Table 4-3). As patients must change at least 5 points on the Roland Scale in order to demonstrate meaningful clinical change from initial evaluation to follow-up, the MCID is 5 points.

The sensitivity and specificity of the 5-point disability change score in the demonstration data were 0.97 and 0.87, respectively (see Table 4-3). This means that the change score threshold of 5 points is highly sensitive for identifying imaginary patients who are likely to return to work and highly specific for classifying imaginary patients unlikely to return to work.

The +LR is 7.22 **(Table 4-4)** with a 95% confidence interval that does not hold 1 (a meaningless value for LR). A nomogram can be used to determine post-test probability of return to work. The essential statistics are:

Prevalence = 41%
+LR = 7.22
−LR = 0.03

These values are entered into the nomogram in **Figure 4-6**.

In summary, this demonstration shows that a clinician can be about 85% certain that a patient who changes +5 Roland-Morris points is likely to return to work. The −LR of 0.03 (also with a confidence interval that does not hold 1) complements the finding from the +LR. The −LR in this case indicates that an imaginary person who returns to work is not likely to have a disability change score of less than 5 Roland-Morris points.

Interpretation of ROC Curve Analysis for the Anchor Method

The contingency table data at the optimal change score of 5 Roland-Morris Disability points (see Table 4-3) are placed in a 2×2 contingency table for further analysis **(Fig. 4-7)**. The cut-point in this contingency table (5 disability points) is the MCID. The diagram in Figure 4-7 shows that:

- 35 subjects who improved by 5 or more disability points returned to work (cell A—true positive);
- 45 patients who did *not* improve by at least 5 disability points did *not* return to work (cell D—true negative);
- 7 patients met the change threshold of 5 disability points, but did not return to work (cell B—false-positive);
- 1 subject did not meet the threshold change score for improvement, but managed to return to work (cell C—false-negative).

The MCID from this analysis is interpreted according to the design of the anchor. In this case, the anchor is return to work or not. This means that patients who *improve* 5 or more points from initial evaluation to follow-up have meaningful positive change and those who improve less than 5 points are classified as no change or decline.

Distribution Method

The distribution method derives meaningful clinical change based on the statistical characteristics of the patient sample. The distribution method encompasses

Video Tutorial 4-1

Anchor Method for Determining *Meaningful Clinical Change* Using Statistical Software

Application:

- Illustrates how to reproduce ROC numeric outputs for all possible cut-points (see Table 4-3) and plot a ROC curve (see Fig. 4-5)

Demonstration Data Set:

- *Ch4_Roland_Morris_Disability_Scale.**S0*** (for NCSS)
- *Ch4_Roland_Morris_Disability_Scale.**Sav*** (for SPSS and PSPP freeware)

Steps:

1. Open the disk and navigate to this chapter.
2. Select the Video Tutorial 4-1: Anchor Method that is appropriate for the software you are using.
3. View how to run the analysis-using software.

Use of Software:

1. Verify that you have either NCSS, SPSS, or PSPP freeware statistical software loaded on your computer.
2. Run the analysis illustrated in the video using the appropriate data set for the statistical software that you have installed.

Table 4-3	**NCSS Data for Contingency Tables at Multiple Cut-Points Generated From ROC Analysis of Roland-Morris Change Scores.**
	Optimal cut-point based on MCID is highlighted. Output is truncated.

HYPOTHETICAL DATA

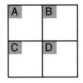

RM-change score Cutoff

Value	A	B	C	False+ D	Specificity A/(A + C)	C/(A + C)	Sensitivity B/(B + D)	D/(B + D)
−3.00	36	41	0	11	1.00000	0.00000	0.78846	0.21154
−2.00	36	34	0	18	1.00000	0.00000	0.65385	0.34615
−1.00	36	28	0	24	1.00000	0.00000	0.53846	0.46154
0.00	36	24	0	28	1.00000	0.00000	0.46154	0.53846
1.00	36	18	0	34	1.00000	0.00000	0.34615	0.65385
2.00	36	17	0	35	1.00000	0.00000	0.32692	0.67308
3.00	35	13	1	39	0.97222	0.02778	0.25000	0.75000
4.00	35	12	1	40	0.97222	0.02778	0.23077	0.76923
5.00	35	7	1	45	0.97222	0.02778	0.13462	0.86538
6.00	31	6	5	46	0.86111	0.13889	0.11538	0.88462
7.00	28	2	8	50	0.77778	0.22222	0.03846	0.96154
8.00	22	1	14	51	0.61111	0.38889	0.01923	0.98077
9.00	18	1	18	51	0.50000	0.50000	0.01923	0.98077
10.00	14	1	22	51	0.38889	0.61111	0.01923	0.98077
11.00	10	1	26	51	0.27778	0.72222	0.01923	0.98077
12.00	9	0	27	52	0.25000	0.75000	0.00000	1.00000

numerous statistical manipulations and each provides a measure of change.[2] For the purposes of this text, the distribution-based measure of meaningful clinical change will be minimal detectable change (MDC; also called *reliable change* or *smallest real difference*; see also Table 4-1).[7,8,30,31] The MDC is the smallest change in outcome that likely reflects true improvement or true worsening.[7,30]

An example of the distribution method is the use of the MDC on the Berg Balance Scale to evaluate changes in balance ability.[20] The Berg Balance Scale consists of 14 tasks that test balance and mobility. Each task is rated from 0 (unable to perform or requiring maximal assistance) to 4 (normal performance). The composite score across 14 tasks can vary from 0 to 56.[32] When the MDC was calculated for the Berg Scale, the meaningful clinical change threshold for people with multiple sclerosis who improved their balance was

+3 points *(follow-up score minus initial assessment score)*, whereas those with a change of at least −3 points (or negative change scores with an absolute value greater than 3) were classified as "worse."[20]

Patients with a change in the Berg score *less than* +3 points *but greater than* -3 points can be classified as "unchanged." An illustration of this convention is shown in **Figure 4-8**.

In practice, factors like potential ambiguity of the questions on any clinical assessment scale could draw a different response from the patient at initial versus follow-up visits independently of any change in self-perceived health status. *Measurement error, therefore, is the amount of change that is seen in the outcome scores that is due to factors other than a change in disability.* In other words, the MDC represents the minimal amount of change that is not likely due to chance variations of outcome scores with repeated measures.

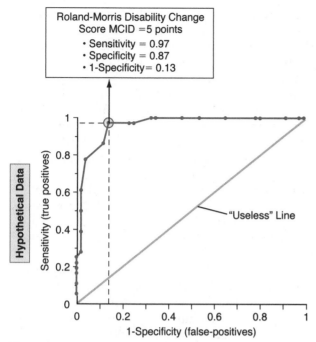

Figure 4-5 ROC plot for meaningful clinical change. The plot shows the distribution of true versus false-positives for all possible cut-points generated from the change scores on the clinical assessment tool. The data point highlighted illustrates the optimal cut-point based on the highest accuracy (tally of true positive and true negative results in the data set). This cut-point is the MCID. The plot is derived from hypothetical data in Table 4-3.

Demonstration of Distribution Method

The hypothetical data set for the Roland-Morris disability scores used for the anchor method demonstration is also used here for a demonstration of the distribution method. There are several steps to calculating the MDC. Before arriving at the value of the MDC, the standard error of measure (SEM) must be calculated. This statistic

| Table 4-4 | 95% Confidence Intervals for the 5-point Roland-Morris Disability Change Score in the Hypothetical Roland-Morris Data Set (Calculated Using the 95% Confidence Interval Calculator in Chapter 3 of the bound-in disk). |

Diagnostic Statistic	Lower Limit 95% Confidence Interval	Upper Limit 95% Confidence Interval
+Likelihood Ratio = 7.22	3.62	14.22
−Likelihood Ratio = 0.03	0.00	0.22

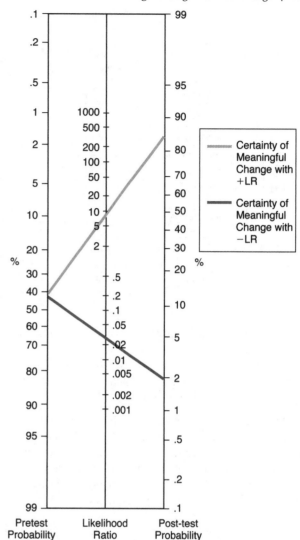

Figure 4-6 Nomogram used to determine the level of certainty for return to work in the demonstration of MCC using the anchor method in a hypothetical data set.

has been used as a measure of MCC in its own right and is one index of the amount of measurement error in a clinical assessment tool.[1,4] In any case, the SEM is a central component of the MDC calculation.

$$SEM = SD\ initial\ \sqrt{1-r} \qquad \textbf{eq 4-1}$$

where SD is the standard deviation of the scores on the initial evaluation (refer to the appendix to this chapter for a definition of SD) and "r" is the test-retest reliability coefficient.[33]

There are several methods of calculating "r":

- Correlate the initial scores with the follow-up scores using a Pearson Product Moment or Spearman rank order correlation coefficient (Chapter 6).[33]
- Compare the initial scores with the follow-up scores using analysis of variance (ANOVA) and

Meaningful Clinical Change Research

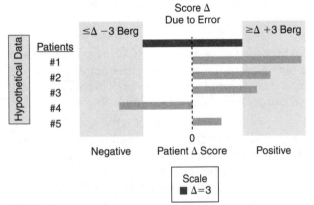

Figure 4-7 Contingency table for the Roland-Morris optimal change score in the demonstration data set. The cutpoint (5 points of change) is the minimal clinically important difference (MCID) in this demonstration.

then calculate an intraclass correlation coefficient (Chapter 6).
- Measure internal consistency of the clinical assessment tool using Cronbach's alpha as the reliability coefficient (Chapter 7).[34]

It has been suggested that the SEM can be used as a "proxy" for estimating MCID and thus would constitute an additional measure of change that might be useful in the absence of a robust criterion-reference for global change.[19,33,35] A comparison of SEM and MCID will be demonstrated later in this chapter.

ⁱⁱ SEM can also be estimated by using the square root of the mean square error term in an ANOVA (Fleiss 1986). Refer to Chapter 6.

Haley et al.[1] recommend the use of a measure of test-retest reliability as the reliability coefficient in the SEM equation. For the demonstration exercise in this chapter, a Spearman rank order correlation coefficient is used to determine the strength of the association between the hypothetical initial and follow-up Roland-Morris disability scores. Correlation coefficients can vary from +1 to −1. The closer the coefficient is to the absolute value of 1, the stronger the direct (+) or indirect (−) relationship between the scores on repeated administration of the disability scale. In the demonstration example, the correlation between initial and follow-up disability scores is $r_{Spearman}$ = 0.45 (abbreviated r_s). The association between initial and follow-up scores is illustrated in **Figure 4-9**.

The MDC may now be calculated by multiplying the SEM by 1.65 (the z-score associated with 90% level of confidence) and the square root of 2, reflecting the additional uncertainty introduced by using difference scores from measurements at two points in time.[31] The z-score is defined in the appendix to this chapter. A summary of the MDC formula from Haley et al.[1] with notations is shown in **Figure 4-10**.

The MDC has the notation MDC_{90}, indicating that the MDC is based on a 90% CI. For the demonstration example, the MDC_{90} is 11 and is derived as follows:

Standard deviation of initial disability scores (SD) = 6.48

Test-retest correlation coefficient (r) = 0.45

$$SEM = SD_{initial}\sqrt{1-r} = 6.48\sqrt{1-0.45} = \mathbf{4.8}$$

$$MDC_{90} = \text{Critical z-score}_{level\ of\ confidence} * SEM * \sqrt{2} = 1.645 * 4.8 * 1.41 = \mathbf{11}$$

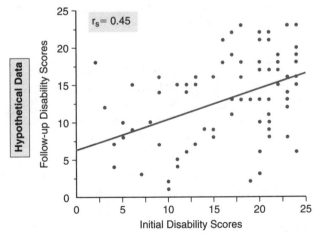

Figure 4-8 Illustration of MDC = ±3 for the Berg Balance Scale. Patients #1 through #3 show meaningful improvement in balance, whereas patient #4 shows clinically significant worsening. Patient #5 does not meet the meaningful change threshold for improvement even though Δ is in the positive direction. Data shown are hypothetical.

Figure 4-9 Scatter plot of initial versus follow-up hypothetical Roland-Morris disability scores. Line of best fit (least squares regression line) is shown projecting through the data points.

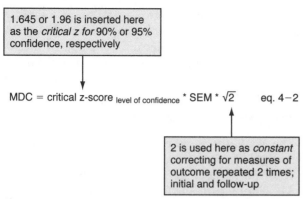

$$MDC = critical\ z\text{-}score_{\text{level of confidence}} * SEM * \sqrt{2} \qquad \text{eq. } 4\text{--}2$$

Figure 4-10 Illustration of calculation of MDC. SEM = standard error of measure. Critical z-score is defined in the appendix to this chapter.

The interpretation for this result is that there is 90% confidence that patients who change at least ±11 points on the Roland-Morris Scale show true change in disability. Note that the SEM shows 5 disability points before conversion to the MDC statistic. As a proxy measure of meaningful clinical change,[19,33,35] the SEM in this demonstration shows essentially the identical threshold derived by the anchor method using the return-to-work global criterion (MCID = 5 disability points).

Generalization of MCC Findings to a Clinical Setting

Once meaningful clinical change is established in the peer-reviewed literature, clinicians utilize this information to guide their practice in several ways. If the hypothetical demonstration data could be generalized to real patients with low back dysfunction, changes of 5 points in the Roland-Morris Disability Scale over the course of intervention would have great prognostic value. However, there are several issues that should be considered before using a single MCC point estimate in a clinical environment.

The anchor and distribution methods are not mutually exclusive and can be used in combination to enhance the analysis of meaningful clinical change.[4,20,36] Ideally, there should be consensus among MCC indices to establish confidence in the change threshold for clinical application. In practice, however, the anchor and distribution methods address different aspects of MCC. In order to avoid the problem of forcing the selection of a single point estimate, Haley et al. suggest reporting a range of MCC values based on multiple methods of calculating MCC.[1]

In the demonstration analysis, the large discrepancy between the MCID and SEM compared to the

Video Tutorial 4-2

Distribution Method for Determining Meaningful Clinical Change Using Statistical Software

Application:
• Illustrates how to use statistical software to calculate SDs and an Excel spreadsheet calculator for standard error of measure (SEM) and minimum detectable change (MDC)

Demonstration Data:
• *Ch4_Roland_Morris_Disability_Scale.**S0*** (for NCSS)
• *Ch4_Roland_Morris_Disability_Scale.**Sav*** (for SPSS and PSPP freeware)

Application:
MDC (minimal detectable difference) Calculator (P_Calculator-MDC.xls)
Excel is needed to view and use the P calculator)

Steps:
1. Open the disk and navigate to this chapter.
2. Select Video Tutorial 4–2: Distribution Method
3. View how to run the analysis-using software.

Use of Software:
1. Verify that you have either NCSS, SPSS, on PSPP freeware statistical software as well as Microsoft Excel loaded on your computer.
2. Run the analysis illustrated in the video using the appropriate data set for the statistical software that you have installed.

MDC_{90} highlights the importance of using multiple indices to characterize meaningful clinical change. The MDC_{90} is large in the demonstration because there is not a strong relationship between initial and follow-up scores (note the wide scatter of points around the line of best fit in Fig. 4-9). Therefore, the range of possible MCC thresholds varies from 5 (anchor method) to 11 Roland-Morris points (distribution method). This wide range would leave much to clinician judgment when selecting the threshold MCC as a treatment goal or to researchers seeking to base outcome on MCC. New statistical methods such as triangulation are being tested to determine how the anchor and distribution methods can be combined with other data describing the patient's response,[37] but definitive work on this topic is pending and is beyond the scope of this text.

---

iii If clinical researchers selected a 95% confidence interval instead of a 90% confidence interval as shown, then the critical z for the MDC calculation would be 1.96, resulting in a MDC = 13.

Also, the severity of disease of patients studied in the literature must be known so that MCC thresholds can be applied to the appropriate target group. Some studies limit the assessment of patients to a specific stage of deficit so that the MCC reported applies only to patients with a particular level of dysfunction (e.g., early versus severe Parkinson's disease[38]). Others analyze meaningful change in the context of disease severity by using a percentage of change from baseline rather than an absolute scale value. For example, Jordan et al.[39] found that patients with low back pain who improved 30% from their baseline Roland-Morris score had clinically significant change. This method allowed the authors to provide a MCC threshold for improvement regardless of each patient's initial disability status. Stratford et al.[40] reported several different MCC scores, each corresponding to a particular level of initial severity for self-reported disability.

Reviews of literature to find the best MCC for a particular clinical application should also focus on the target population of interest. The finding that a change in gait speed of 0.10 m/s for nonimpaired elders living in the community[4] might not apply to the institutionalized elderly or to those diagnosed with a neurological disorder that impairs gait. Similarly, the MCC score for a functional assessment of people with mild Parkinson's disease might not apply to those with a severe form of the disorder.[38]

MCC: Clinical Versus Statistical Significance

Statistical significance means that findings of a difference or an association are not likely due to chance (significance testing is covered in the appendix to this chapter). Statistical significance is not the same as clinical significance. If it is known that 5 disability points on the Unified Parkinson's Disease Rating Scale motor section is the MCC threshold,[38] then the finding that a treatment group was 2 or 3 disability points better than a control group after intervention might be statistically significant, but clinically meaningless. Thus, the MCC might be larger than the magnitude of change that is found to be statistically significant.[36]

SUMMARY

- The MCC threshold can vary depending on the method of calculation.
- A review of literature is required to identify the MCC for a particular clinical assessment prior to initiating patient evaluation and treatment in the clinic.
- Clinicians should consider the target population and degree of disease severity at the time of initial evaluation in studies reporting MCC threshold before applying thresholds in the clinical setting.
- For the anchor method, criterion standards for meaningful clinical change are an essential component for identifying the MCC threshold.
- The ROC curve provides a statistical method that dichotomizes the change scores for the clinical assessment tool and helps identify the optimal cut-point for meaningful clinical change.
- The distribution method for assessing MCC relies on statistical characteristics of the outcome scores, such as standard deviation, correlations between initial and discharge scores, and z-scores, to establish confidence intervals; hence the term *distribution* (see appendix).
- While calculated from a 2×2 contingency table in similar fashion, the *interpretation* of sensitivity, specificity, and likelihood ratios for meaningful clinical change research differs from diagnostic validity research.
- Consideration of several MCC statistics (e.g., MCID and MDC) may be necessary to establish an appropriate range of MCC thresholds for a particular clinical assessment tool.

Key Terms

- z-scores
- Critical z-score
- z-score sample
- z-score universe
- Standard deviation (SD)
- Estimate of the standard error of the mean (SEM)

The Normal Distribution and Standard Deviation

The normal ("bell-shaped") curve is a frequency distribution (it is also referred to as a gaussian distribution). Think of the normal curve as a model, a template, or a theoretical frequency distribution where the same number of cases or scores occurs at specified distances above and below the mean. The normality assumption allows generalizations to be made from the sample to the population. These generalizations usually take the form of confidence intervals and hypothesis tests.[41]

The model for a normal curve is the same regardless of the type of outcome measure being evaluated. For example, it does not matter if the outcome measure is range of motion (degrees), walking distance (meters), or disability scale points. If these measures are assumed to be normally distributed, then the model for their corresponding frequency distributions is that:

- 34% of the cases or scores will occur within 1 SD from the mean;
- 48% of the cases or scores will occur within 2 SDs from the mean;
- 49.9% of the cases or scores will occur within 3 SDs from the mean.

Because the normal curve is symmetrical, the same pattern of case occurrence is found on either side of the mean. The template or model of the normal distribution is illustrated in **Figure 4-11**.

The SD is a measure of variability and is derived from the distance of each point in the data set from the mean:

$$SD = \sqrt{SS / n - 1} \qquad \text{eq A4-1}$$

where

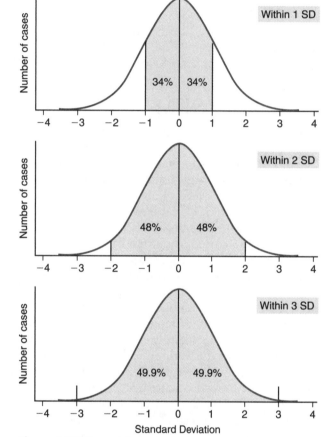

Figure 4-11 Normal (gaussian) curve where the number of cases in the sample is assumed to occur at specified distances from the mean.

SS = sum of the squared deviations from the mean
n = number of data points

Thus, if the mean = 6 and a point in the data = 2, the deviation of that point from the mean is 6 − 2 = 4. The squared deviation from the mean is 4², or 16. When each point in the data set is treated this way, the SS is simply the sum of squared deviations from the mean.

Larger SDs indicate larger variance of scores around the mean. However, case occurrence on the normal distribution is not altered by the size of the SD. For example, if mean shoulder abduction range of motion is 20 degrees with an SD of 5 degrees (expressed as 20 degrees ± 5 degrees), then according to **Figure 4-11,** 68% of the scores will occur between 15 and 25 degrees:

34% of scores between 20 and 25 (+1 SD);
34% of scores between 20 and 15 (–1 SD);
Total of 68% of scores ±1 SD.

In contrast, if the same mean has a SD of 10 degrees of motion, then 68% of the scores will occur between 10 and 30 degrees:

34% of scores between 20 and 30 (+1 SD);
34% of scores between 20 and 10 (–1 SD);
Total of 68% of scores ±1 SD.

Estimating SEM

When clinicians collect outcome measures, they typically do so on a relatively small number of patients. For example, if a practitioner evaluated visual neglect in patients with stroke, the patients of interest might be from a local clinic or a small number of clinics. This group of patients is a *sample* of the larger universe of patients across the globe. The SD represents the variability around the mean visual neglect scores for the *sample* of patients with stroke.

It is not possible to collect information about every patient in the universe. Using statistical theory, however, there is a way to estimate the SD of scores in the universe of patients.[41] If random samples of patients with stroke were theoretically evaluated over and over again throughout the world, then each sample would produce a mean visual neglect score. When the mean visual neglect scores are plotted, in theory they form a normal distribution. Thus, the SD of the sampling distribution of mean visual neglect scores for patients with stroke is the standard error of the mean (σ_{mean}).

Direct measurements of the population or universe of patients are not possible, but the σ_{mean} can be estimated using the SD and the number of patients (N) in the sample. The formula for estimating σ_{mean} is

Estimated $\sigma_{mean}=$ $\qquad SE = \dfrac{SD}{\sqrt{N}}$ **eq A4-2**

SE and Confidence Intervals

As the SE is an estimation of a population statistic (not a sample statistic), it allows inferences about the outcome measure in the universe of patients. Thus, when the SE is used in some form to calculate a confidence interval surrounding a point estimate, the practitioner is inferring that the true value of the point estimate (read "the value of the population statistic") likely occurs within the confidence interval estimated from sample statistics (**Fig. 4-12**).

Measures of Variability

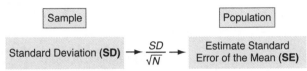

Figure 4-12 Comparison of measures of variability in a sample versus the population.

The SE Versus SEM

The SE is not the same as the SEM. The SEM addresses consistency of repeated clinical measures and can be thought of as a SD adjusted for reliability. The concept of consistency is highlighted by the inclusion of a correlation coefficient in the calculation of SEM (see **eq. 4-1**). The correlation in the SEM calculation usually measures the association baseline versus follow-up outcome scores (see Fig. 4-9). High correlations indicate greater consistency (and less measurement error) in repeated assessments of patient function by producing a small SEM. Conversely, low correlations between repeated patient assessments will expand the SEM, illustrating that larger measurement error must be at the root of inconsistent evaluation scores over time. There is no correlation coefficient in the calculation of the SE.

z-Scores for Individual Patients

A z-score measures the distance (in the number of SDs) that a subject's score is from the mean of the sample (**eq. A4-3**) or the population (**eq. A4-4**). The z-score is calculated by taking the original score minus the mean and normalizing that difference to the SD:

$$z\ score\ (sample) = \frac{Patient\ Score - Mean}{SD} \qquad \textbf{eq A4-3}$$

For example, if the mean+/–SD of the Roland-Morris disability score is 10 ± 5 disability points in a sample of 25 patients ($N = 25$), and the subject of interest has a Roland score of 19 points, then that subject has a z-score of

$$z\ score\ (sample) = \frac{Patient\ Score - Sample\ Mean}{SD}$$
$$= \frac{19-10}{5} = \frac{9}{5} = 1.8$$

In other words, this subject's score is 1.8 SDs above the mean of the sample. *If the scores represent a scale like the Roland-Morris Disability Scale (where higher scores indicate more disability), then the patient in this example has worse disability than the average patient.*

A z-score for the universe of patients requires a population mean (estimated by the sample mean) and a population SD (estimated by the SE).

eq A4-4

$$\text{z score (population)} = \frac{Patient\ Score - Population\ Mean}{SE}$$

For the Roland-Morris example above, the z-score when referring to the population of patients with low back dysfunction is

$$SE = \frac{SD}{\sqrt{N}} = \frac{5}{\sqrt{25}} = \frac{5}{5} = 1$$

$$\text{z score (population)} = \frac{Patient\ Score - Population\ Mean}{SE}$$

$$= \frac{19-10}{1} = 9$$

An average score of 19 obtained from 25 imaginary patients world be 9 SDs, above the mean of the population of all samples of similar sample sizes and similar patient characteristics.

The use of z-score (sample) versus z-score (population) depends upon the application. If clinicians are interested in measuring patient performance with respect to the immediate sample, then the SD is used at the denominator of the z-score. Alternatively, if the goal is to estimate patient status with respect to the population of similar patients, then the SE is used as the denominator of the z-score. This distinction (sample versus population) is highlighted in **Figure 4-12**.

Change Scores (Δ) for Individual Patients

When using disability scales like the Roland-Morris Scale, where higher scores represent more self-perceived disability, the change score (Δ = initial − discharge score) is positive when the patient *improves*. For example:

Patient Change Score (Δ):

Patient score at initial evaluation = 20 Roland points (high disability)
Patient score at discharge = 5 Roland points (lower disability)
Δ score = 20 − 5 = **+15 (improvement)**

Sample Statistics for Demonstration (given the following values)

Mean Δ score = 13
SD of change scores = 5 change points
SE of change scores = 1 change point

Change scores enter the z-score equations the same way as raw scores. However, the numerator and denominators of the z-score are now Δ scores rather than raw scores.

Change scores must be interpreted relative to the scale of the outcome measure. A patient with a positive Δ score in this example has a functional level that is *better* than average (reference z-score = 0). The hypothetical patient had a change from initial to follow-up evaluation that was 0.4 SD above the mean change for the sample (**eq. A4-5**) and 2 SDs above the mean change score for the population (**eq. A4-6**). Note that if the subtraction of initial and follow-up Δ scores were reversed, a negative change score would represent improvement. Regardless of the method used to calculate a z-score or the outcome measure that is converted to a z-score (e.g., strength measure, cognitive index, or disability score), the distribution of z-scores will always have a mean = 0 and a SD = 1 (**Fig. 4-13**).

eq A4-5

$$\text{z score (sample)} = \frac{Patient\ \Delta\ Score - Sample\ Mean\ \Delta\ Score}{SD\ \Delta\ scores}$$

$$= \frac{15-13}{5} = \frac{2}{5} = 0.4$$

eq A4-6

$$\text{z score (population)} = \frac{Patient\ \Delta\ Score - Population\ Mean\ \Delta\ score}{SE\ \Delta\ scores}$$

$$= \frac{15-13}{1} = \frac{2}{1} = 2$$

Critical z Values for Confidence Intervals

Critical z values are constants and delineate the boundaries of confidence intervals or decision thresholds for hypothesis testing (discussed in Chapter 5). There are two critical z values that are most commonly used for these purposes: 1.645 and 1.96 (**Table 4-5**).

For example, a 90% confidence interval (CI) surrounding a statistic will show how confident one can be that the true statistic occurs within the interval. When MDC is calculated using a critical z-score of 1.645, this constant establishes a 90% CI surrounding the MDC (see Fig. 4-10). If a higher level of confidence is desired (e.g., 95% CI) then z = 1.96 would be used (see Table 4-5). Note that the 95% confidence level would result in a larger MDC (using **equation 4-2**):

90% Confidence: MDC = critical z-score $_{\text{level of confidence}}$ * SEM * $\sqrt{2}$ = **1.65** * 4.8 * 1.41 = **11**

95% Confidence: MDC = critical z-score $_{\text{level of confidence}}$ * SEM * $\sqrt{2}$ = **1.96** * 4.8 * 1.41 = **13**

This shows that the interval likely containing the true score widens (i.e., from 11 to 13 disability points of change from initial to follow-up evaluations) when the CI increases to 95%. The change in

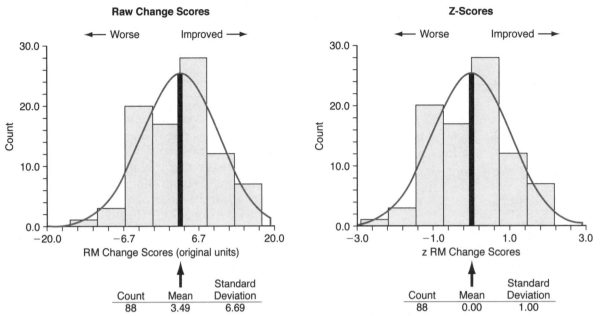

Figure 4-13 Hypothetical data used to demonstrate a comparison of change scores in original disability units and the conversion of those change scores to z-scores. Note the mean for the z-score distribution is always 0 and the SD is always 1.

the width of the CI is illustrated in **Figure 4-14.** With all other factors in the MDC equation fixed, the increase in MDC at 95% confidence occurs because more area under the normal curve is covered (1.96 SD vs. 1.645 SD).

Once a constant is selected to establish the level of confidence, then the variable that has the greatest influence on the MDC is the SEM **(equation 4-1).** As a general rule, *for a given CI,* it is desirable to have a small MDC. For either the 90% or 95% confidence level, it would be better to have a point estimate change score on the order of 5 disability points, for example, as opposed to 11 or 13 points because the MDC represents the smallest score that is an *error-free measure of clinical change.*

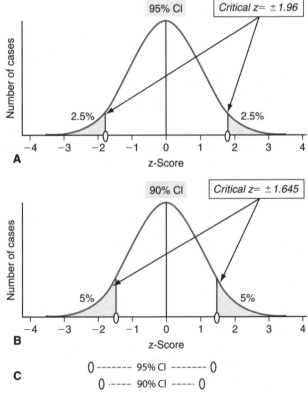

Figure 4-14 Comparison of confidence intervals (CI) with different critical z. (A) 95% CI, (B) 90% CI, and (C) interval width for 95% CI versus 90% CI.

Table 4-5	Critical z Values (Constants) for Confidence Intervals. Standard Deviations (SD) or Standard Errors (SE).	
SD (or SE) on Normal Curve	**Percent of Cases Between Mean and SD (or SE)**	**Confidence Interval**
1.645	45%	Constant for 90% confidence interval (45% * 2)
1.96	47.5%	Constant for 95% confidence interval (47.5% * 2)

PRACTICE

1. The assessment tool of interest is a new clinical tool where the clinician directly observes motor function in patients with stroke. The tool assesses 50 motor functions (e.g., grasping, standing ability) and the score range is 0 (minimal disability) to 100 (maximal disability). Patients were evaluated initially and during a 4-week follow-up post-treatment. A review of literature reveals the following data from a study assessing MDC in this clinical assessment tool:
   SD of initial assessment scores = 14
   Correlation (r) between initial and discharge scores = 0.69
   a. Using a 90% CI (in other words MDC_{90}), what is the MDC?
   b. Does the MDC change if the authors use a 95% CI (MDC_{95})? If so, what are the new values?
   c. Given an MDC_{90} = 18, what does this mean?
   d. If the authors wanted to determine an estimate of MCID without using a ROC analysis, which statistic would they use?
   e. What is the value of the statistic approximating the MCID, given SD of assessment scores at the initial evaluation = 14 and the correlation between initial versus follow-up scores is r = 0.69?
   f. Given an estimated MCID = 8 points, what does this mean?
2. Given a +LR = 14 (95% CI 2–31),
   a. How is this value interpreted in the context of diagnostic validity?
   b. How is this value interpreted in the context of meaningful clinical change?
3. The following output is from a hypothetical study using the anchor method to determine MCC. The "change score" is the change of patient performance from initial evaluation to follow-up after 2 weeks of treatment. Plot the ROC curve using Excel or any other graphing program, and identify the optimal MCID on the curve.

Change Score	A	B	C	D	Sensitivity	1 – Specificity
1.00	36	18	0	34	1.00000	0.34615
2.00	36	17	0	35	1.00000	0.32692
3.00	35	13	1	39	0.97222	0.25000
4.00	35	12	1	40	0.97222	0.23077
5.00	35	7	1	45	0.97222	0.13462
6.00	31	6	5	46	0.86111	0.11538
7.00	28	2	8	50	0.77778	0.03846
8.00	22	1	14	51	0.61111	0.01923
9.00	18	1	18	51	0.50000	0.01923
10.00	14	1	22	51	0.38889	0.01923

4. Which contingency table is appropriate for studying MCC using the anchor method?

a.

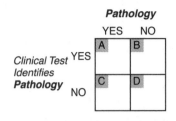

b.

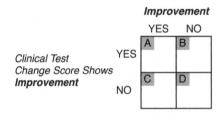

c.

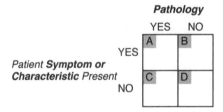

5. Clear identification of the target population (the population of patients on which MCC research is focused) is required to ensure appropriate generalization of the MCC threshold to specific patients undergoing rehabilitation interventions. The demonstration data set with hypothetical Roland-Morris disability scores includes patients with a wide range of self-perceived disability. Use the demonstration data set along with the statistical software loaded in your computer to compare the MDC_{90} for patients who have initial disability scores ≤12 versus those with initial disability scores > 12.

NCSS KEY ACTIONS

Locate filter dialog box.

Run the NCSS filter to analyze only patients with initial RM scores ≤ 12 (patients with low self-perceived disability).

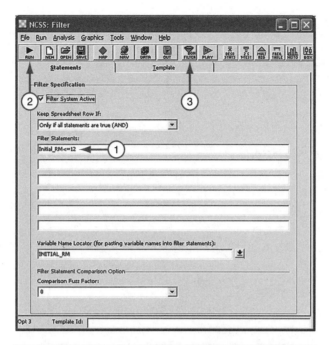

1. Type in filter statement ("Initial_RM" is the variable name for initial RM score and "< = **12**" signifies analysis; includes only subjects with less than or equal to 12 RM points (**low disability scores**).

2. RUN activates filter.

3. Filter confirmed with "on Filter" button turning yellow.

Run the NCSS filter to analyze only patients with initial RM scores > 12 (patients with high self-perceived disability).

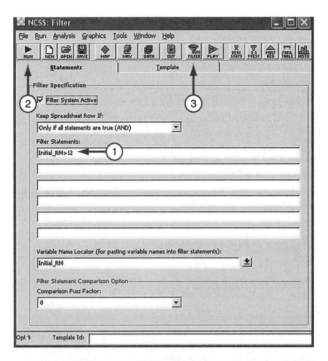

1. Type in filter statement ("Initial_RM" is the variable name for initial RM score and "> **12**" signifies analysis; includes only subjects with greater than 12 RM points (**high** disability scores).

2. RUN activates filter.

3. Filter confirmed with "on Filter" button turning yellow.

SPSS KEY ACTIONS

Locate filter dialog box.

Run the SPSS filter to analyze only patients with initial RM scores ≤ **12** (patients with low self-perceived disability).

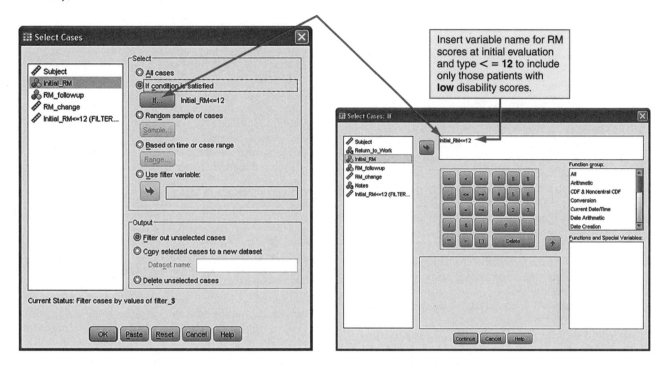

Insert variable name for RM scores at initial evaluation and type < = **12** to include only those patients with **low** disability scores.

Run the SPSS filter to analyze only patients with initial RM scores > **12** (patients with high self-perceived disability).

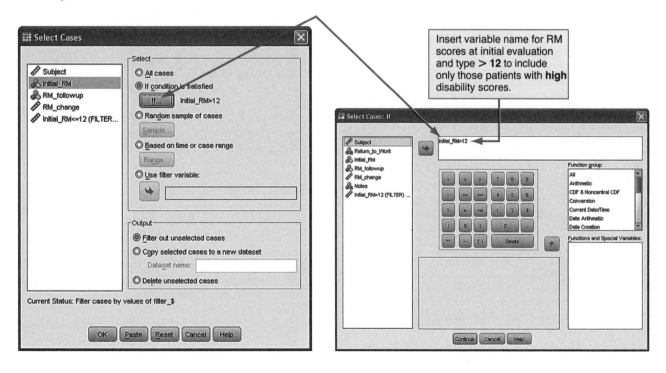

Insert variable name for RM scores at initial evaluation and type > **12** to include only those patients with **high** disability scores.

ANALYSIS IN NCSS AND SPSS

After a filter is activated, follow procedures in *Video Tutorial 4-2: Distribution Method*.

REFERENCES

1. Haley SM, Fragala-Pinkham MA. Interpreting change scores of tests and measures used in physical therapy. Phys Ther 2006; 86:735–743.
2. Crosby RD, Kolotkin RL, Williams GR. Defining clinically meaningful change in health-related quality of life. Clin Epidemiol 2003; 56:395–407.
3. Jaeschke R, Singer J, Guyatt GH. Measurement of health status. Ascertaining the minimal clinically important difference. Control Clin Trials 1989; 10:407–415.
4. Palombaro KM, Craik RL, Mangione KK, et al. Determining meaningful changes in gait speed after hip fracture. Phys Ther 2006; 86:809–816.
5. Lydick F, Epstein RS. Interpretation of quality of life changes. Qual Life Res 1993; 2:221–226.
6. Schmitt J, Di Fabio RP. The validity of prospective and retrospective global change criterion measures. Arch Phys Med Rehabil 2004; 86:2270–2276.
7. Schmitt J, Di Fabio RP. Reliable change and minimum important difference (MID) proportions facilitated group responsiveness comparisons using individual threshold criteria. J Clin Epidemiol 2004; 57:1008–1018.
8. Stratford PW, Binkley JM, Riddle DL. Health status measures: strategies and analytic methods for assessing change scores. Phys Ther 1996; 76:1109–1123.
9. Herrmann D. Reporting current, past, and changed health status. What we know about distortion. Med Care 1995; 33:AS89–94.
10. Norman GR, Stratford P, Regehr G. Methodological problems in the retrospective computation of responsiveness to change: the lesson of Cronbach. J Clin Epidemiol 1997; 50:869–879.
11. BenDebba M, Heller J, Ducker TB, et al. Cervical spine outcomes questionnaire: its development and psychometric properties. Spine 2002; 27:2116–2124.
12. L'Insalata JC, Warren RF, Cohen SB, et al. A self-administered questionnaire for assessment of symptoms and function of the shoulder. J Bone Joint Surg Am 1997; 79:738–748.
13. Stucki G, Liang MH, Fossel AH, et al. Relative responsiveness of condition-specific and generic health status measures in degenerative lumbar spinal stenosis. J Clin Epidemiol 1995; 48:1369–1378.
14. Wright JG, Young NL. A comparison of different indices of responsiveness. J Clin Epidemiol 1997; 50:239–246.
15. van der Windt DA, van der Heijden GJ, de Winter AF, et al. The responsiveness of the Shoulder Disability Questionnaire. Ann Rheum Dis 1998; 57:82–87.
16. Iyer LV, Haley SM, Watkins MP, et al. Establishing minimal clinically important differences for scores on the Pediatric Evaluation of Disability Inventory for inpatient rehabilitation. Phys Ther 2003; 83: 888–898.
17. Hoving JL, Koes BW, de Vet HC, et al. Manual therapy, physical therapy, or continued care by a general practitioner for patients with neck pain. A randomized, controlled trial. Ann Intern Med 2002; 136:713–722.
18. Smidt N, van der Windt DA, Assendelft WJ, et al. Corticosteroid injections, physiotherapy, or a wait-and-see policy for lateral epicondylitis: a randomised controlled trial. Lancet 2002; 359: 657–662.
19. Wells G, Beaton D, Shea B, et al. Minimal clinically important differences: review of methods. J Rheumatol 2001; 28:406–412.
20. Paltamaa J, Sarasoja T, Leskinen E, et al. Measuring deterioration in international classification of functioning domains of people with multiple sclerosis who are ambulatory. Phys Ther 2008; 88:176–190.
21. Brach JS, Perera S, Studensk S, et al. Meaningful change in measures of gait variability in older adults. Gait and Posture 2010; 31:175–179.
22. de Vet HCW, Bouter LM, Bezemer PD, et al. Reproducibility and responsiveness of evaluative outcome measures. Int J Tech Assess in Health Care 2001; 17:479–487.
23. Deyo RA, Centor RM. Assessing the responsiveness of functional scales to clinical change: an analogy to diagnostic test performance. J Chronic Dis 1986; 39:897–906.
24. Guyatt GH, Sullivan MJ, Thompson PJ, et al. The 6-minute walk: a new measure of exercise capacity in patients with chronic heart failure. Can Med Assoc J 1985; 132:919–923.
25. Roland M, Fairbank J. The Roland–Morris Disability Questionnaire and the Oswestry Disability Questionnaire. Spine 2000; 25:3115–3124.
26. Roland M, Morris R. A study of the natural history of back pain part l: development of a reliable and sensitive measure of disability in low-back pain. Spine 1983; 8:141–144.
27. Cherkin DC, Deyo RA, Battie M, et al. A comparison of physical therapy, chiropractic manipulation, and provision of an educational booklet for treatment of patients with low back pain. N Engl J Med 1998; 339:1021–1029.
28. Ostelo RWJG, deVet HCW, Knola DL, et al. 24-item Roland-Morris Disability Questionnaire was preferred out of six functional status questionnaires for post-lumbar disc surgery. J Clin Epidemiol 2004; 57:268–276.
29. Wiesinger GF, Nuhr M, Quittan M, et al. Cross-cultural adaptation of the Roland-Morris Questionnaire for German-speaking patients with low back pain. Spine 1999; 24:1099–1103.
30. Jacobson NS, Truax P. Clinical significance: a statistical approach to defining meaningful change in psychotherapy research. J Consult Clin Psychol 1991; 59:12–19.
31. Ottenbacher KJ, Johnson MB, Hojem M. The significance of clinical change and clinical change of significance: issues and methods. Am J Occup Ther 1988; 42:156–163.

32. Riddle DL, Stratford PW. Interpreting validity indexes for diagnostic tests: an illustration using the Berg Balance Test. Phys Ther 1999; 79:939–948.

33. Wyrwich KW, Nienaber NA, Tierney WM, et al. Linking clinical relevance and statistical significance in evaluating intra-individual changes in health-related quality of life. Med Care 1999; 37:469–478.

34. Wyrwich KW. Minimal important difference thresholds and the standard error of measurement: is there a connection? J Biopharm Stat 2004; 14:97–110.

35. Wyrwich KW, Tierney WM, Wolinsky FD. Further evidence supporting standard error of measurement based criterion for identifying meaningful intra-individual change in health-related quality of life. J Clin Epidemiol 1999; 52:861–873.

36. Kupferberg DH, Kaplan RM, Slymen DJ, et al. Minimal clinically important difference for the UCSD Shortness of Breath Questionnaire. J Cardiopulmon Rehab 2005; 25:370–377.

37. Leidy NK, Wyrwich KW. Bridging the gap: using triangulation methodology to estimate minimal clinically important differences (MCIDs). COPD 2005; 2:157–165.

38. Schrag A, Sampaio C, Counsell N, et al. Minimal clinically important change on the Unified Parkinson's Disease Rating Scale. Movement Disorders 2006; 21:1200–1207.

39. Jordan K, Dunn KM, Lewis M, et al. A minimal clinically important difference was derived for the Roland-Morris Disability Questionnaire for low back pain. J Clin Epidemiol 2006; 59:45–52.

40. Stratford PW, Binkley JM, Riddle DL, et al. Sensitivity to change of the Roland-Morris Back Pain Questionnaire: part 1. Phy Ther 1998; 78: 1186–1196.

41. Hinze J. NCSS Help System. Kaysville, UT: NCSS, 2007.

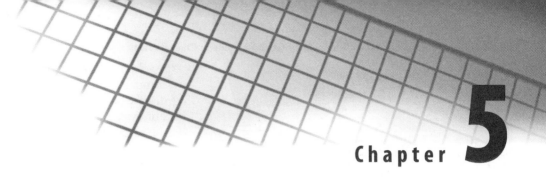

Comparing Clinical Assessments: Which Is Better?

Clinical Questions
- Does my clinical assessment adequately identify changes in the patient's status?
- Is the assessment tool the best that is available when considering the burden on the patient and the population, severity, and chronicity of the disorder that is being evaluated?

Multiple clinical assessments are often used to provide a comprehensive view of the patient's function. The tools that are included in a test battery require careful consideration because there is a burden on the patient and therapist when too many tools are used to evaluate patient progress over time. The level of symptom severity can limit the choice of tools because some assessments might not be sensitive to clinical change when the target population encompasses severely involved people or, conversely, patients with mild involvement. Also, as a practical matter, the amount of training required to administer the test should be considered prior to clinical implementation.[1] Many characteristics of assessment tools can be measured to allow comparisons between tools or within different versions of the same tool. These measured characteristics include[1]:

- Time to administer the test
- Validity (does the tool accurately measure the presence of pathology or dysfunction as discussed in Chapter 3)
- Meaningful clinical change (what is the amount of change measured by the tool that has functional significance, as covered in Chapter 4)
- Reliability
- Floor/ceiling effects
- Responsiveness

The focus in this chapter is on responsiveness of assessments and floor/ceiling effects. Research addressing these characteristics provides important pieces of evidence to justify the selection of tool(s) to assess a particular population of patients.

An assessment tool that is responsive must first detect meaningful change when it has occurred, and second, it must remain stable when no change has occurred.[2-4] There are many different statistical approaches to measuring responsiveness,[2,4-7] but there is little agreement in the literature on how to calculate and report responsiveness to clinical change.[2-8] In addition, the results of responsiveness research will often be influenced by the selection of a particular responsiveness index, the design of the study to assess responsiveness, and the target population.[2,4]

Applications of Responsiveness Research

The literature evaluating responsiveness addresses several topics that have direct application to a clinical setting (Fig. 5-1):

- *Determine if the responsiveness of long versus short forms of the same tool are similar so that abbreviated forms might be used to decrease patient and therapist burden.*[9] For example, the Berg Balance Scale is a widely used assessment tool for balance function.[1] The scale consists of 14 functional behaviors scored from 0 (needs assistance or poor function) to 4 (independent or does not need assistance).[10] The composite score summed across the 14 items can vary from 0 to 56, with higher scores indicating better performance (Fig. 5-2). Chou et al.[9] studied patients with stroke and evaluated their

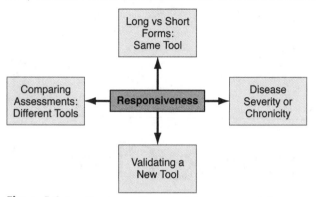

Figure 5-1 Applications of responsiveness research in clinical settings.

change scores (14 vs. 90 days poststroke). They used the Berg Balance Scale (14 items) as well as shortened versions of this tool. When the original Berg Scale was shortened to 7 items and the scale for each item was shortened to a new 3-point Berg Scale (0–2–4), the outcome had similar responsiveness compared to the original tool.[9] The authors recommended the shorter tool for use in the clinic because it was simpler and faster to use and produced impairment scores similar to the longer Berg Balance Scale.

- *Compare the responsiveness among assessments.*[11] Do generic health-related assessments detect change as effectively as disease-specific assessments? The advantage of using a generic health-related assessment in the clinic, such as the SF-36,[12] SF-12,[13] or the OPTIMAL tool,[14] is that the same tool can be used with all patients regardless of diagnosis. Generic assessments simplify the evaluation of patient status so that clinic-centered outcomes can be monitored without incorporating additional disease-specific or region-specific assessment tools. However, in order to use generic health-related assessments with confidence, the

psychometric properties of these tools should be comparable to the properties of high-quality disease-specific assessments.

- For example, Schmitt and Di Fabio[11] compared the responsiveness of the DASH[15] (Disabilities of the Arm, Shoulder, and Hand) and the SPADI (Shoulder Pain and Disability Index)[16,17] (both disease-specific tools) to the SF-12. They found greater responsiveness of the disease-specific tools when used with patients who had proximal arm pathology compared to the generic assessment. These findings might support the use of disease-specific tools rather than generic assessments in this population of patients. However, findings in favor of either type of assessment can vary with the target population, and a literature review is required before selecting the battery of assessment tools that will be used in the clinic.

- *Evaluate the responsiveness of the same tool when applied to different aspects of a target population of patients.* Is the tool equally responsive to patients with different levels of disease severity or chronicity? For example, Mao et al[18] compared the change in Berg balance scores across several stages of recovery from stroke and found acceptable levels of responsiveness across all stages. The best responsiveness, however, was during the early stages of recovery.[18]

- *Validate a new tool with the goal of establishing similar responsiveness between new and established tools.* For example, the responsiveness of a newly derived balance scale called the PASS (Postural Assessment Scale for Stroke Patients) was compared to established balance assessments (the Berg and the Fugl-Meyer Balance Scales).[18] The discovery that all three assessments had similar responsiveness gives the clinician some latitude in selecting one of three tools based on this psychometric property.

Figure 5-2 Items on the Berg Balance Scale. The short version of this tool is comprised of the first 7 items as reported by Chou et al.[9] using a 3-point scale per item (highlighted). ES = effect size based on different scales. Refer to Kornetti et al.[10] to view the 5-point scale per item. (Adapted from Chou CY, Chien CW, Hsueh IP, et al. Developing a short form of the Berg Balance Scale for people with stroke. Phys Ther 2006; 86:195–204 with permission of the American Physical Therapy Association. This material is copyrighted and any further reproduction or distribution requires written permission from APTA.)

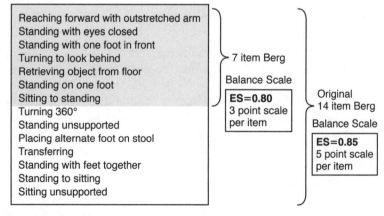

Group Versus Individual Patient Responsiveness Indices

There are two levels of responsiveness indices: the individual patient level and the group level. The individual-level responsiveness indices provide information about the *proportion of patients* in the study that had true meaningful change (positive or negative). The group-level responsiveness indices, in contrast, provide a summary of the performance of an *entire group of patients* without reference to individual patients.[11]

Individual Patient Indices

Currently, there is no accepted standard for measuring test responsiveness on the individual-patient level. However, one feature that is common to all "individual-patient" measures of test responsiveness is the clinical change threshold. A clinical change threshold is the amount of change in the patient's assessment from the initial evaluation to the follow-up that represents meaningful or true change (see Chapter 4). For example, if the clinical change threshold is 10 points on a disability questionnaire, then patients who improve by 10 points have demonstrated meaningful positive change. Those who change less than 10 points have not reached the threshold for meaningful positive change. Those who change in the direction of worse function by 10 or more points have meaningful negative change. The clinical change threshold is represented by the minimum clinically important difference (MCID) or the minimal detectable change (MDC). The process for determining both of these thresholds is outlined in Chapter 4.

A study of disability questionnaires[19] proposed that determining the proportion of patients who changed at least as much as a change threshold would provide an index of test responsiveness. In other words, by comparing several different assessment tools applied to the same group of patients at the same time, the tools showing the largest proportion of patients exceeding the clinical change threshold would be the tools that were most responsive.

Reliable Change Proportions

The reliable change proportion is based on the MDC. As the MDC represents the smallest score change that likely reflects true change rather than measurement error, the reliable change proportion is the proportion of patients who have a true positive or negative change

in their clinical performance. The reliable change proportion is calculated:[11]

$$\text{Reliable Change Proportion} = \frac{(\#{\geq}MDC) + (\#{\leq}{-}MDC)}{N} \quad \textbf{eq 5-1}$$

where # is a count of patients meeting or exceeding the MDC ("≥") or meeting or falling below the *negative* MDC ("≤ "), N is the total number of patients assessed, and the **MDC** is used as the change threshold.

For example, Stevenson[20] reported the MDC_{90} was ±6 Berg balance points for patients with stroke. Using **equation 5-1**, the MDC for the Berg scale, and the following hypothetical numbers, the reliable change proportion is:

$N = 48$
$\#{\geq}6 = 29$
$\#{\leq}{-}6 = 10$

$$\text{Reliable Change Proportion}^a = \frac{(\#{\geq}MDC) + (\#{\leq}{-}MDC)}{N}$$
$$= \frac{(29) + (10)}{48} = 0.81 \ or \ 81\%$$

MCID Proportions

The MCID proportion is the proportion of patients who exceed the MCID change threshold to show improvement. If a receiver operating characteristic (ROC) curve and associated 2×2 contingency table are used to calculate MCID,[b] then the number of patients classified as true positive (cell A) and true negative (cell D) is known. Since the definition of responsiveness is that a clinical tool will show change when change truly occurs and not show change when the patient is stable,[2-4] it is reasonable to include the counts from cells A and D in the MCID proportion.

The MCID was calculated in Chapter 4. The MCID *proportion* is calculated:

$$\text{MCID Proportion} = \frac{(\#\text{cell A}) + (\#\text{cell D})}{N} \quad \textbf{eq 5-2}$$

where # is a count of patients in cells A and D of the contingency table, N is the total number of patients assessed, and the **MCID** is used as the change threshold.

Group Indices

Responsiveness of an assessment tool can also be measured by group-level statistics such as effect size ($ES_{responsiveness}$),[21] standardized response mean (SRM),[22]

---

[a]Note that there are 9 patients in this hypothetical demonstration that did not meet or exceed 6 points or fall below –6 or more points.
[b]When a contingency table is not used to calculate MCID, then the number of patients exceeding the MCID threshold is counted as patients with meaningful improvement.

and Guyatt's Responsiveness Index (GRI).[23] These statistics are called "group level" because change is measured in reference to scores of the group as opposed to scores of the individual patients.

Effect size is the average change from initial to follow-up divided by the standard deviation of the initial evaluation score (baseline score) for a group of patients judged to have changed over time.[21] The SRM[22] and GRI[23] are variations on the concept of an effect size.

- $ES_{responsiveness}$ [21,24]:

$$\frac{\text{Average Change from Initial to Follow-up Evaluation}}{\text{SD Initial Evalution Scores}} \quad \textbf{eq 5-3}$$

- SRM[25]:

$$\frac{\text{Average Change from Initial to Follow-up Evaluation}}{\text{SD of Change scores}} \quad \textbf{eq 5-4}$$

- GRI [4,23]:

$$\frac{\text{Average Change observed in a group expected to undergo change}}{\text{SD of Change scores in stable patients}} \quad \textbf{eq 5-5}$$

Evaluating the Statistical Significance of Responsiveness Indices

The point estimates of responsiveness provide a descriptive account of which tool has the best responsiveness to clinical change. Overall, a larger responsiveness index indicates greater sensitivity to change. Clinicians simply view the results and focus on the assessment tool with the higher index. The $ES_{responsiveness}$ is a commonly used measure of responsiveness.[1,11,14,18,26] The descriptive interpretation of the absolute value of the ES is made using an arbitrary convention proposed by Cohen;[24] ES on the order of 0.8 is considered large, 0.5 is moderate, and 0.2 is small. The SRM also has been interpreted using Cohen's description.[19]

The limitation when using a descriptive scale of ES magnitude is the lack of clear boundaries delineating statistically significant difference. If different assessment tools are evaluated for responsiveness, does an ES of 0.8 for tool "A" really differ from an ES of 0.6 for tool "B"? When it is necessary to determine if differences in responsiveness among assessment tools are statistically significant (e.g., when responsiveness indices give inconsistent results) a comparison of confidence intervals[11] or a receiver operating characteristic (ROC) analysis can potentially resolve conflicts by testing the significance of difference between two or more clinical assessment tools.[2,4]

Confidence Intervals for Responsiveness Indices

The calculation of 95% confidence intervals (CIs) surrounding the point estimates of responsiveness indices provides a way to determine the range of possible true values of the point estimate. When comparing two assessment tools, there will be a pair of point estimates (e.g., an ES for tool A and an ES for tool B). If *the CIs for responsiveness point estimates overlap, there is no statistical difference between assessment tools for this index.*[11]

It is assumed that the responsiveness indices are normally distributed so that statistical theory related to probability and the normal curve can be applied to compare the variability of scores surrounding the point estimate (see appendix to Chapter 4). When these assumptions are applied to proportions (individual responsiveness indices), the formulas advanced by Wilson[27] and cited by Agresti and Coull[28] are used. In the case of group responsiveness indices, the difference scores in the numerator are assumed to be normally distributed for ES, SRM,[29] and GRI.[c,30]

Hand calculation of 95% CIs for the point estimates of responsiveness is cumbersome, but the CIs can be readily computed using the bound-in disk calculator for this chapter.

Demonstration: Assessing Responsiveness

The Roland-Morris Disability Questionnaire (Chapter 4), is compared to the Oswestry Disability Questionnaire in a demonstration using hypothetical data to determine which clinical assessment tool has better responsiveness. The results of this demonstration, therefore, are entirely imaginary.

The Oswestry Disability Questionnaire measures self-perceived disability for people with low-back dysfunction. The tool has 10 questions (or "sections") and each section score is tallied and converted to a composite score of 100% **(Fig. 5-3)**. As with the Roland-Morris assessment, higher scores on the Oswestry indicate greater disability compared to lower scores.

Demonstration Design

The design of the demonstration exercise for responsiveness is shown in **Figure 5-4**. Note that all subjects

---

[c]In the case of group indices, the distribution of difference scores was assumed to have a mean of 0 and a SE = (1/sqrt (N)). Refer to Beaton et al.[29] The estimated SE is then multiplied by the critical z = ±1.96 to estimate the 95% CI surrounding the point estimate.

Oswestry Disability Index 2.0

Could you please complete this questionnaire? It is designed to give us information as to how your back (or leg) trouble has affected your ability to manage in everyday life. Please answer every section. Mark one box only in each section that most closely describes you today.

Section 1: Pain intensity
__ I have no pain at the moment.
__ The pain is very mild at the moment.
__ The pain is moderate at the moment.
__ The pain is fairly severe at the moment.
__ The pain is very severe at the moment.
__ The pain is the worst imaginable at the moment.

Section 2: Personal care (washing, dressing, etc.)
__ I can look after myself normally without causing extra pain.
__ I can look after myself normally but it is very painful.
__ It is painful to look after myself and I am slow and careful.
__ I need some help but manage most of my personal care.
__ I need help every day in most aspects of self care.
__ I do not get dressed, wash with difficulty, and stay in bed.

Section 3: Lifting
__ I can lift heavy weights without extra pain.
__ I can lift heavy weights but it gives extra pain.
__ Pain prevents me from lifting heavy weights off the floor but I can manage if they are conveniently positioned, *e.g.*, on a table.
__ Pain prevents me from lifting heavy weights but I can manage light to medium weights if they are conveniently positioned.
__ I can lift only very light weights.
__ I cannot lift or carry anything at all.

Section 4: Walking
__ Pain does not prevent me walking any distance.
__ Pain prevents me walking more than 1 mile.
__ Pain prevents me walking more than a quarter of a mile.
__ Pain prevents me walking more than 100 yards.
__ I can only walk using a stick or crutches.
__ I am in bed most of the time and have to crawl to the toilet.

Section 5: Sitting
__ I can sit in any chair as long as I like.
__ I can sit in my favorite chair as long as I like.
__ Pain prevents me from sitting for more than 1 hour.
__ Pain prevents me from sitting for more than half an hour.
__ Pain prevents me from sitting for more than 10 minutes.
__ Pain prevents me from sitting at all.

Section 6: Standing
__ I can stand as long as I want without extra pain.
__ I can stand as long as I want but it gives me extra pain.
__ Pain prevents me from standing for more than 1 hour.
__ Pain prevents me from standing for more than half an hour.
__ Pain prevents me from standing for more than 10 minutes.
__ Pain prevents me from standing at all.

Section 7: Sleeping
__ My sleep is never disturbed by pain.
__ My sleep is occasionally disturbed by pain.
__ Because of pain I have less than 6 hours sleep.
__ Because of pain I have less than 4 hours sleep.
__ Because of pain I have less than 2 hours sleep.
__ Pain prevents me from sleeping at all.

Section 8: Sex life (if applicable)
__ My sex life is normal and causes no extra pain.
__ My sex life is normal but causes some extra pain.
__ My sex life is nearly normal but is very painful.
__ My sex life is severely restricted by pain.
__ My sex life is nearly absent because of pain.
__ Pain prevents any sex life at all.

Section 9: Social life
__ My social life is normal and causes me no extra pain.
__ My social life is normal but increases the degree of pain.
__ Pain has no significant effect on my social life apart from limiting my more energetic interests, *e.g.*, sport, *etc.*
__ Pain has restricted my social life and I do not go out as often.
__ Pain has restricted social life to my home.
__ I have no social life because of pain.

Section 10: Traveling
__ I can travel anywhere without pain.
__ I can travel anywhere but it gives extra pain.
__ Pain is bad but I manage journeys over 2 hours.
__ Pain restricts me to journeys of less than 1 hour.
__ Pain restricts me to short necessary journeys under 30 minutes.
__ Pain prevents me from traveling except to receive treatment.

Scoring the ODI

For each section of six statements the possible total score is 5; if the first statement is marked, the score is 0; if the last statement is marked, it is 5. Intervening statements are scored according to rank. If more than one box is marked in each section, take the highest score. If all 10 sections are completed the score is calculated as follows: if 16(total scored) out of 50 (total possible score)x100=32%. If one is missed (or not applicable) the score is calculated: Example: 16 (total scored)/45 (total possible score) x 100 = 35.5% Therefore, the final score may be summarized as: (total score/(5 x number of questions answered)x 100%. The authors suggest rounding the percentage to a whole number for convenience.

Figure 5-3 Oswestry Disability Index 2. (Reprinted from Roland M, Fairbank J. The Roland-Morris Disability Questionnaire and the Oswestry Disability Questionnaire. Spine 2000; 25:3115–3124).

in this hypothetical example are scored on both the Roland-Morris and Oswestry disability scales at the initial evaluation and then again at follow-up. The criterion standard for improvement is return to work (all imaginary patients were not working at the time of initial evaluation). Part of the hypothetical data set for

this demonstration exercise is illustrated in **Figure 5-5** (29 of 88 subjects).

The presumption is that those who returned to work will show important clinical change on the assessment tool, whereas those who do not return to work will not demonstrate important clinical change.

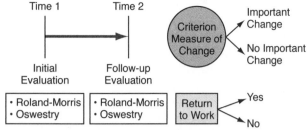

Figure 5-4 Design of the demonstration exercise for responsiveness. (Adapted from Stratford PW, Binkley JM, Riddle DL. Health status measures: strategies and analytic methods for assessing change scores. Phys Ther 1996; 76:1109–1123 with permission of the American Physical Therapy Association. This material is copyrighted and any further reproduction or distribution requires written permission from APTA.)

Calculation Demonstration for Responsiveness Indices

Individual Patient Indices

Reliable Change Proportion Demonstration

Step 1: Calculate the SEM for (see Chapter 4, equation 4-1) each assessment tool:

- Roland-Morris
  - $SD_{initial} = 6.48$
  - $r_s = 0.45$
  - SEM = 4.81~5 points (units are questions on the scale)
- Oswestry
  - $SD_{initial} = 24.5$
  - $r_s = -0.083$
  - SEM = 25.5% disability

Step 2: Calculate the MDC_{90} for (see Chapter 4, equation 4-2) for each assessment tool:

- Roland-Morris MDC_{90} = 11 disability points (units are questions on the scale)
- Oswestry MDC_{90} = 59% disability

Step 3: Calculate the point estimate for the reliable change proportion (**eq. 5-1**) for each assessment tool:

- Roland-Morris Reliable Change Proportion
  - # $\geq MDC_{90} = 11$
  - # $\leq -MDC_{90} = 1$
  - RM Reliable Change Proportion = 11 + 1/88 = **0.14**
- Oswestry Reliable Change Proportion
  - # $\geq MDC_{90} = 9$
  - # $\leq -MDC_{90} = 0$
- Oswestry Reliable Change Proportion = 9 + 0/88 = **0.10**

Subject	Return_to_Work	Initial_RM	RM_followup	RM_change	Initial_Oswestry	Oswestry_followup	Oswestry_change
1	No	16	18	−2	54	29	25
2	No	18	18	0	65	12	53
3	Yes	20	3	17	64	25	39
4	Yes	20	17	18	30	19	11
5	No	2	18	−16	82	38	44
6	No	5	8	−3	93	42	51
7	No	20	22	−2	6	48	−42
8	No	18	23	−5	15	35	−20
9	No	21	21	0	12	42	−30
10	Yes	23	16	7	42	27	15
11	No	20	21	−1	40	46	−6
12	Yes	10	2	8	62	39	23
13	No	9	7	2	19	49	−30
14	Yes	23	8	15	89	23	66
15	Yes	23	8	15	86	32	54
16	No	17	19	−2	8	42	−34
17	No	11	15	−4	52	36	16
18	No	12	15	−3	82	29	53
19	No	8	10	−2	48	28	20
20	Yes	20	10	10	63	9	54
21	Yes	24	15	9	78	11	67
22	Yes	12	6	6	57	16	41
23	No	4	7	−3	88	12	76
24	Yes	23	12	11	64	20	44
25	No	23	23	0	31	47	−16
26	Yes	23	13	10	89	8	81
27	No	21	17	4	25	25	0
28	Yes	21	11	10	75	47	28
29	Yes	10	2	8	38	5	33

Figure 5-5 Hypothetical data set for comparing responsiveness of two disability scales. RM = Roland-Morris disability score. Data for 29 of 88 patients are shown. See the data file "Ch5_Responsiveness" for Excel, NCSS or SPSS, on the bound-in disk.

Step 4: Calculate the 95% CIs for each reliable change proportion (see calculator associated with Chapter 5 on bound-in disk) for each assessment tool, given $N = 88$:

- 95% CI Roland-Morris *Reliable Change* Proportion = 0.08 to 0.22
- 95% CI Oswestry *Reliable Change* Proportion = 0.05 to 0.18

MCID Proportion Demonstration

Step 1: ROC curve analysis produces output showing the change scores for clinically meaningful difference (review the method in Chapter 4). The MCID is the optimal cut-point where the change score correctly classifies the largest number of patients who improved plus those who had clinically significant worsening.

- Roland-Morris Scale MCID = 5 disability points
- Oswestry Scale MCID = 25% disability[d]

[d]Two points on the ROC curve for hypothetical Oswestry data showed equal accuracy at detecting meaningful clinical change. The change scores of 25% and 26% each correctly classified the most true positive (cell A) plus true negative (cell D) patients. For purposes of illustration, the 25% change score was used.

Video Tutorial 5-1

Reliable Change Proportion: Using an Excel Spreadsheet

Application:
- Illustrates how to use an Excel spreadsheet with hypothetical patient data to calculate:
  - standard deviations (SDs)
  - correlations (*r*)
  - the standard error of measure (SEM)
  - minimum detectable change (MDC)
  - reliable change proportion

Demonstration Data:
- Ch5-Responsiveness.xls

Steps:
1. Open the disk and navigate to this chapter.
2. Select the Video Tutorial 5-1: Calculating Individual Measures of Assessment Responsiveness: Reliable Change Proportion.
3. View how to run the analysis using an Excel spreadsheet.

Use of Software:
1. Verify that you have Excel software loaded on your computer.
2. Run the analysis illustrated in the video.

Step 2: Calculate the point estimate for the MCID proportion (**eq. 5-2**) for each assessment tool. This requires a count of the number of patients who have change scores that meet or exceed the MCID as true positive (# ≥ MCID) and a count of those who truly did not experience change (true negative).

- MCID proportion for Roland-Morris Scale
  - Cell A 35 + Cell D 45/N 88 = **91%**
- MCID proportion for Oswestry Scale
  - Cell A 28 + Cell D 38/N 88 = **75%**

Step 3: Calculate the 95% CIs for each MCID proportion (disk calculator for Chapter 5) for each assessment tool, given $N = 88$:

- 95% CI Roland-Morris *MCID* Proportion = 0.83 to 0.95
- 95% CI Oswestry *MCID* Proportion = 0.65 to 0.83

Group Indices

Effect Size for Responsiveness (ES$_{responsiveness}$) Demonstration

Step 1: Use Excel to average the change scores for a given assessment tool (initial minus follow-up) and repeat for each assessment tool:

- Roland-Morris average change score = 3.5 points (units are questions on the scale)
- Oswestry average change score = 22% disability

Video Tutorial 5-2

MCID Proportion: Using Statistical Software

Application:
- Illustrates how to use statistical software with hypothetical patient data to:
  - determine the optimal change score using ROC analysis
  - calculate MCID proportions for each assessment tool

Demonstration Data:
- Ch5-Responsiveness.s0 (NCSS)
- Ch5-Responsiveness.sav (SPSS)
- Ch5-Responsiveness.xls (Excel)

Steps:
1. Open the disk and navigate to this chapter.
2. Select the Video Tutorial 5-2: Calculating Individual Measures of Assessment Responsiveness: Minimal Clinically Important Difference.
3. View how to run the analysis first in NCSS and then in SPSS. Additional analyses are shown in Excel.

Use of Software:
1. Verify that you have either NCSS or SPSS, along with Excel loaded on your computer.
2. Run the analysis illustrated in the video.

Step 2: Use Excel to calculate the standard deviation (SD) of the *initial* scores in each assessment tool:

- Roland-Morris SD of *initial* scores = 6.5 points
- Oswestry SD of *initial* scores = 24.5% disability

Step 3: Calculate $ES_{responsiveness}$ (**eq. 5-3**):

- Roland-Morris $ES_{responsiveness}$ = 3.5/6.5 = **0.54**
- Oswestry $ES_{responsiveness}$ = 22%/24.5% = **0.90**

Step 4: Calculate the 95% CIs for each ES (see calculator associated with Chapter 5 on bound-in disk) for each assessment tool, given $N = 88$:

- 95% CI Roland-Morris $ES_{responsiveness}$ = 0.33 to 0.75
- 95% CI Oswestry $ES_{responsiveness}$ = 0.69 to 1.11

SRM Demonstration

Step 1: Average the change scores for a given assessment tool (initial minus follow-up) and repeat for each assessment tool (same numerator as $ES_{responsiveness}$):

- Roland-Morris average change score = 3.5 points (units are questions on the scale)
- Oswestry average change score = 22% disability

Step 2: Use Excel to calculate the SD of the *change* scores in each assessment tool:

- Roland-Morris SD of *change* scores = 6.7 points (units are questions on the scale)
- Oswestry SD of *change* scores = 29.3% disability

Step 3: Calculate SRM for Responsiveness (**eq. 5-4**):

- Roland-Morris SRM = 3.5/6.7 = **0.52**
- Oswestry SRM = 22%/29.3% = **0.75**

Step 4: Calculate the 95% CIs for each SRM (see calculator associated with Chapter 5 on bound-in disk) for each assessment tool, given $N = 88$:

- 95% CI Roland-Morris SRM = 0.31 to 0.73
- 95% CI Oswestry SRM = 0.54 to 0.96

Guyatt's Responsiveness Index (GRI) Demonstration

Step 1: *For only those who returned to work[e]* use Excel to average the change scores for a given assessment

tool (initial minus follow-up) and repeat for each assessment tool:

- Roland-Morris average change score = 9.4 points
- Oswestry average change score = 39.6% disability

Step 2: *For only those who did **not** return to work[f]* use Excel to calculate the SD of the *change* scores in each assessment tool:

- Roland-Morris SD of *change* scores = 4.7 points (questions on the scale)
- Oswestry SD of *change* scores = 29.1% disability

Step 3: Calculate GRI for Responsiveness (**eq. 5-5**):

- Roland-Morris GRI = 9.4/4.7 = **2**
- Oswestry GRI = 39.6/29.1 = **1.36**

Step 4: Calculate the 95% CIs for each GRI (see calculator) for each assessment tool, given $N = 88$:

- 95% CI Roland-Morris SRM = 1.79 to 2.21
- 95% CI Oswestry SRM = 1.15 to 1.57

Resolving Discrepancies Among Responsiveness Indices With CIs

The results up to this point in the analysis of hypothetical data are summarized in **Table 5-1** and **Figure 5-6**. *It can be seen that the determination of responsiveness will vary according to the type of responsiveness statistic used.* If the 95% CIs are ignored and the point estimates are evaluated in a descriptive manner, the individual responsiveness for RM appears to be better than Oswestry. However, the Oswestry Questionnaire might appear to have greater responsiveness than the Roland-Morris Scale in terms of the $ES_{responsiveness}$ (0.90 vs. 0.54) and the SRM (0.75 vs. 0.52). The opposite, however, was found for the GRI (1.36 vs. 2).

When incorporating the 95% CIs into the summary, there is no difference in the responsiveness between the Roland and Oswestry scores because the CIs for all responsiveness indices (except for the

---

[e]Use the SORT function in Excel to reorder the rows according to the "Return_to_Work" variable column. Once sorted, highlight the change scores for RM or Oswestry only for those returning to work (indicated by "YES" in the return-to-work column, and calculate the mean. This can also be done in NCSS or SPSS using a filter.

[f] Use SORT function in Excel to reorder the rows according to the "Return_to_Work" variable column. Once sorted, highlight the change scores for RM or Oswestry only for those not returning to work (indicated by "NO" in the return to work column, and calculate the SD. This can also be done in NCSS or SPSS using a filter.

Table 5-1	Summary of the Responsiveness Analysis Using Hypothetical Data Comparing the Roland-Morris Versus Oswestry Disability Questionnaires. (ES = Effect Size, SRM = Standardized Response Mean, GRI = Guyatt's Responsiveness Index.)		

DEMONSTRATION: RESPONSIVENESS ANALYSIS WITH HYPOTHETICAL DATA		Roland-Morris	Oswestry
		Index [95% CI]	Index [95% CI]
Individual Responsiveness Indices			
	Reliable Change Proportion	0.14 [0.08–0.22]	0.10 [0.05–0.18]
	MCID Proportion	0.91 [0.83–0.95]	0.75 [0.65–0.83]
Group Responsiveness Indices			
	$ES_{responsiveness}$	0.54 [0.33–0.75]	0.90 [0.69–1.11]
	SRM	0.52 [0.31–0.73]	0.75 [0.54–0.96]
	GRI	2 [1.79–2.21]	1.36 [1.15–1.57]

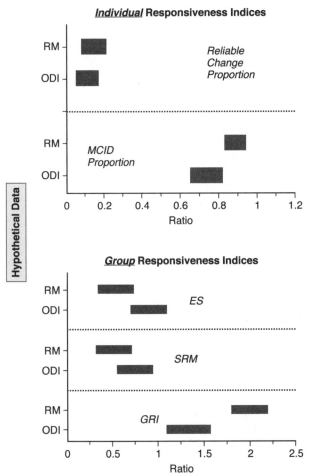

Figure 5-6 Comparison of 95% confidence intervals for responsiveness indices in the demonstration analysis of hypothetical data. RM = Roland-Morris scale, ODI = Oswestry Disability Index. Double horizontal arrow shows area of nonoverlapping GRI CIs.

GRI) overlap (see Fig. 5-6). *The GRI, therefore, is the only measure that indicates a significant difference between the assessment scales with the Roland-Morris Scale hypothetically showing better responsiveness than the Oswestry.*

It is not uncommon for multiple responsiveness indices to differ.[4,11] Change at the group level may not be reflected at the individual level. In turn, average effects across a group may not be meaningful to the individual patient. The design of the responsiveness study can also influence the determination of sensitivity to change (refer to Stratford for an additional review[4]). The demonstration used in this text is a pre–post design with the assumption that those meeting an external criterion (return to work) will have greater improvement than those who do not (see Fig. 5-4). The GRI is compatible with the design of the demonstration exercise, because this index separates the response of those expected to change from those expected to remain stable **(eq. 5-5)**. This characteristic is not found in the $ES_{responsiveness}$ or SRM.[5]

ROC Curve Analysis to Resolve Discrepancies Among Responsiveness Indices

The basic features of ROC curve analysis were presented in Chapter 3. A ROC analysis on change scores was presented in Chapter 4. In this chapter, the ROC analysis has been repeated using the data set illustrated in **Figure 5-5** to obtain the optimal cut-points for the MCID (see Video Tutorial: 5-2). The ROC output from this procedure is shown in **Figure 5-7**.

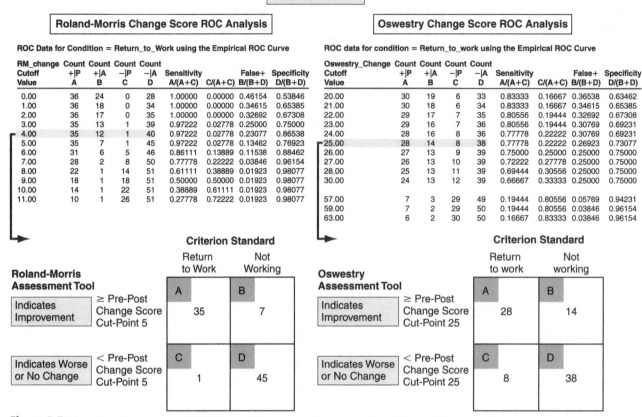

Figure 5-7 Transfer of cut-points in ROC analysis to a contingency table. All possible cut-points for the change scores on the Roland-Morris and Oswestry Disability Questionnaires are not shown due to space limitations. The cut-point for the optimal change score is highlighted for each assessment tool. The ROC curve analysis is translated into a contingency table (below each table of numbers). For purposes of illustration, the Oswestry change score cut-point at 25% was selected even though 26% also represents a valid change score cut-point (both points have the same total values for identifying true positives in Cell A plus true negatives in Cell D). Output is from NCSS v 2007.

This new aspect of the ROC analysis involves hypothesis testing of the area under the ROC curve ("AUC") when the change scores from 2 or more clinical assessment tools are plotted. Stratford et al.[4] recommend that two basic hypotheses be tested. In the demonstration exercise, these hypotheses are:

Null Hypothesis (1): There will be *no difference* in the capacity of Roland-Morris and Oswestry Disability Scales to assess clinical change.

Alternative Hypothesis (1): There will be a difference in the ability of the Roland-Morris and Oswestry Disability Scales to assess clinical change.

Null Hypothesis (2): The AUC of each scale will be less than or equal to the theoretical "useless" AUC.

Alternative Hypothesis (2): Each scale will have significantly more capacity than a theoretical "useless" scale to assess clinical change (>AUC than useless).

Testing AUC Hypothesis (1): Roland-Morris Versus Oswestry

The ROC curve analysis can be used to test these hypotheses and thus determine if the sensitivity to change in one clinical assessment tool is *significantly higher* compared to the other tool. If there is no difference in AUC among the assessment tools, then it is concluded that there is no significant difference in responsiveness to clinical change. The test of statistical significance using the ROC analysis determines if the difference between tools occurs beyond chance differences. This method of statistical significance testing can be used in conjunction with inspection of CI overlap or as a stand-alone method of evaluating responsiveness.

The ROC is a comprehensive analysis from the point of view that all possible cut-points for change scores on each clinical assessment tool are evaluated for sensitivity and specificity to clinical change. Each row in the output from **Figure 5-7** represents a contingency table with cells A, B, C, and D, as denoted in Chapter 4. Quantities representing the percentage of true positives (cell A) and false-positives (cell B) are plotted as illustrated in **Figure 5-8**.

Results of AUC Hypothesis Test (1)

Are the AUCs generated by the change scores for the Roland-Morris and the Oswestry questionnaires in this demonstration exercise significantly different (see Fig. 5-8)? The output of this hypothesis test, generated from statistical software, is shown in **Figure 5-9**. The relevant components of the statistical output are:

- The AUCs for each clinical assessment tool using hypothetical data are listed (0.80 for Oswestry and 0.96 for Roland-Morris)
- The hypothetical CIs for each tool are inspected for overlap. If there is overlap, then the AUCs are not statistically different. In this case, however, there is no overlap and it can be seen that the hypothetical RM change score plot covers a greater area in the CI than the Oswestry change score plot. Thus, in this imaginary demonstration, the Roland-Morris Scale is significantly more responsive **(Fig. 5-10)**.

Testing AUC Hypothesis (2): Does the Responsive Measure Differ From a "Useless" Tool?

Verification analysis is done to determine if the assessment tool of choice is significantly better than a hypothetical "useless" tool. The useless line (Chapter 3) is a line on the ROC curve that represents an equal occurrence of true and false positives. This is referred to as "useless" because change scores approximating this line have no value and are not responsive to clinical change.

The AUC under the useless line is 0.5 (bottom half of the plot area). When a plot of change scores produces an AUC that is not significantly different from 0.5, then the assessment tool producing those change scores is "useless" (e.g., as the sensitivity of the tool increases, so does the false-positive rate).

Results of AUC Hypothesis Test (2): Assessment Tools Versus Theoretical "Useless" Tool

Statistical output comparing the area under the useless line with the area generated by each assessment tool

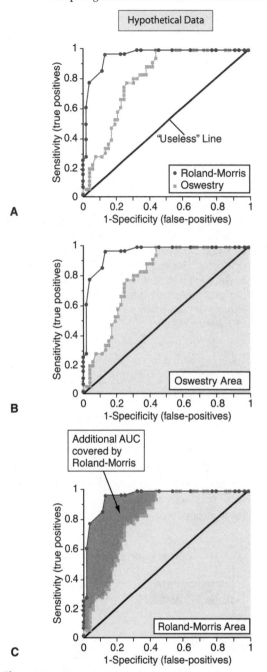

Figure 5-8 (A) ROC plots comparing responsiveness of the Roland-Morris versus Oswestry disability measures (hypothetical data). (B) Area under the curve (AUC) covered by the Oswestry change scores. (C) AUC covered by the Roland-Morris change scores.

in this demonstration is shown in Figure 5-9. The relevant components of the statistical output are:

- The AUC for each clinical assessment tool was compared to the theoretical "useless tool" (AUC useless = 0.5).
- In order to be significantly different from the AUC of the useless line, the clinical assessment

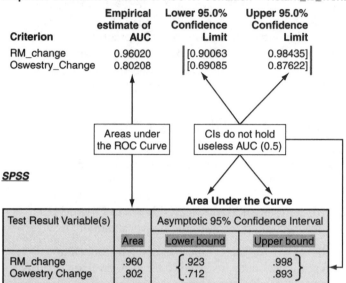

Figure 5-9 Hypothesis tests comparing (1) AUC for Roland-Morris hypothetical data versus Oswestry hypothetical data and (2) a comparison of the AUC for each tool versus the "Useless" AUC. NCSS output is illustrated in the top panel and SPSS output is shown in the bottom panel. Outputs differ slightly due to different methods of calculation and have been edited to show only relevant results.

tool AUC must show a 95% CI that does *not* contain the useless value.

The outcome in Figure 5-9 and Figure 5-10 indicates that the useless AUC = 0.5 does not appear in the 95% CI for either tool. Therefore, the alternative for hypothesis (2) (each clinical assessment tool will have significantly more capacity than a theoretical "useless" scale to assess clinical change) using hypothetical data is supported.

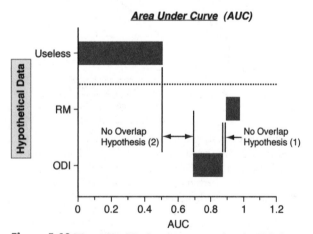

Figure 5-10 The 95% CIs for the area under the ROC curve are shown for hypothetical data comparing the Roland-Morris (RM) and Oswestry Scale outputs. Note that the imaginary data shows that both 95% CIs do not overlap with each other (hypothesis 1) or the useless area (hypothesis 2). RM = Roland-Morris, ODI = Oswestry Disability Index, AUC = area under curve. See text for discussion.

Overall Summary of Hypothetical Responsiveness Demonstration

The results using imaginary data showed that point estimates of individual and group responsiveness indices were contradictory. When CIs were evaluated, only one group index (GRI) showed nonoverlapping 95% CIs among clinical assessment tools (see Fig. 5-6), in favor (hypothetically) of the Roland-Morris Scale. Further analyses using ROC methods and hypothesis testing showed that the Roland-Morris Scale covered more area in the ROC curve than the Oswestry (again hypothetically) but that both tools provided responsiveness capacity significantly better than "useless" (see Fig. 5-10).

Floor and Ceiling Effects and Target Population

When selecting an assessment tool, the target population along with floor and ceiling effects should be considered together with responsiveness. The floor effect is the percentage of patients who score the minimum possible points. In contrast, the ceiling effect is the percentage of patients who score the maximum possible points on the assessment tool. When assessment has a high percentage of ceiling or floor effects ($\geq 20\%$),[1,31] then the tool is not fully measuring the differences in function among patients. Floor and ceiling deficits mean that when many patients have the lowest or highest possible score, the clinician does not know the true level of patient function. How much worse (or better) would patients have performed if they did not reach the limit of the test? This question cannot be answered with assessment tools that have floor or ceiling deficits. If the practitioner prefers the use of an assessment tool with floor or ceiling effects, it is recommended that the assessment be supplemented with other clinical evaluations.[1]

For example, the Berg Balance Scale discussed earlier has a composite score that can vary from 0 to 56, with higher scores indicating better performance. The Berg Balance Scale was originally developed to assess the function of community-dwelling elderly persons (the target population).[32] Since its development, the tool has been used for many different patient populations, including those with Parkinson's disease,[33] multiple sclerosis,[34] and stroke.[1] When used with patients who had a stroke, the Berg Balance Scale had floor effects during the acute phase of convalescence (24% at 14 days poststroke)[9] and ceiling effects 38 days poststroke (26%).[35] These findings highlight the fact that the measurement characteristics of assessment tools can change when used with different populations of patients or with patients who have changing levels of severity. In this case, the literature cited suggests that when clinicians use the Berg Balance Scale for the target population with stroke, it will be difficult to measure the true functional level of patients scoring at the extremes of the assessment scale during the recovery times noted.[1]

The nature of the scale must be considered when floor and ceiling effects are described in the literature. For example, low scores on the Berg Scale indicate poor performance,[10] whereas low scores on other assessment tools (e.g., OPTIMAL,[14] see Chapter 9) indicate high function. When scales with these differences are compared, it is essential to define floor and ceiling effects (**Fig. 5-11**). Does a floor effect, which indicates the percentage of patients who scored the lowest possible points, indicate poor function or best function?

Referring to Figure 5-11, a floor effect could indicate that low scores mean there is a cluster of low-functioning patients (Berg) or high-functioning patients (OPTIMAL). In order to compare floor and ceiling effects among different assessment tools, *it is recommended that the clinician convert all results so that a floor effect indicates poorest function and a ceiling effect indicates best function (eq5-6 and 5-7).*

Floor Effect = # of Patients with Worst Possible Score/Total Number of Patients **eq 5-6**
Ceiling Effect = # of Patients with Best Possible Score/Total Number of Patients **eq 5-7**

Generalization of Findings

As with diagnostic validity research and work addressing meaningful clinical change, once responsiveness and

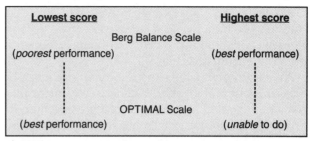

Figure 5-11 Comparison of floor and ceiling effects in scales with different end points. The Berg Balance Scale[32] and the OPTIMAL[14] Scale are used as examples.

floor/ceiling effects of the clinical assessment tool are established, clinicians can use this information to complement the rationale for selecting a tool to evaluate the status of their patients over time. Research addressing responsiveness and floor/ceiling effects is specific to a target population, and the results, if applied to other patient groups, should be interpreted with caution.

Responsiveness outcomes can differ depending on several factors, including selection of a particular responsiveness index, the design of the study to assess responsiveness, and the target population.[2,4] In addition, the severity of disease or dysfunction in the target population will influence generalization of responsiveness results. When searching the literature to support a decision to utilize a particular assessment tool, a match of these characteristics with the population seen in the clinic would provide an optimal, evidence-based rationale for use of a particular tool.

Effect Size, Power, and Estimation of Meaningful Clinical Change

The $ES_{responsiveness}$ is useful for the determination of statistical power. In clinical research with two groups, power is the ability to find a difference between treatment and control groups (or between two sessions within the same group) if a difference truly exists. The standard for acceptable power is 80%. In other words, we accept type II error 20% of the time.[g]

The ES is used as a basis for determining statistical power by entering a statistical table where the body of the table holds power values.[h] If a published study comparing the mean scores of two groups (or the

[g]Type II error is referred to as beta and it is the probability that a researcher will find no difference between groups when a difference, in fact, exists.

[h]Follow the column with ES 0.6 down until the standard of 80% power is approximated. Then move laterally to the left to view *n*: the number of patients per group required to achieve that level of power.

mean change scores) reported an ES = 0.6, then that study should have included at least 45 patients/group to have enough power to detect a difference between groups if one existed (**Fig. 5-12**).

When research addressing the responsiveness of a measurement tool identifies a clinical assessment that has a high level of sensitivity to change, the clinician knows the amount of change that can be detected by the clinical assessment. This information can be used to identify the number of patients that should be included in clinical research to achieve the standard level of statistical power.

For example, if two assessments of outcome were under consideration for use in a clinical study and their $ES_{responsiveness}$ were 0.6 and 0.94, respectively, then the preferred tool (considering only power) would be the

Table 5-2	Comparison of Two Effect Sizes on the Number of Subjects Needed in a Study to Achieve the Standard Level of Statistical Power	
$ES_{responsiveness}$	Power	# Ss per Group Needed (from Power Table)
0.60	81	45
0.94 (~1.00)	80	17

tool with ES = 0.94. The reason for this preference is that given a fixed number of patients, the tool with ES = 0.94 has more power compared with ES = 0.60 (**Table 5-2**).

In a different context, some studies use $ES_{responsiveness}$ to estimate meaningful clinical change. However, $ES_{responsiveness}$ is not a direct measure of meaningful clinical change and is difficult to interpret in that context.[36]

SUMMARY

- A responsive assessment tool is one that detects meaningful change when it has occurred and remains stable when no change has occurred.
- There are different responsiveness indices that reflect either the proportion of patients who have improved (individual patient-level responsiveness) or provide a summary measure of responsiveness related to an entire group of patients.
- The choice of responsiveness indices depends on the design of the research used to study responsiveness.
- Group responsiveness measures should be coupled with individual patient-level measures to provide a battery of indices that show a consistent pattern of responsiveness.
- When responsiveness indices are not consistent, an examination of the 95% CI and a ROC curve analysis can be used to determine if statistically significant differences in responsiveness exist between two or more assessment tools. This method can also determine if the assessment tool of choice has significantly more responsiveness than a theoretically "useless" tool.
- Excessive floor/ceiling effects can obscure the assessment of patient function, so selection of assessment tools should be matched to severity, stage of convalescence, and target population in order to minimize these effects.

					Effect Size						
n	.10	.20	.30	.40	.50	.60	.70	.80	1.00	1.20	1.40
8	05	07	09	11	15	20	25	31	46	60	73
9	05	07	09	12	16	22	28	35	51	65	79
10	06	07	10	13	18	24	31	39	56	71	84
11	06	07	10	14	20	26	34	43	61	76	87
12	06	08	11	15	21	28	37	46	65	80	90
13	06	08	11	16	23	31	40	50	69	83	93
14	06	08	12	17	25	33	43	53	72	86	94
....											
35	07	13	23	38	54	70	82	91	98		
36	07	13	24	39	55	71	83	92	99		
37	07	14	25	39	56	72	84	92	99		
38	07	14	25	40	57	73	85	93	99		
39	07	14	26	41	58	74	86	94	99		
40	07	14	26	42	60	75	87	94	99		
42	07	15	27	44	62	77	89	95	99		
44	07	15	28	46	64	79	90	96	*		
46	08	16	30	48	66	81	91	97			
48	08	16	31	49	68	83	92	97			

Figure 5-12 Power when comparing the differences in patient performance from initial evaluation to follow-up evaluation for a two-tailed test ($\alpha2$) at $p = 0.05$. ($\alpha2$) indicates a two-tailed test of difference where it is possible to have a result that shows improvement at one tail of a probability distribution or a decline at the opposite tail. Power tables like this one are set up to estimate power for two independent groups. When studying the same group of patients tested twice, the ES is adjusted by multiplying $ES*\sqrt{2}$. See Chapter 10 for additional details. (Adapted from Statistical power analysis for the behavioral sciences by Cohen, J. Copyright 1988 in the format Textbook via Copyright Clearance Center.[24] The complete table is shown in Chapter 13, Table 13-7.)

PRACTICE

1. In a study of $N = 250$ patients, if the number of patients meeting or exceeding the MDC was 50 and none of the patients in the sample fell below the MDC threshold, then what is the point estimate of the corresponding individual responsiveness index?

2. For the scenario in question 1, what is the range of responsiveness values that could be expected 95% of the time with an infinite number of study replications?

3. When comparing the 95% CIs of two clinical assessment tools, which of the following responsiveness indices shows a significant difference across the tools?
  a. Reliable change proportion: tool #1 [0.4–0.6], tool #2 [0.5–0.7]
  b. MCID proportion: tool #1 [0.25–0.75], tool #2 [0.80–0.90]
  c. $ES_{responsiveness}$: tool #1 [0.52–0.73], tool #2 [0.19–0.43]
  d. SRM: tool #1 [0.52–0.73], tool #2 [0.19–0.53]
  e. GRI: tool #1 [0.69–0.78], tool #2 [0.22–0.59]

4. In question 3, assuming that the point estimates are in the middle of the CI, which responsiveness indices provide contradictory results with respect to point estimates?

5. The optimal cut-point on a ROC curve of assessment tool *change scores* is linked with which responsiveness index?

6. When the responsiveness of two assessment tools are compared using a ROC analysis, the comparison involves 95% CIs of the area under the curve (AUC) for each tool. The AUC CI in this instance determines the statistical difference between what?

7. Assume that a clinical assessment tool used for patient motor function provides a range of scores from 1 (best performance) to 10 (unable to perform) for each of 10 items. The composite score minimum is 10 and the maximum is 100. In this example, 22 out of 50 patients scored 100 and 3 out of 50 scored 10. Using the recommended calculation, what are the values for the:
  a. floor effect?
  b. ceiling effect?

8. Is the tool described in question 7 too easy or too difficult for the patients in the study? Why?

REFERENCES

1. Blum L, Korner-Bitensky N. Usefulness of the Berg Balance Scale in stroke rehabilitation: a systematic review. Phys Ther 2008; 88:559–566.
2. de Vet HCW, Bouter LM, Bezemer PD, et al. Reproducibility and responsiveness of evaluative outcome measures. Int J Tech Assess in Health Care 2001; 17:479–487.
3. Fritz JM. Sensitivity to change [Letter]. Phys Ther 1999; 79:420–422.
4. Stratford PW, Binkley JM, Riddle DL. Health status measures: strategies and analytic methods for assessing change scores. Phys Ther 1996; 76:1109–1123.
5. Crosby RD, Kolotkin RL, Williams GR. Defining clinically meaningful change in health-related quality of life. Clin Epidemiol 2003; 56:395-407.
6. Norman GR, Stratford P, Regehr G. Methodological problems in the retrospective computation of responsiveness to change: the lesson of Cronbach. J Clin Epidemiol 1997; 50:869–879.
7. Schmitt J, Di Fabio RP. The validity of prospective and retrospective global change criterion measures. Arch Phys Med Rehabil 2004; 86:2270–2276.
8. Stratford PW, Riddle DL, Binkley JM, et al. Sensitivity to change [Letter]. Phys Ther 1999; 79:420–422.
9. Chou CY, Chien CW, Hsueh IP, et al. Developing a short form of the Berg Balance Scale for people with stroke. Phys Ther 2006; 86:195–204.
10. Kornetti DL, Fritz SL, Chiu Y-P, et al. Rating scale analysis of the Berg Balance Scale. Arch Phys Med Rehabil 2004; 85:1128–1135.
11. Schmitt J, Di Fabio RP. Reliable change and minimum important difference (MID) proportions facilitated group responsiveness comparisons using individual threshold criteria. J Clin Epidemiol 2004; 57:1008–1018.
12. Ware JE, Sherbourne CD. A 36-item short form health survey (SF-36): I. Conceptual framework and item selection. Med Care 1992; 30:473–483.
13. Jenkinson C, Layte R, Jenkinson D, et al. A shorter form health survey: can the SF-12 replicate results from the SF-36 in longitudinal studies? J Public Health Med 1997; 19:179–86.
14. Guccione AA, Mielenz TJ, DeVellis R, et al. Development and testing of a self-report instrument to measure actions: Outpatient Physical Therapy Improvement in Movement Assessment Log (OPTIMAL). Phys Ther 2005; 85:515–530.
15. Hudak PL, Amadio PC, Bombardier C. The Upper Extremity Collaborative Group (UECG). Development of an upper extremity outcome measure: the DASH (disabilities of the arm, shoulder and hand). Am J Ind Med 1996; 29:602–608.
16. Roach KE, Budiman-Mak E, Songsiridej N, et al. Development of a shoulder pain and disability index. Arthritis Care Res 1991; 4:143–149.

17. Williams JW Jr, Holleman DR Jr, Simel DL. Measuring shoulder function with the Shoulder Pain and Disability Index. J Rheumatol 1995; 22:727–732.

18. Mao HF, Hsueh IP, Tang PF, et al. Analysis and comparison of the psychometric properties of three balance measures for stroke patients. Stroke 2002; 33:1022–1027.

19. Davidson M, Keating JL. A comparison of five low back disability questionnaires: reliability and responsiveness. Phys Ther 2002; 82:8–24.

20. Stevenson TJ. Detecting change in patients with stroke using the Berg Balance Scale. Austral J Physiother 2001; 47:29–38.

21. Kazis LE, Anderson JJ, Meenan RS. Effect sizes for interpreting changes in health status. Med Care 1989; 27(Suppl 3):S178–89.

22. Liang MH, Fossel AH, Larson MG. Comparisons of five health status instruments for orthopedic evaluation. Med Care 1990; 28:632–642.

23. Guyatt GH, Walter S, Norman G. Measuring change over time: assessing the usefulness of evaluative instruments. J Chronic Dis 1987:171–178.

24. Cohen J. Statistical Power Analysis for the Behavioral Sciences. Hillsdale, NJ: Lawrence Erlbaum Associates, 1988.

25. Stucki G, Liang MH, Fossel AH, et al. Relative responsiveness of condition-specific and generic health status measures in degenerative lumbar spinal stenosis. J Clin Epidemiol 1995; 48:1369–1378.

26. English CK, Hillier SL. The sensitivity of three commonly used outcome measures to detect change amongst patients receiving inpatient rehabilitation following stroke. Clin Rehab 2006; 20.

27. Wilson EB. Probable inference, the law of succession, and statistical inference. J Amer Stat Assoc 1927; 22:209–212.

28. Agresti A, Coull B. Approximate is better than "exact" for interval estimation of binomial proportions. Amer Statistician 1998; 52:119–126.

29. Beaton DE, Hog-Johnson S, Bomburdier C. Evaluating changes in health status: reliability and responsiveness of five generic health status measures in workers with musculoskeletal disorders. J Clin Epidemiol 1997; 50:79–93.

30. Tuley MR, Mulrow CD, McMahan CA. Estimating and testing an index of responsiveness and the relationship of the index to power. J Clin Epidemiol 1991; 44:417–421.

31. Andresen EM. Criteria for assessing the tools of disability outcomes research. Arch Phys Med Rehabil 2000; 81:S15–S20.

32. Berg KO, Wood-Dauphinée SL, Williams JI, et al. Measuring balance in the elderly: validation of an instrument. Can J Public Health 1992; 83:S7–S11.

33. Qutubuddin AA, Pegg PO, Cifu DX, et al. Validating the Berg Balance Scale for patients with Parkinson's disease: a key to rehabilitation evaluation. Arch Phys Med Rehabil 2005; 86:789–792.

34. Paltamaa J, Sarasoja T, Leskinen E, et al. Measures of physical functioning predict self-reported performance in self-care, mobility, and domestic life in ambulatory persons with multiple sclerosis. Arch Phys Med Rehabil 2007; 88:1649–1657.

35. Salbach NM, Mayo NE, Higgins J, et al. Responsiveness and predictability of gait speed and other disability measures in acute stroke. Arch Phys Med Rehabil 2001; 82:1204–1212.

36. DiCenso A, Guyatt G, et al. Evidence-Based Nursing: A Guide to Clinical Practice. St Louis, MO: Elsevier Mosby, 2005.

Chapter 6

Consensus on Patient Assessment

Clinical Questions

- When different clinicians evaluate the same patient, do they reach the same conclusion?
- If outcome of patient evaluation guides the choice of rehabilitation interventions, then will unreliable assessments lead to inappropriate or ineffective treatments?

There are growing instances where patient classification guides the therapist to use a specific treatment protocol (e.g., classifications of facial neuromotor disorders,[1] people with clinical signs of knee osteoarthritis,[2] stroke,[3] or carpal tunnel syndrome[4]). The treatment that patients receive will depend upon the signs and symptoms that place the patient in a certain category of intervention. If agreement about the patient's functional level is poor, then the possibility of misclassification is magnified. In some instances it has been shown that misclassification (or no classification) reduces efficacy of care,[5,6] but this assumption has yet to be validated in many classification schemes.

One example of a specific treatment protocol linked to patient classification was reported by Currier et al.[2] They discovered a group of clinical variables that were important for identifying patients likely to respond to hip mobilization therapy (including limited passive range of motion in selected joints and pain with hip distraction). The finding of only one sign during the patient's evaluation was reported to increase the success of mobilization treatment from a pretest probability of 68% to a posttest probability of 92%. Clinical measures tend to vary with repeated testing.[2,a]

If consensus is good, then different therapists would consistently agree on the patient's signs and symptoms. However, if consensus is poor, one therapist might indicate that the patient has a sign (e.g., limited range of motion that is predictive of therapeutic success) and proceed with a specified intervention, whereas another therapist might find a different profile and proceed with a different course of therapy. This logic applies to any sign and symptom in any classification rule. The overarching question facing practitioners who review the literature addressing patient classification is "How much agreement between clinicians is enough to establish confidence in the classification system of interest?"

Agreement is a form of reliability where consensus is measured.[7,8] The practitioner should have confidence that the assessment tool(s) has been shown to have good agreement including, where appropriate,

- agreement between two clinicians administering the same standardized assessment;
- agreement between patient and caregiver; and
- a single clinician's agreement with self when assessing the same patient over time or a patient's self-assessment when repeated over time.[b]

Several examples of the clinical application of agreement are illustrated in **Table 6-1.**

---

[a]Refer to the standard error of measure in the authors' Table 6-3.

[b]When determining agreement with self, the test-retest interval is set at a duration where the patient's status is presumed to remain unchanged and recall of the initial test result is not likely. There is controversy in the statistical literature regarding the appropriateness of measuring agreement to estimate test-retest reliability because the responses from subjects over time might not be independent data points. Refer to Tooth and Ottenbacher[8] and Sim and Wright[14] for expanded discussions.

Table 6-1	Examples of Consensus Assessment in the Rehabilitation Literature		
Authors	**Target Population**	**Primary Clinical Assessment Tool**	**Agreement Among Whom?**
Sander et al.[9]	Adults with traumatic brain injury	Community Integration Questionnaire	Inter rater (Patients vs. family members)
Verheyden et al.[10]	Multiple sclerosis	Trunk Impairment Scale	Inter rater (between two clinicians) Intra rater (test-retest agreement for the same clinician)
Akinwuntan et al.[11]	Stroke	Driving Test	Inter rater (between two evaluators)
Razmjou et al.[12]	Low-back dysfunction	McKenzie Diagnostic Classifications	Inter rater (between two clinicians)

Assumptions for Conducting Consensus Analysis

There are a group of statistical tests that provide a comprehensive assessment of agreement.[8,13-15] The assumptions underlying the use of agreement statistics[8,14] are that:

- the outcome measure is categorical or ordinal[c] (see **Table 6-2**);
- the assessment provided by the raters is independent; and
- the responses provided by the patients are independent.

When two clinicians assess patient performance (inter rater agreement), each rater must do so independently. Sim and Wright emphasize that consensus assessment "... is not appropriate for a situation in which one observer is required to either confirm or disconfirm a known previous rating from another observer."[14,p.263] In this case, the data are not independent because the first rating is known by the clinician who is providing the second rating.

In situations where the assessment of the same clinician is compared to self across two different sessions of patient evaluation (intra rater agreement), caution is required in interpreting agreement statistics because the rater or the patient may recall the first measure (which could influence subsequent ratings of patient performance). The recall phenomenon tends to inflate the amount of agreement observed.[14,5]

Some experts maintain that the assessment of intra rater agreement (also referred to as test-retest agreement) is not appropriate because it violates the assumptions of independence.[8] Others, while acknowledging that any intra rater study has some degree of dependence

Table 6-2	Types of Data	
Data Type	**Description**	**Examples**
Categorical *(Categories with no inherent order of magnitude)*	Dichotomous (only two categories)	Sex (Male/Female), Pass/Fail
	Polytomous (multiple categories)	Patient classifications with more than two categories (e.g., deficits in gait rhythm vs. speed vs. endurance)
	Nominal (synonymous with categorical)	Any dichotomous or polytomous variable
	Discrete (synonymous with categorical)	Any dichotomous or polytomous variable
Ordinal *[Numbers indicate ordered magnitude (rank) but intervals may not be equal]*	Rank-ordered	Rating of function Poor (1) Fair (2) Excellent (3) Rating of pain Absent (0) Minimal (1) Moderate (2) Severe (3)
Continuous *(Numbers indicate order of magnitude with meaningful intervals)*	Scaled or numeric*	Timed Up and Go Test (seconds) Quality of Life score (0 to 100%)

*Note: Some statistical software programs include rank-ordered data under the "Numeric" data label.

[c]Experts do not agree on the use of ordinal data when measuring agreement. Tooth and Ottenbacher[8] caution against this practice while Sim and Wright (2005) endorse the practice.

among test and retest ratings, suggest that dependence can be minimized by implementing various design strategies, such as increasing the time between ratings (provided that the clinical trait being evaluated is stable and not expected to change) and randomizing the order of patient assessment.[14,16]

Measurement of Consensus Using Dichotomous Categorical Data

Percent Agreement

Categorical data that are dichotomous have only two categories (e.g., yes/no, pass/fail, faller/nonfaller; Table 6-2). A common and intuitive measure of consensus for dichotomous categorical data is the percent agreement among raters. A 2×2 contingency table is typically used to sort agreements and disagreements in order to calculate percent agreement (Fig. 6-1). For example, if the goal was to determine the consensus between two clinicians who assessed driving ability in patients recovering from a stroke (similar to the method used by Akinwuntan et al.[11]), a contingency table with four cells could be used. Counting the patients where both evaluators agreed that patients either passed or failed the motor vehicle

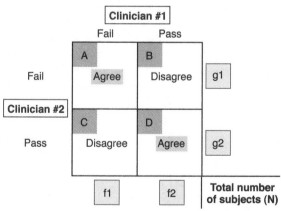

Figure 6-1 A 2×2 contingency table set up to sort agreements and disagreements of two raters. Agreement is found on the diagonal of the contingency table (see shaded cells A and D for "agreement diagonal"). Marginal totals for each column are designated f1 and f2; marginal totals for each row are designated g1 and g2.

ᶠThe conventions for labeling totals for each row ("g") and each column ("f") were adapted from Sim J, Wright CC. The kappa statistic in reliability studies: use, interpretation, and sample size requirements. Phys Ther 2005; 85:257-268 with permission of the American Physical Therapy Association. This material is copyrighted and any further reproduction or distribution requires written permission from APTA.

driving test can be expressed as the proportion of agreement (Po):

$$Po = \frac{(cell\,A) + (cell\,D)}{N} \qquad \text{eq 6-1}$$

where the counts in cells A + D are summed and divided by the total number of observations (N). The percent agreement is then

Percent Observed Agreement $= Po * 100$ **eq 6-2**

Disagreement among the raters occurs when

- rater #1 indicates the patient passed the road test but rater #2 failed the client (cell B) or
- rater #1 indicates the patient failed the road test, but rater #2 passed the client (cell C).

Kappa: Chance-Corrected Agreement

Some authors have indicated that percent observed agreement alone as a measure of consensus has limited value because it does not account for chance agreements.[15] In other words, one rater could guess the status of any patient and just happen to agree with their paired rater.

The kappa statistic ("k") is designed to account for chance agreement between evaluators.[17,18] The values of kappa range from 0 (agreement no different than chance) to 1 (perfect agreement). In some cases, kappa can be less than 0 (agreement worse than chance).[8] Kappa is calculated by **equation 6-3**:

$$K = \frac{Po - Pc}{1 - Pc} \qquad \text{eq 6-3}$$

where Po is the proportion of observed agreements and Pc is the proportion of chance agreements.[18]

Chance Agreements

The number of agreements that occur by chance for each cell is calculated by dividing the product of the column total × the row total where the cell resides by N. For example, consider a hypothetical readiness-to-drive study. Here, the data from two imaginary clinicians is outlined in **Figure 6-2**.

The chance agreement frequency for cells in the *agreement diagonal* (cells A and D) in Figure 6-2 is

Number of Chance Agreements for
Cell A = (f1 * g1)/N **eq 6-4**
= (59 * 66)/84
= ~ 46
Number of Chance Agreements
for Cell D = (f2 * g2)/N **eq 6-5**
= (25 * 18)/84
= ~ 5

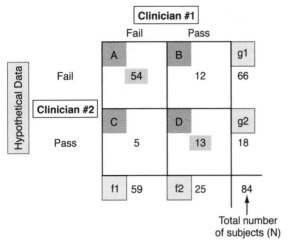

Figure 6-2 Hypothetical data used in the comparison of a readiness-to-drive assessment from two imaginary evaluators. The number in each cell is the patient count for 84 imaginary patients. Agreement is found on the diagonal of the contingency table (see shaded cells A and D for "agreement diagonal"). Totals for each column are designated f1 and f2; totals for each row are designated g1 and g2.

This means that the two hypothetical evaluators could have agreed by chance that 46 imaginary patients failed the driver test (true positive) or that 5 patients passed the test (true negative).[d] The proportion of chance agreements (Pc) is the sum of chance agreements *along the agreement diagonal* divided by *N* **(eq. 6-6)**. For the 2×2 contingency table shown in Figure 6-2, the format described by Sim et al.[14] is used to determine the proportion of chance agreements (Pc, eq. 6-6; cell counts from Fig. 6-2):

$$Pc = \frac{(f1 * g1/N) + (f2 * g2/N)}{N} \qquad \textbf{eq 6-6}$$

$$Pc = \frac{(59 * 66/84) + (25 * 18/84)}{84} = \sim 0.62$$

Observed Agreements

The proportion of *observed agreements* (Po) along the agreement diagonal is

$$Po = \frac{(cell\,A) + (cell\,D)}{N} \quad \text{(using eq 6-1)}$$

$$Po = \frac{(54) + (13)}{84} = \sim 0.80$$

Thus, kappa is the proportion of "chance corrected" agreements:

$$K = \frac{Po - Pc}{1 - Pc} \qquad \text{(using eq 6-3)}$$

$$K = \frac{0.80 - 0.62}{1 - 0.62} = 0.47 = 47\%$$

[d]Note that failing the driver's test is considered a positive result for the presence of dysfunction, thus true positive.

The result means that when corrected for chance agreements, the imaginary clinicians agreed on driving ability in 47% of the cases. In this example, there is a discrepancy between observed agreement (Po = 0.80 = 80%) versus the chance corrected agreement ($k = 0.47 = 47\%$). These discrepancies occur frequently and several reasons are well documented in the literature to account for this phenomenon.[8,14,15,19]

When the distribution of counts is skewed in the contingency table, then k and Po may yield contradictory results.[20] Viewing the counts in Figure 6-2, for example, the agreement diagonal has 54 cases in Cell A, but only 13 cases in cell D. If cells A and D were more uniform (say 34 and 33, respectively), then the skew would be minimized. Po would still equal 0.80, but k increases to 0.60. Thus, the value of kappa is sensitive to a skew in the count distribution within the cells of the contingency table.

Resolving Conflicts Between Kappa and Observed Agreement

In order to resolve contradictions between the magnitude of observed agreement and kappa, Cicchetti and Feinstein[20] recommend reporting kappa along with two additional measures of *observed agreement*: "Ppos" and "Pneg."[20] Ppos is the proportion of agreement on a positive rating of the clinical test, whereas Pneg is the proportion of agreement on a negative rating of the clinical test. These statistics are analogous to sensitivity and specificity (respectively) described previously for diagnostic validity testing (see Chapter 3):

$$Ppos = \frac{2 * A}{f1 + g1} \qquad \textbf{eq 6-7}$$

$$Pneg = \frac{2 * D}{f2 + g2} \qquad \textbf{eq 6-8}$$

where cells A, D, and marginal totals f1, f2 and g1, g2 are defined in Figure 6-1.

Example (using hypothetical data from Fig. 6-2):

$$Ppos = \frac{2 * A}{f1 + g1} = \frac{2 * 54}{59 + 66} = 0.86 = 86\%$$

$$Pneg = \frac{2 * D}{f2 + g2} = \frac{2 * 13}{25 + 19} = 0.60 = 60\%$$

The values for Ppos and Pneg in the example show that the imaginary evaluators have better agreement when identifying those who failed the driving test (Ppos ~"consensus sensitivity") compared to agreement when determining who passed the driving test (Pneg ~"consensus specificity"). This information helps to explain why observed agreement (Po) differed substantially from kappa. In essence, the imaginary raters had considerably more agreement on patients with positive driving tests compared to their agreement on patients with negative tests. This imbalance or skew influences the magnitude of kappa.[20] As a general rule, both Ppos and Pneg should approximate similar magnitudes in order to establish kappa as a valid consensus statistic.

Kappa, Prevalence, and Bias

The value of kappa is also influenced by both prevalence and bias.[8,14] Prevalence is estimated by the frequency of the target condition in the sample (see Chapter 3, eq. 3-4; cells A + C/N). Given the same percent agreement, a prevalence that departs substantially from 50% in either direction (higher or lower) can alter kappa compared to a prevalence closer to 50%.[14] *This scenario reflects the condition where agreements (cell A versus D) are asymmetrical.* A prevalence index has been proposed to measure the prevalence magnitude in the contingency table[14]:

$$prevalence\ index = \frac{|a-d|}{N} \qquad \textbf{eq 6-9}$$

where *a* and *d* are the cell counts from the contingency table and *N* is the total number of patients counted.[e] Example (using hypothetical data from Fig. 6-2):

$$prevalence\ index = \frac{|54-13|}{84} = 0.49$$

Bias also reflects a skew in the distribution of cases throughout the contingency table, but in this case *the disagreements are asymmetrical (cell B versus C).* A bias index has been proposed to measure the bias magnitude in the contingency table[14]:

$$bias\ index = \frac{|b-c|}{N} \qquad \textbf{eq 6-10}$$

Example (using hypothetical data from **Fig. 6-2**):

$$bias\ index = \frac{|12-5|}{84} = 0.08$$

The ideal prevalence and bias index is 0.[f] A suggested arbitrary rule is that when either index is >0.40, this indicates a skewed distribution of cases

in the contingency table that should be noted as a potential challenge to the validity of kappa.

Descriptive Significance of Kappa

The magnitude of kappa can be evaluated descriptively or through the use of statistical significance testing. Landis and Koch[18] proposed an arbitrary descriptive scale for assessing the magnitude of kappa that had six levels (increments from "poor" to "almost perfect"). Clinical researchers have considered the practical context when judging the magnitude of kappa.[14,21,22] Suggested thresholds for low kappas have varied from 0.40[14] to 0.60.[22] A simplified (but un-validated) rating scale can serve as a general guide for clinical use (**Table 6-3**). This clinical scale can also be applied to Po, Ppos, and Pneg (**Table 6-4**). While the minimum level of acceptable agreement can vary depending upon context, it seems reasonable to propose that the use of assessment tools or protocols in the clinic have at least "good" reliability.

Interpretation of Consensus Measures Using a Descriptive Scale

The summary of statistical tests reflecting consensus measures derived from the hypothetical data in Figure 6-2 is shown in Table 6-4. In this example, kappa is not a robust index of consensus because the prevalence index is high. In other words, the skew of counts in the contingency table detracts from the validity of kappa. This leaves measures of observed agreement for a better interpretation of outcome (Po, Ppos, and Pneg). The imaginary raters in this demonstration had good observed agreement overall (Po) with excellent agreement on patients who were not ready to drive (Ppos). Even though Pneg is low, the hypothetical method for determining driver readiness errs on the side of patient and public safety. All of the statistics in Table 6-4 provide information about

[e]Taking the absolute value of the difference between Cells A and D in the prevalence index addresses the scenario where prevalence might be substantially less than 50%, thereby removing the possibility of a negative index value.

[f]Pc, bias index, and prevalence index were adapted from Sim J, Wright CC. The kappa statistic in reliability studies: use, interpretation, and sample size requirements. Phys Ther 2005; 85:257–268 with permission of the American Physical Therapy Association. This material is copyrighted and any further reproduction or distribution requires written permission from APTA.

Table 6-3	Example of an Arbitrary Scale to Describe the Strength of Agreement
Kappa Statistic	**Strength of Agreement**
0.00–0.40	Poor
0.41–0.60	Fair
0.61–0.80	Good
0.81–1.00	Excellent

Table 6-4	Summary of Consensus Measures for Hypothetical Dichotomous Categorical Data Illustrated in Figure 6-2	
Consensus Measure	Value in *Hypothetical* Readiness-to-Drive Example ++	Description
Proportion Observed Agreement (**Po**)	0.80	*Good observed* agreement (*not* corrected for chance)
* **Ppos** (consensus "sensitivity")	0.86	*Excellent* agreement on patients who are not ready to drive
* **Pneg** (consensus "specificity")	0.60	*Fair* observed agreement on patients who should be allowed to drive
Kappa (*k*)	0.47	*Fair* agreement corrected for chance
* **Prevalence Index**	>0.40	Unacceptable skew: distribution of cases with agreement (cell A vs. D)
* **Bias Index**	<0.40	Acceptable skew: distribution of cases with disagreement (cell B vs. C)

++Refer to Figure 6-2.

consensus. *Clinicians reviewing the literature should be encouraged to calculate the battery of consensus statistics on 2×2 tables (where possible) to complete their review of the literature, especially when published manuscripts do not contain this information.*[g]

Statistical Significance of Kappa

The kappa statistic is a "point estimate" (i.e., a single value). Drawing different samples of patients from the target population would likely yield a different kappa on each occasion simply due to sampling error. Variation of kappa across many experiments on the same target population is estimated by a z-score and confidence interval (CI) to determine if the "true" value of kappa falls in a range that indicates statistical significance[14] (see the appendix to Chapter 4 for z-score review).

Consensus Calculator

Application:
• Use an Excel spreadsheet to calculate kappa and other statistical measures of consensus

Steps:
1. Verify that you have Microsoft Excel software loaded on your computer.
2. Open the disk and navigate to this chapter.
3. Select the P_Consensus CALCULATOR.xls and click on the tab (worksheet) for kappa.
4. Enter contingency table counts for Cells A, B, C, and D in the area shown.
5. Consensus results are automatically calculated once cell values are entered by the reader.

Use of Calculator:
The calculator can be used to verify hand calculations of consensus statistics or to compare reported results in the literature to the spreadsheet results.

The calculation of CI surrounding a kappa point estimate requires:

• z-score (constants) corresponding to the % of the confidence interval
  • 1.96 for a 95% CI or
  • 1.645 for a 90% CI
• the standard error (SE) of kappa (calculated using statistical software or the bound-in disk)

and is based on the formulas developed by Fleiss et al.[23] (cited in Hanley[24]).[h] The 95% CI for kappa is calculated:

$$95\% \text{ CI} = \text{kappa} \pm (z_{95\%} * \text{SE}) \quad \textbf{eq 6-11}$$

The 90% CI for kappa is calculated:

$$90\% \text{ CI} = \text{kappa} \pm (z_{90\%} * \text{SE}) \quad \textbf{eq 6-12}$$

If the classification system in Table 6-3 is used, kappa values ≤ 0.40 represent poor agreement; thus, if the confidence interval includes a kappa value of 0.40 or less, agreement among raters could be considered poor regardless of the magnitude of the point estimate. In the demonstration example for two imaginary raters evaluating readiness to drive:

kappa = 0.47
SE_{kappa} = 0.10 (calculated from the disk),
which yields

$$95\% \ CI = kappa \pm (z_{95\%} * SE) = 0.47 \pm (1.96 * 0.10),$$
or the interval
$$95\% \ CI = [0.27\text{———}(0.47)\text{———}0.67]$$
$$90\% \ CI = kappa \pm (z_{90\%} * SE) = 0.47 \pm (1.645 * 0.10)$$
or the interval
$$90\% \ CI = [0.31\text{———}(0.47)\text{———}0.63]$$

The results of this demonstration analysis using hypothetical data indicate that the clinician can be 95% certain that with repeated testing in the target population, kappa will fall in a range between 0.27 and 0.67. Alternatively, the clinician can be 90% certain that kappa will fall in a range between 0.31 and 0.63.

Further interpretation of the CI depends upon the minimum value of kappa that is considered meaningful. A clinician might decide that instead of a kappa threshold of 0.40, a higher threshold is needed to establish meaningful agreement among raters. If kappa = 0.60 is used as the threshold of chance-corrected agreement, then CIs including this value would not be considered a meaningful consensus among raters (see Verheyden et al.[22] for an example).

Also, the width of the CI can alter the interpretation of kappa statistical significance. Note that the width of the 90% CI is smaller than the width of the 95% CI. This means that it is possible to find the threshold value of kappa in one interval but not the other. The choice of which CI to use is generally based on the preference of the researcher. However, the 95% CI provides a more rigorous analysis compared to the 90% CI. The results of the demonstration example show that a kappa = 0.47 would not be statistically meaningful under either CI.

Measurement of Consensus Using Polytomous Categorical Data

Kappa can be calculated for any balanced or "square" contingency table (i.e., 2×2, 3×3, 4×4 ... $k \times k$). When there are more than two categories in the categorical data, then the data are called "polytomous."[8] Consensus on polytomous data from the perspective of rehabilitation research often involves the measurement of agreement on diagnostic classifications. Examples of polytomous classifications include people with stroke[3] ("force production deficit," "fractionated movement deficit," and "perceptual deficit"), patients with low-back pain dysfunction[12] ("postural movement pattern," "derangement movement pattern," or "tissue adhesion pattern"), or patients with facial neuromotor disorders ("initiation deficits," "facilitation," "movement control," "relaxation" classifications).[1]

Demonstration of Consensus Analysis Using Polytomous Data

For the demonstration of kappa calculation, a hypothetical data set was created for people with stroke (Fig. 6-3) using the classification system proposed by Scheets et al.[3] These data are imaginary and used here only to promote an understanding of statistical process. In this demonstration, two imaginary clinicians simultaneously classify each of 42 imaginary people with stroke. The goal is to measure the level of consensus among the raters when classifying patients within three possible movement diagnoses.

Statistical software applied to the hypothetical data set uses a cross-tabulation procedure to re-create a table similar to Table 6-5 in order to compute kappa and the standard error (SE) of kappa.

The validity indices applied to kappa in a 2×2 contingency table (Table 6-4) do not easily translate to square tables of different sizes. It is recommended, therefore, that kappa be reported along with the SE_{kappa}, a 95% CI, and the percent agreement among raters (not corrected for chance agreements) when contingency tables are larger than 2×2. In this demonstration example:

kappa = 0.71
SE_{kappa} = 0.11
95% CI = [0.49———(0.71)———0.93] (*via hand calculation using* equation 6-11)
Po = 0.80%

Video Tutorial 6-1

Calculating Kappa and SE_{kappa} for Polytomous Data Using Statistical Software

Application:
- Illustrates how to use statistical software to calculate the kappa statistic and the standard error of kappa for polytomous categorical data

Demonstration Data:
- *Ch6-Polytomous Kappa.**S0*** (for NCSS)
- *Ch6-Polytomous Kappa.**Sav*** (for SPSS)

Steps:
1. Open the disk and navigate to this chapter.
2. Select Video Tutorial 6-1: Calculating Measures of Consensus: Polytomous Kappa.
3. View how to run the analysis using software.

Use of Software:
1. Verify that you have either NCSS or SPSS statistical software loaded on your computer.
2. Run the analysis illustrated in the video using the appropriate data set for the statistical software that you have installed.

Patient_num	Rater_1	Rater_2
1	force	force
2	fractionated mvt	fractionated mvt
3	fractionated mvt	fractionated mvt
4	perceptual	perceptual
5	perceptual	perceptual
6	perceptual	perceptual
7	perceptual	perceptual
8	perceptual	perceptual
9	fractionated mvt	fractionated mvt
10	fractionated mvt	fractionated mvt
11	perceptual	perceptual
12	perceptual	perceptual
13	force	force
14	force	force
15	fractionated mvt	fractionated mvt
16	fractionated mvt	fractionated mvt
17	fractionated mvt	fractionated mvt
18	fractionated mvt	fractionated mvt
19	force	fractionated mvt
20	force	fractionated mvt
21	force	fractionated mvt
22	force	fractionated mvt
23	fractionated mvt	fractionated mvt
24	fractionated mvt	fractionated mvt
25	fractionated mvt	fractionated mvt

Figure 6-3 Hypothetical data set up for a consensus analysis on polytomous data to generate a kappa statistic. Twenty-five of 42 rows are displayed here. The full data set is available on the bound-in disk (use "Ch6-Polytomous Kappa" and choose the file with either the NCSS or SPSS extension).

Refer to the Video Tutorial 6-1 to view the relevant statistical outputs from NCSS and SPSS.

Some experts believe that the assessment of consensus using the kappa statistic with polytomous data is not appropriate.[8] Tooth and Ottenbacher[8] point out that kappa essentially averages the measure of agreement across multiple categories. In Table 6-5, for example, the calculation of kappa is a single statistic that includes the agreement between imaginary raters on their diagnosis of force deficit versus fractionated movement, force deficit versus perceptual deficit, and fractionated movement versus perceptual deficit. Tooth and Ottenbacher[8] recommend polytomous data be subdivided into a series

of dichotomous tables where separate kappa statistics can be derived (i.e., separate the analysis of force versus fractionated movement classification, etc.). This approach, while statistically sound, can be cumbersome when many categories exist in the data set.

Measurement of Consensus Using Ordinal Data: Weighted Kappa

The kappa statistic is unweighted. This means that all disagreements among raters have the same impact on the value of kappa. When the data are ordinal (or categorical "where there is an *a priori* clinical or theoretical rationale for valuing disagreements differently" [8, p.1373]), then it may be desirable to assign weights to the disagreements. For example, in a hypothetical study of rehabilitation potential, 27 imaginary patients were evaluated with a standardized battery of clinical assessments. Clinicians were asked to rate the patients' rehabilitation potential on a scale of 1 to 3 (1 = "good", 2 = "fair", and 3 = "poor"). If the likelihood of being referred to a rehabilitation service diminishes with a "fair" rating and is unlikely if the patient receives a "poor" rating, then it would seem appropriate to penalize a "good" versus "poor" disagreement more than a "good" versus "fair" disagreement.

The formula for calculating the weighted kappa statistic is[8]

$$kappa\ (w) = 1 - \frac{\sum wfo}{\sum wfc} \qquad \textbf{eq 6-13}$$

where fo is the observed frequency, fc is the chance frequency, w is the cell weight, wfo is the weighted frequency of observed disagreements, and wfc is the weighted frequency of chance disagreements.

There are several methods of weighting disagreements.[8,14,25,26] The quadratic method was selected for illustration here; it uses the square of the amount of

Table 6-5	Demonstration of a 3×3 Contingency Table to Analyze Polytomous Data for Classifying Imaginary Patients with Stroke Using the Classification Scheme Proposed by Scheets et al.[3]

		HYPOTHETICAL DATA			
		Rater 1			
		Force Deficit	Fractionated Movement	Perceptual Deficit	Totals
Rater 2	Force Deficit	7	0	0	7
	Fractionated Movement	5	11	1	17
	Perceptual Deficit	2	0	16	18
	Totals	14	11	17	42

discrepancy between ratings.[27] Thus, with perfect agreement the discrepancy is 0, so the weight is $(0)^2 = 0$. The discrepancy between "good" versus "fair" is 1 point, so $(1)^2 = 1$. Finally, the discrepancy between "good" versus "poor" rehabilitation potential is 2, which is weighted $(2)^2 = 4$ points. In this example the multipliers that are used to weight for each cell are summarized in **Table 6-6**.

Hypothetical data for 27 patients are illustrated in **Figure 6-4**. The first three columns of data show the patient number, the rating from clinician #1, and the rating from clinician #2, respectively. A numeric score is entered for each clinician in the next two columns. Finally, the weighted disagreement is entered (square of the difference in ratings between clinicians).

Using this hypothetical data set, a cross-tabulation procedure is run with statistical software to generate observed counts in each cell of the table (fo) and the counts that would be expected by chance (fc). Many statistical software packages calculate only the **unweighted** kappa. In order to apply the quadratic method of weighting disagreements among raters, selected parts of the output (f_o and f_c) are copied to an Excel spreadsheet for further processing **(Fig. 6-5)**.

Once Σfo and Σfc are calculated in Excel (circled numbers in step 3, **Fig. 6-5**), these results are entered into **equation 6-13**:

$$kappa\ (w) = 1 - \frac{\sum wfo}{\sum wfc} = 1 - \left(\frac{26}{38.1}\right) = 0.32$$

The weighted kappa shows that with quadratic weights applied to the disagreements among imaginary clinicians assessing rehabilitation potential in the demonstration data set, there is 32% agreement when corrected for chance agreements. The magnitude of the weighted kappa is interpreted in the same way as kappa. However, the SE_{kappa} derived from many statistical programs is based on unweighted data. Thus, the CIs for weighted kappa may not be accurate.[24]

As clinicians apply weighting schemes to consensus data, they introduce a subjective and arbitrary element to the outcome.[8,27] Different weighting schemes may produce different results. The **unweighted** kappa for the demonstration example in Figure 6-5 ($k = 0.12$; calculation not shown) indicates that when near agreements are not given credit, chance corrected agreement is lower than the weighted kappa. Soeken and Prescott[27] caution that unless there is a strong theoretical or clinical rationale for using a particular weighting scheme, the selection of weighted kappa as a measure of consensus should be avoided. Under certain conditions (described in the next section), an intraclass correlation coefficient can serve as an alternative to the weighted kappa statistic.

Intraclass Correlation Coefficients as Measures of Consensus

The advantage to using an *intraclass correlation coefficient* (ICC) for measuring consensus is that there is no need to assign arbitrary weights to disagreements.[i] The

[i]When a quadratic weighting method is used on ordinal data to weight disagreements, the results closely approximate the ICC (Rae, Educ Psychol Meas 1988; 48:367-374). However, other weighting schemes may not yield similar results.

Video Tutorial 6-2

Calculating Weighted Kappa Using Statistical Software

Application:
• Illustrates how to use statistical software and Microsoft Excel to calculate a weighted kappa statistic.
Demonstration Data:
• *Ch6-Weighted Kappa.***S0** (for NCSS)
• *Ch6-Weighted Kappa.***Sav** (for SPSS)
Steps:
1. Open the disk and navigate to this chapter.
2. Select Video Tutorial 6-2: Calculating Measures of Consensus: Weighted Kappa.
3. View how to run the analysis using NCSS and SPSS statistical software. Then view a completion of the weighted kappa calculation using the Consensus Calculator in Excel.
Use of Software:
1. Verify that you have either NCSS or SPSS statistical software and Excel loaded on your computer.
2. Run the analysis illustrated in the video using the appropriate data set for the statistical software that you have installed.

Table 6-6	Multipliers (Constants) for Weighting Disagreements Using a Quadratic Weighting Scheme		
		Clinician 1	
	Good	Fair	Poor
Clinician 2 Good	0	1	4
Fair	1	0	1
Poor	4	1	0

Note that exact agreement among clinicians (the shaded "agreement diagonal") is weighted 0 because there is no disagreement. Each constant is multiplied by the value in the contingency table with the corresponding location.

Patient	Clinician_1	Clinician_2	Score_Clinician_1	Score_Clinician_2	Wt_Disagreement
1	A_Good	B_Fair	1	2	1
2	A_Good	A_Good	1	1	0
3	A_Good	A_Good	1	1	0
4	B_Fair	C_Poor	2	3	1
5	A_Good	A_Good	1	1	0
6	C_Poor	B_Fair	3	2	1
7	A_Good	A_Good	1	1	0
8	A_Good	A_Good	1	1	0
9	C_Poor	B_Fair	3	2	1
10	A_Good	A_Good	1	1	0
11	A_Good	A_Good	1	1	0
12	B_Fair	C_Poor	2	3	1
13	A_Good	B_Fair	1	2	1
14	A_Good	A_Good	1	1	0
15	C_Poor	C_Poor	3	3	0
16	A_Good	B_Fair	1	2	1
17	A_Good	C_Poor	1	3	4
18	C_Poor	B_Fair	3	2	1
19	A_Good	A_Good	1	1	0
20	C_Poor	A_Good	3	1	4
21	C_Poor	C_Poor	3	3	0
22	A_Good	C_Poor	1	3	4
23	A_Good	A_Good	1	1	0
24	B_Fair	A_Good	2	1	1
25	A_Good	A_Good	1	1	0
26	C_Poor	A_Good	3	1	4
27	A_Good	B_Fair	1	2	1

Figure 6-4 Hypothetical data set up for a consensus analysis to generate a weighted kappa statistic. All 27 rows are displayed here. The data set is available in the bound-in disk (use "Ch6-Weighted Kappa" and choose the file with either the NCSS or SPSS label). Column headings show the labels of variables used in the analysis. Scores: 1 = Good rehabilitation potential, 2 = Fair, 3 = Poor. The variable column labeled "Wt_Disagreement" is the difference between the scores of clinicians 1 and 2 *squared* (weighted disagreements).

ICC is actually a family of three different correlation coefficients described by Fleiss[28] that can be used with continuous[28] or ordinal data[29] (see Table 6-2 for data levels). The ICC in all cases varies from 0 (poor agreement) to 1 (excellent agreement; the same descriptive measures as kappa in Table 6-3).

- When the goal is to determine if a single clinician (or rater) consistently assesses the same patients at two or more points in time, an in*tra* rater ICC is used ($ICC_{intra rater}$). In this scenario, the consensus assessment comes from a single person performing repeated measures (hence, in*tra* rater agreement). It is assumed that the patients are randomly selected.

For the assessment of in*ter* rater agreement, there are two distinct ICCs. The selection of an in*ter* rater ICC depends upon how the raters were selected.

- *Raters Fixed:* When the clinicians are *not* selected randomly from a larger pool of raters, then the fixed group of clinicians are the only clinicians of interest. There is no desire to generalize the results to other raters (e.g., a consensus study confined to a single clinic to determine how well clinicians at that site agree on the assessment of patients at the

initial evaluation). The assessment of consensus under this scenario is referred to as $ICC_{inter\,rater\,fixed}$ because the raters comprise a fixed group.

- *Raters Random:* When clinicians are selected randomly from a pool of raters, the raters are assumed to be representative of a larger group of clinicians who might be involved in patient assessment at some point in the future. In this case, there is a desire to generalize the ability to agree on clinical assessments to other raters (e.g., a multicenter consensus study to determine how well clinicians agree on the assessment of patients at the initial evaluation). The assessment of consensus under this scenario is referred to as $ICC_{inter\,rater\,random}$ because the raters are selected randomly.

Calculate ICC Through Analysis of Variance

All ICCs are derived from a statistical process called repeated measures analysis of variance (RM-ANOVA). The summary table generated from a RM-ANOVA provides the values necessary to calculate an ICC. It is helpful to remember that consensus is all about the concept of variance. Variance is simply the variability

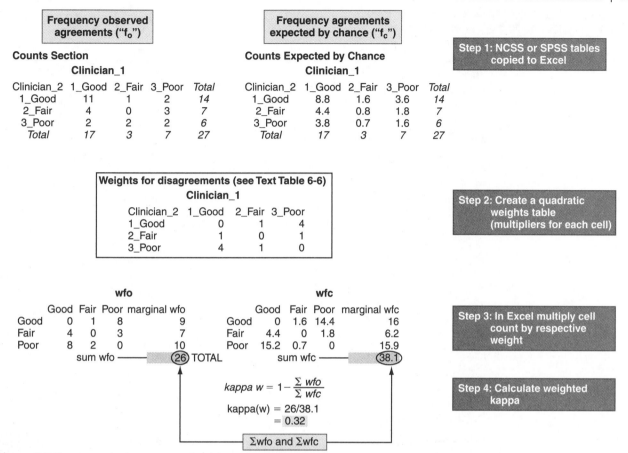

Figure 6-5 Steps in calculating a weighted kappa statistic using the quadratic method of weighting disagreements among raters. Σwfo and Σwfc are highlighted by arrows in step 3.

of scores. In previous chapters, the concept of standard deviation, standard error, and standard error of measure were described as different ways to measure variability (see eq. 4-1, eq. A4-2, and eq. A4-3). In the ANOVA summary table generated by statistical software, variability is measured by terms like "sum of squares" and "mean square" (**Table 6-7**). An illustration of how these terms reflect variability of scores is shown in **Figure 6-6**.

The term *sum of squares* indicates the sum of squared deviations of scores from the mean.[j] As can be seen in Figure 6-6, when sum of squares are averaged, this yields a "mean square." The term *mean square* is used in the formulas for ICC to create a measure of consensus. Since ANOVAs partition or separate variance for different sources (e.g., variance among patients versus variance among raters), each mean square term represents the variance for its respective source (Table 6-7). When the mean square

is small, there is low variability of scores from a mean (Fig. 6-6A). By contrast, when the mean square is larger, departure of scores from a mean is greater (Fig. 6-6B).

The partitions of variance in an ANOVA include

- Between Patient Variance (Patient Mean Square or PMS)
- Between Trial Variance (Trial Mean Square)
- Between Rater Variance (Rater Mean Square or RMS)
- Error Variance (the amount of score variation due to factors such as unskilled raters or ambiguous assessment tools; referred to as Error Mean Square or EMS. The EMS is also referred to as "unexplained variance" because error variability cannot be explained by other sources of variance.)

In order to facilitate an understanding of the derivation of each ICC, the appendix to this chapter reviews selected aspects of the ANOVA process. A review of the appendix is recommended before continuing with the demonstrations of ICC calculations.

---

[j]Or in some cases, variation of a group of means from the grand mean.

Table 6-7	Interpretation of ANOVA Summary Terms		
ANOVA Term	**Interpretation**	**Explanation**	**Example**
"Source"	Source of variance	The variance is partitioned or separated by specific sources in the analysis	• variance due to Patient • variance due to Rater • variance due to Trial • variance due to Error
"Df"	Degrees of freedom	Reflects number of observations, patients, raters, or trials	• Patient df = # patients – 1 • Rater df = # raters – 1 • Trial df = # trials – 1 • Interaction Patient × Trial = Patient df * Trial df • Total df = total number of observations
"SS" or "Sums of Squares"	Sum of squared deviations from the mean of a group or the "grand" (overall) mean	• SS among individual scores deviate from the group mean ("within group") • SS among groups are deviations of each group mean from the grand mean ("between group")	See Figure 6-6
"MS" or "Mean Squares"	Mean of the sum of squares (variance)	Mean square is the "variance" for a particular source in the ANOVA summary table	See Figure 6-6

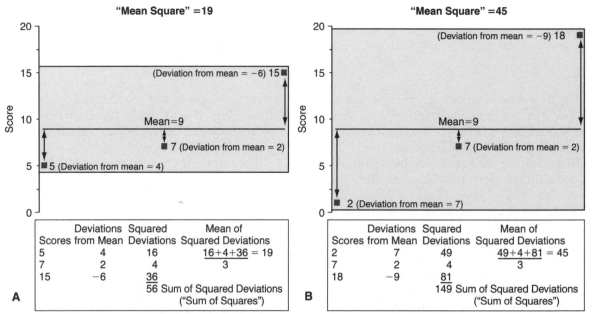

Figure 6-6 Conceptual illustration of sums of squares and mean squares. (A) Variations of scores from the mean yield a "mean square" term of 19. (B) With the same mean, larger variations of scores from the mean yield a larger mean square term of 45. The extent of variance in both panels is represented by the shaded rectangles. Note: variance = mean square. If the calculations presented in this figure were based on sample statistics, the variance calculation would use $N - 1$ in the denominator (in this case, 2 instead of 3).

Demonstration of ICC Calculation for *Intra* Rater Agreement

Intra rater agreement for continuous or rank-ordered data is calculated from a simple replication study where one clinician assesses a group of patients multiple times.[28] The RM-ANOVA is one-way (the single factor is "Trials" because multiple trials are collected for each patient). The factor "Patient" is always included in a RM-ANOVA because we are interested in how consistent these multiple ratings are for each patient. The classification of the RM-ANOVA remains a "one-way" or "one-factor" ANOVA because the "patient" factor is universal and is not included in the factor count. The number of levels in the "Patient" group for this ANOVA is equal to the number of patients.

The demonstration data set for calculation of $ICC_{intra\ rater}$ is illustrated in **Figure 6-7**. These data are hypothetical. Sixty-nine imaginary patients with gait deficits were evaluated 3 times (trials)

by a single imaginary clinician (Fig. 6-7A). The outcome measure is meters walked in 6 minutes (the variable column named "Walk_6min_m"). The design of the study has a focus on "Patients" and how patient ratings vary across trials (Fig. 6-7B).[k] The RM-ANOVA compares variance of walk distance between patients and within patients (across trials 1, 2, and 3). For the purpose of this demonstration, the imaginary patients were selected randomly.

ANOVA Summary Table for $ICC_{intra\ rater}$

The concept underlying the use of selected RM-ANOVA summary terms in the calculation of $ICC_{intra\ rater}$ facilitates an understanding of what is actually measured by the ICC statistic. For *intra* rater agreement, the numerator of the ICC is conceptually the difference among patient ratings with error removed (PMS – EMS). This represents the "true variance" of ratings on the 6-minute walk test across patients. The denominator is the "total variance" between ratings since this value combines the between patient effect (conceptually, how much the mean of each patient's scores varies from the mean of all patients) with the error term (conceptually, how much each patient's

[k]The "Trial" factor is ignored because the clinician is interested in the within and between patient variance, not the "within trial" variance per se. The number of trials, however, is used in the formula for this ICC to adjust the magnitude of the denominator of the ICC, and the trial × patient interaction is used to compute the error term.

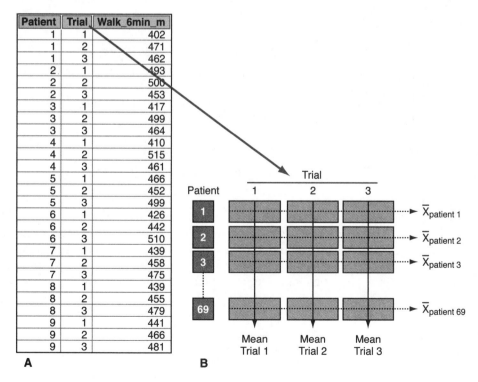

Patient	Trial	Walk_6min_m
1	1	402
1	2	471
1	3	462
2	1	493
2	2	500
2	3	453
3	1	417
3	2	499
3	3	464
4	1	410
4	2	515
4	3	461
5	1	466
5	2	452
5	3	499
6	1	426
6	2	442
6	3	510
7	1	439
7	2	458
7	3	475
8	1	439
8	2	455
8	3	479
9	1	441
9	2	466
9	3	481

A

B

Figure 6-7 (A) Hypothetical data set up to generate a one-way repeated measures ANOVA for calculation of $ICC_{intra\ rater}$. Twenty-seven of 207 rows are displayed here. The full data set is available on the bound-in disk (use "Ch6-ICC Intrarater" and choose the file with either the NCSS or SPSS extension). (B) Study design showing the format of each patient's performance across trials and the collapse of 6-minute walk distance across trials to yield a mean score for each patient.

scores vary from their own repeated trials plus all other variance).

The $ICC_{intra\ rater}$ represents *true variance* of 6-minute walk test scores among patients divided by *total variance* of walk test scores. The conceptual formula for all ICCs, including $ICC_{intra\ rater}$ is

$$ICC = \frac{\text{True Variance Among Patient's score}}{\text{Total Variance Among Scores}} \quad \textbf{eq 6-14}$$

For any patient, error ("within group"; or EMS) is the variability viewed across each row for each patient (Fig 6-7B; trial 1 vs. trial 2 vs. trial 3). This aspect of the consensus analysis (the error term) is essentially the interaction between patients × trials (the variance of each patient's score across each trial; see the appendix to this chapter for additional detail). The hope is that the measures for each patient across the trials are consistent, thereby producing a small error term (i.e., a small EMS).

When comparing across patients (e.g., patient 1 versus patient 2, etc.), the "between patient variability" (PMS) is viewed down the column of patient means; $X_{Patient1}$ through $X_{Patient69}$. If patients are rated with consistent values across their own trials, but ratings differ from the mean of all patients (larger between patient variability), the ICC will tend to be higher compared to situations where error variability is relatively large. The one-way RM-ANOVA summary table generated from the hypothetical data is illustrated in **Figure 6-8.**

The formula for $ICC_{intra\ rater}$ is[28]

$$\frac{ICC}{\text{intrarater}} = \frac{PMS - EMS}{PMS + (ko - 1) * EMS} = \frac{\text{True Variance}}{\text{True Variance}} \quad \textbf{eq 6-15}$$

where PMS = between patient mean square (between "group" mean square), EMS = within group mean square (read "Error" mean square or the interaction between patients and their scores on each trial; the "AB" term in NCSS or the "Residual" term in SPSS), and ko = number of replicate readings taken for any individual patient.

All of the terms for calculating $ICC_{intra\ rater}$ in this demonstration are derived from Figure 6-8. The calculation is shown below:

$$
\begin{aligned}
ICC\ intrarater &= \frac{PMS - EMS}{PMS + (ko - 1) * EMS} \\
&= \frac{3785 - 845}{3785 + (3 - 1) * 845} = 0.54
\end{aligned}
$$

The mean square terms from an ANOVA summary table are entered into a handheld calculator or Microsoft Excel to determine the ICC.[l] Refer to the bound-in disk for an ICC calculator created in Excel. The intra rater agreement is ICC = 0.54 on a scale of 0 to 1. Applying the descriptive scale used for kappa (Table 6-3), an ICC = 0.54 shows a "fair" level of agreement for a single rater evaluating patients across three trials.

Standard Error of Measure (SEM) and 95% CI for ICC

Equation 6-15 generates a point estimate for **intra** rater reliability. However, when evaluating the statistical significance of an ICC there are several methods of calculating confidence intervals[m] surrounding the point estimate.[28] One approach reviewed by Fleiss[28] uses a confidence interval that is established around an individual patient's score. This approach retains the original units of the outcome measure and relies on the standard error of measure (SEM).

$$SEM = SD\sqrt{1-r} \quad \textbf{eq 6-16} \text{ (similar to eq 4-1)}$$

or

$$SEM = \sqrt{EMS} \quad \textbf{eq 6-17}$$

where SD = standard deviation and r = the test-retest correlation coefficient (Chapter 4, eq. 4-1).

Alternatively, the square root of the mean square error term (EMS) from the ANOVA summary table may be used.

Calculation of SEM: Example

For $ICC_{intra\ rater\ fixed}$, a particular patient for this example scored 433 meters in a 6-minute walk test when averaged across three different trials (data from Fig. 6-7A):

Selected patient's score (averaged across 3 raters)
= 433 meters
EMS (from Fig. 6-8) = 845
$SEM = \sqrt{845} = 29$ meters

The SEM is one measure of accuracy. In this sense, the SEM can be used as a "proxy" for estimating the margin of error in much the same manner as the SEM was used as a proxy to estimate meaningful clinical change (see Chapter 4). For this demonstration,

---

[l]SPSS calculates various forms of the ICC. For this text, the presentation of ICCs is demonstrated by hand calculations derived from the appropriate ANOVA summary table.

[m]Some statistical software also calculates the SE of ICC so that symmetrical CIs can be created on a normal distribution. When this is the case, the CI for ICC is interpreted in the same way as the CI for kappa.

NCSS

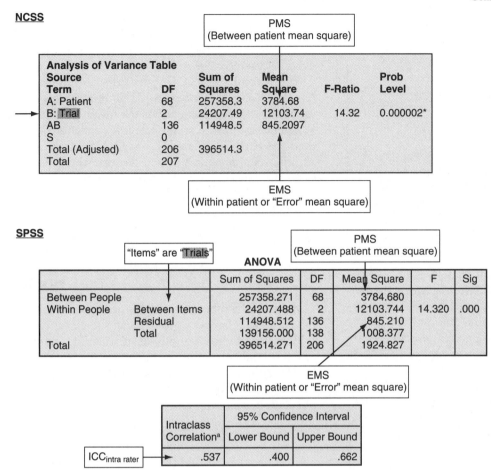

PMS
(Between patient mean square)

Analysis of Variance Table Source Term	DF	Sum of Squares	Mean Square	F-Ratio	Prob Level
A: Patient	68	257358.3	3784.68		
B: Trial	2	24207.49	12103.74	14.32	0.000002*
AB	136	114948.5	845.2097		
S	0				
Total (Adjusted)	206	396514.3			
Total	207				

EMS
(Within patient or "Error" mean square)

SPSS

"Items" are "Trials"

PMS
(Between patient mean square)

ANOVA

		Sum of Squares	DF	Mean Square	F	Sig
Between People		257358.271	68	3784.680		
Within People	Between Items	24207.488	2	12103.744	14.320	.000
	Residual	114948.512	136	845.210		
	Total	139156.000	138	1008.377		
Total		396514.271	206	1924.827		

EMS
(Within patient or "Error" mean square)

	Intraclass Correlation[a]	95% Confidence Interval	
		Lower Bound	Upper Bound
ICC$_{intra\ rater}$	.537	.400	.662

Figure 6-8 ANOVA summary table for a one-way RM-ANOVA to calculate ICC$_{intra\ rater}$ from a hypothetical data set. The outcome measure is meters walked in 6 minutes. Top panel is the NCSS output; the SPSS output appears below. Outputs are truncated to show the most relevant results.

repeated measures of 6-minute walk distance are estimated to be accurate to within ±29 meters. The 95% CI (a more comprehensive index of the margin of error), however, is preferred.

The confidence interval surrounding the patient's walk test score is [28]

$$95\%\ CI = Patient's\ Mean\ Score \pm 1.96 * (SEM) \div \sqrt{m}$$

eq 6-18

where SEM is the standard error of measurement, m = number of observations per patient contributing to the mean = $433 \pm 1.96 * (29)/\sqrt{3} = 33$,

Upper Confidence Limit = 433 + 33 = 466 meters, and Lower Confidence Limit = 433 − 33 = 400 meters.

This 95% confidence shows that for a patient with a score of 433 (averaged across three different trials assessed by a single rater), the true score will vary from 400 meters to 466 meters. As the 95% CI for the ICC becomes larger, the stability of the measure (and, hence, the agreement among raters) becomes worse. Refer to the Consensus Calculator on the bound-in disk for automatic calculation of the ICC once the ANOVA summary table is generated.

ICC for *Inter* rater Agreement

Inter rater agreement for continuous or rank-ordered data is calculated from a study designed to have two or more clinicians assess a group of patients multiple times.[28] The conceptual formula for ICCs (eq. 6-14) applies to each type of ICC$_{inter\ rater}$. The RM-ANOVA is used to generate the ANOVA summary table. The RM-ANOVA here is one-way (one factor, which is "Rater") and the ICC derived

Video Tutorial 6-3

Calculating ICC Int*ra* Rater Using Statistical Software

Application:
• Illustrates how to use statistical software and Excel to calculate the int*ra* rater ICC.

Demonstration Data:
• *Ch6-ICC intrarater.**SO*** (for NCSS)
• *Ch6-ICC intrarater.**Sav*** (for SPSS)

Continued

Steps:
1. Open the disk and navigate to this chapter.
2. Select Video Tutorial 6-3: Calculating Measures of Consensus: Intra rater ICC.
3. View how to run the analysis using NCSS and SPSS statistical software. Then view a completion of the ICC calculations using the Consensus Calculator in Excel.

Use of Software:
1. Verify that you have either NCSS or SPSS statistical software and Excel loaded on your computer.
2. Run the analysis illustrated in the video using the appropriate data set for the statistical software that you have installed.

from this RM-ANOVA is either $ICC_{inter rater fixed}$ or $ICC_{inter rater random}$. The distinction between the two types of inter rater ICCs depends solely on the method used to select the raters (randomly versus selected as a sample of convenience, as described earlier). *In both scenarios, it is assumed that patients were selected randomly.*

The primary concern for clinicians regarding random versus nonrandom selection of raters is an ICC that can be generalized. As a rule, if raters are selected randomly, then the coefficient can be generalized to a similar population of raters (e.g., therapists with at least 5 years of experience in geriatrics). In contrast, if raters are *not* selected randomly and represent a sample of convenience (e.g., the therapists working in a particular clinic), then the ICC results apply only to that group of raters.

The demonstration data set for calculation of $ICC_{inter rater fixed}$ and $ICC_{inter rater random}$ is illustrated in **Figure 6-9**. These data are hypothetical. Sixty-nine randomly selected imaginary patients were evaluated independently by three clinicians ("raters"). For the purpose of this demonstration, it is first assumed that the *raters* were chosen as a sample of convenience (fixed) to enable the calculation of $ICC_{inter rater fixed}$. Then it will be assumed that the clinicians were randomly selected from a larger group of clinicians for the calculation of $ICC_{inter rater random}$. The formulas for each type of inter rater ICC use the values in the ANOVA summary, but note that the formulas for each type of inter rater ICC differ slightly.[28] The outcome measure, again, is the distance walked in 6 minutes.

Demonstration of ICC Calculation for Inter rater Agreement: Raters "Fixed"

The one-way RM-ANOVA summary table is illustrated in **Figure 6-10**. By reviewing the DF in this table, the clinician knows that 69 patients (df patient

= 69 − 1 = 68) were assessed by three raters (df rater = 3 − 1 = 2), who made a total of 207 observations (total DF). This verifies that 69 patients were evaluated by 3 raters ($3 \times 69 = 207$).

The formulas for ICC inter rater introduce the "RMS" (Rater Mean Square). This term reflects the variability among raters versus the mean of all raters. When raters disagree on the scores for patients overall, then the RMS is inflated. Larger RMS values, with all other factors constant, will decrease the ICC because the denominator of the ICC equations (reflecting total error) will increase **(eq 6-14)**.

The formula for $ICC_{inter rater fixed}$ is[28]

$$ICC\ Interrater\ fixed\ = \frac{N(PMS - EMS)}{N * PMS + (k-1) * RMS + (N-1)(K-1) * EMS}$$

eq 6-19

where PMS = between group mean square for patients, RMS = between group mean square for raters, EMS = error (within) group mean square, k = number of raters, and N = number of patients.

All of the terms for calculating $ICC_{inter rater fixed}$ in this demonstration are derived from **Figure 6-10**. The calculation is shown below:

$$ICC\ Interrater\ fixed\ = \frac{N(PMS - EMS)}{(N * PMS) + ((k-1) * RMS) + ((N-1)(K-1) * EMS)}$$
$$= \frac{69(3920 - 146)}{69 * 3920 + ((3-1) * 862) + ((69-1)(3-1) * 146)}$$

Thus, the inter rater agreement (where the raters were not selected randomly) is 0.89 on a scale of 0 to 1. Descriptively, this level of agreement is "excellent." The evaluation of accuracy shows:

$$SEM = sqrt(EMS) = sqrt(146) = 12$$
(see eq. 6-17)
$$Selected\ Patient\ Score = 400\ m$$
$$95\%\ CI = 400\ m \pm 1.96 * 12/sqrt(3) = 13.6$$
(see eq. 6-18)

or

[386.4 m———(400m)———413.6 m]

Demonstration of ICC Calculation for Inter rater Agreement: Raters "Random"

The RM-ANOVA summary table when raters are randomly selected is the same as in Figure 6-10. The way that the RM-ANOVA summary values are used to calculate $ICC_{inter rater random}$, however, differs slightly from $ICC_{inter rater fixed}$.

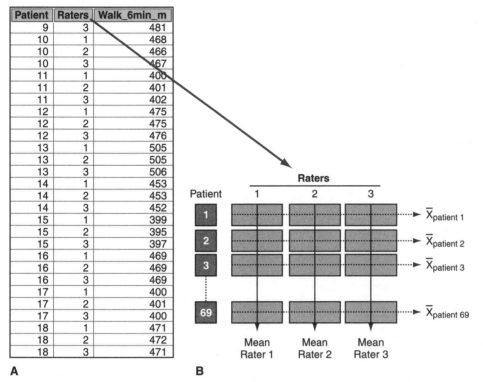

Patient	Raters	Walk_6min_m
9	3	481
10	1	468
10	2	466
10	3	467
11	1	400
11	2	401
11	3	402
12	1	475
12	2	475
12	3	476
13	1	505
13	2	505
13	3	506
14	1	453
14	2	453
14	3	452
15	1	399
15	2	395
15	3	397
16	1	469
16	2	469
16	3	469
17	1	400
17	2	401
17	3	400
18	1	471
18	2	472
18	3	471

A

B

Figure 6-9 (A) Hypothetical data, set up to generate a one-way repeated measures ANOVA for calculation of $ICC_{inter\ rater\ fixed}$ and $ICC_{inter\ rater\ random}$. Values in each cell represent meters walked during the 6-minute walk test. Column headings show that three raters measured each patient's performance. Twenty-eight of 207 rows are displayed here. The full data set is available on the bound-in disk. (Use "Ch6-ICC IntERrater" with either the NCSS or SPSS extension). (B) Study design showing the format of each patient's performance across raters and the collapse of 6-minute walk distance across raters to yield a mean score for each patient.

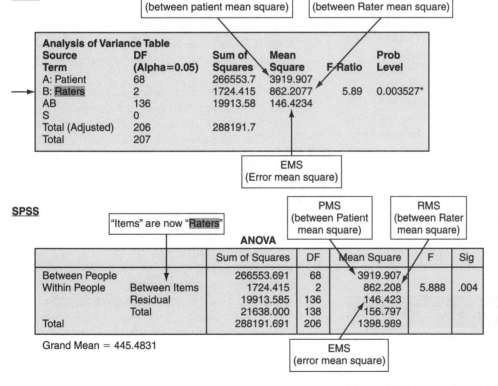

Figure 6-10 Fixed raters[s]: One-way repeated measures analysis of variance summary table to calculate $ICC_{inter\ rater\ fixed}$. The outcome measure is meters walked in 6 minutes. PMS, EMS, and RMS for both NCSS and SPSS statistical software programs have the same rounded values.

[s]Most statistical programs have a check box or variable box to indicate that raters were selected randomly. This maneuver may or may not alter the statistical output. In the demonstration, the output for fixed versus random raters does not change. Differences in the ICC for each type of ICC occur due to slight differences in the formulas for calculating fixed versus random in**er** rater ICCs. Refer to video tutorials for use of this feature in NCSS and SPSS.

The formula for $ICC_{inter\ rater\ random}$ is [28]

$$ICC\ interrater\ random = \frac{N(PMS - EMS)}{(N * PMS) + ((k) * RMS) + ((Nk - N - k) * EMS)}$$

eq 6-20

where PMS = between group mean square for Patients, RMS = between group mean square for Raters, EMS = Error (within) group mean square, k = number of raters, and N = number of patients.

All of the terms for calculating $ICC_{inter\ rater\ random}$ in this demonstration are derived from **Figure 6-10**. The calculation is shown below:

$$ICC\ interrater\ random = \frac{69(3920 - 146)}{69 * 3920 + ((3) * 862) + ((69)(3) - 69 - 3) * 146} = 0.89$$

Thus, the inter rater agreement (where the raters are selected randomly) is 0.89 on a scale of 0 to 1 (in this case the same as inter rater fixed). In descriptive terms, this level of agreement is "excellent." As the EMS is the same as that generated for $ICC_{inter\ rater\ fixed}$, both the SEM and 95% CIs are the same for both types of inter rater ICCs. This might not always be the case.

The concept underlying the use of these selected ANOVA summary terms in the calculation of $ICC_{inter\ rater\ fixed}$ and $ICC_{inter\ rater\ random}$ shows what is actually measured by this ICC statistic. For inter rater agreement, the numerator of the ICC is conceptually the variance among patient ratings recorded by each rater with error removed (PMS – EMS).[n] This represents the "true" variance of ratings on the 6-minute walk test for across the raters since the error term is removed from the patient ratings. The denominator combines the variance between patient scores, the variance among raters, and the error variance so that "total variance" of scores is represented.

[n]Note that the "Patient" effect in this case is essentially the average of walk scores from three raters. That fact makes this numerator appropriate for measuring inter rater agreement. By contrast the ICC intra rater numerator reflects replicate measures for each patient from the same source (a single clinician).

Video Tutorial 6-4

Calculating ICC Inter rater Using Statistical Software

Application:
- Illustrates how to use statistical software and Excel to calculate the inter rater ICC.

Demonstration Data:
- Ch6-ICC interrater.**S0** (for NCSS)
- Ch6-ICC interrater.**Sav** (for SPSS)

Steps:
1. Open the disk and navigate to this chapter.
2. Select Video Tutorial 6-4: Calculating Measures of Consensus: Inter rater ICC
3. The movie shows NCSS analysis followed by SPSS analysis. Then an Excel spreadsheet is shown to complete the ICC calculations (Consensus Calculator on the disk).

Use of Software:
1. Verify that you have either NCSS or SPSS statistical software and Excel loaded on your computer.
2. Run the analysis illustrated in the video using the appropriate data set for the statistical software that you have installed.

SUMMARY

- Agreement among clinicians or raters is a form of reliability that involves the measurement of consensus.
- Selecting the appropriate type of consensus measurement depends on the type of data being analyzed (Table 6-2):
  - Kappa statistics used with categorical data
  - Weighted kappa used with ordinal data where there is a clear and defensible rationale for assigning weights to the level of disagreement among raters
  - Intraclass correlation coefficient used with continuous data (or rank-ordered data where it is not clear how to weight disagreement among raters)
- In a 2×2 contingency table holding categorical data, there are a battery of tests that supplement the interpretation of kappa (Table 6-4).
  There are three varieties of intraclass correlation coefficients (ICCs):
  - Intra rater
  - Inter rater, where the raters are picked from a sample of convenience
  - Inter rater, where the raters are picked randomly from a larger sample of raters
- Kappas and ICCs vary from 0 (agreement no different from chance) to 1 (perfect agreement).
  The consensus measure, whether kappa, weighted kappa, or ICC is a "point estimate" of agreement (a single number representing the degree of consensus).
  Arbitrary descriptive scales provide categories for the amount of consensus provided by the point estimates (Table 6-3).
  Confidence intervals (CIs) surrounding point estimates of kappa or weighted kappa give an

illustration of the amount of variability of these consensus measures expected with repeated experiments.

CIs that include a predefined "poor" value of agreement (e.g., kappa = 0.40) indicate that the amount of agreement is not statistically meaningful.

- Confidence intervals surrounding the point estimates of the ICC are calculated with respect to the individual patient's score.

Larger confidence intervals for any consensus measure indicate poor stability of the measures compared to smaller confidence intervals.

Appendix to Chapter 6
Statistical Foundations for Measuring Consensus on Patient Assessment

Key Terms
- Analysis of Variance (ANOVA)
  - Between Group Variance
  - Within Group ("Error") Variance
  - Statistical Degrees of Freedom
  - Sum of Squares
  - Mean Square
  - F ratio
  - Main Effect
- Repeated Measures Analysis of Variance (RM-ANOVA)
  - Between Subjects Effect
  - Within Subjects Effect
- Type I Error

Introduction: Background on Analysis of Variance

What is analysis of variance (ANOVA)? The ANOVA is a family of statistical procedures that "partitions" or separates the sources of score variance. There are two primary applications for ANOVAs in the rehabilitation literature:

1. Creating an ANOVA summary table that holds partitioned measures of variance ("mean square" terms) that are used to calculate ICCs.
2. Evaluating the difference in means across two or more groups (e.g., Treatment versus Placebo).

ANOVAs for Calculating ICCs
When the purpose of implementing an RM-ANOVA is to calculate an ICC, the idea of hypothesis testing (evaluating the statistical difference among group, treatments, or sessions) is not relevant. Generating the RM-ANOVA summary table is the main interest for calculating ICCs because it holds the mean square values that reflect variance for patients, raters, trials, and the error term. The formulas for ICCs differ markedly from the formulas for F ratio (for example, compare the conceptual formula **equation 6-14** with **equation 6-21**). Therefore, the goal for generating an ANOVA summary table must be clearly established prior to implementing the analysis.

ANOVA for Evaluating Differences Among Groups
ANOVA evaluates the variability of scores (the dependent measure) to help clinicians distinguish variability that is due to a treatment effect versus variability that is due to measurement errors. The assumptions for these statistical procedures are that

- the scores for each group are normally distributed (conform to a bell-shaped curve)
- there is homogeneity of variance among groups (the scores form essentially the same-shaped bell in height and width), and
- for repeated measures designs (discussed later in this appendix), it is assumed that differences between measures on the same subject (e.g., trial 1 vs. trial 2, trial 1 vs. trial 3 and trial 2 vs. trial 3) will be relatively equal and correlated because the measures come from the same person.[30] This assumption is called the assumption of sphericity or circularity.

ANOVAs are generally considered robust tests, which means that assumptions can be violated while preserving the validity of results.[30] Portney and Watkins,[30] however, caution that with repeated measures designs, the assumption of circularity must be addressed because statistical significance can be reached easier when this assumption is violated. Statistical software programs typically correct for violations of this assumption automatically by making adjustments in the statistical degrees of freedom. These adjustments increase the threshold for reaching statistical significance, thereby compensating for lack of circularity in the data.[31,p.214]

ANOVA Example Using 6-Minute Walk Test
Deyle et al.[32] studied the effectiveness of different interventions to treat osteoarthritis of the knee. One outcome measure (dependent variable) in that study was distance walked in 6 minutes on level ground measured in meters.[33] The hypothesis was that an effective intervention would result in longer distances

walked for people in the treatment group vs. a control (placebo) group.

Using distance walked in 6 minutes as the outcome measure, the variability of these "distance scores" was measured from two different perspectives that partition their variance:

- Error (within group) variance
- Between group variance

What Is "Within Group" or "Error Variance"?

In order to optimize the possibility of finding a difference in outcome between treatment and control groups, researchers take steps to minimize measurement error. There are many potential sources of measurement error when performing the 6-minute walk test, including:

- inconsistencies when clinicians start and stop the measurement;
- different instructions to the patients (self-pace? comfortable speed? fastest speed?);
- encouragement to the patients during the test provided unequally;
- subjects tested at different times of day, allowing a differential effect of medications.

While this example addresses the 6-minute walk test, the concept of measurement error is inherent in any outcome measure. Analysis of variance identifies the variability of scores due to measurement error, in general, but does not identify the precise factors contributing to that error.

Synonyms for error variance produced in an ANOVA output are

- within group variance
- unexplained variance

Error variance is the spread of scores around respective group means. In this example, the placebo group has a spread of scores around the placebo mean and the treatment group has a spread of scores around the treatment mean. As the groups represent either the control or treatment condition, then variance of scores *within* these groups cannot be attributed to an intervention effect. In other words, all subjects in the treatment group received the treatment. If their scores vary from their treatment group mean, the reason for this deviation cannot be explained by the effects of the intervention. Similarly, all subjects in the control group received a placebo. If a person's score in the placebo group varies from the placebo group mean, then the reason for this deviation cannot be explained by the placebo intervention. Hence, within group variance is called unexplained variance or error variance. Larger error variance indicates more unexplained variance in the outcome scores compared to smaller error variance. In general, it is optimal to have small error variance. When error variance is low, it suggests that potential sources of error were well controlled.

What Is "Between Group" Variance?

Between group variance is the deviation of group means from the grand mean. The grand mean is the mean of all scores without regard to group designation. Larger between group variance indicates that the average scores from each group varied more from the grand mean compared to a scenario where there is smaller between group variance. It is optimal to have large between group variance because this index reflects the treatment effect. When between group variance is sufficiently large compared to error variance, there will be a significant difference in the outcome measure (e.g., meters walked in 6 minutes) among groups. The expression of variance is in the form of an F ratio:

$$F\ ratio = \frac{Between\ Group\ Variance}{Within\ Group\ Variance} \qquad \textbf{eq 6-21}$$

Interplay of Between and Within Group Variance

The interplay of between group variance and error variance can be visualized in **Figure 6-11**. In the scenario where 6-minute walk data were analyzed for 138 imaginary patients ($n = 69$ in each of two groups: Treatment versus Placebo), in the first case, the distance walked in 6 minutes has a large error variance (Fig. 6-11A) and the means of each group do not differ substantially from the grand mean. Thus, when a small between group difference is coupled with large error variance (Fig. 6-11, dot plot A), the ratio of between group to within group variance will be very small (i.e., a small F ratio) and the result is no significant treatment effect.

In scenario B, however, there is a larger between group and smaller within group variance (Fig. 6-11B). In this case, the ratio of between group to error variance is larger than in the previous scenario. Hence, the distinction among groups becomes more apparent as error variance decreases while between group variance increases (i.e., a larger F ratio). The result is that the group receiving treatment walked significantly further than the control group.

Analysis of variance produces a summary table that is similar among statistical software programs. The ANOVA summary table has the components illustrated in **Figure 6-12**. The table is generated from a "one-way" ANOVA, which means that there is only one independent variable or factor ("Group"). The

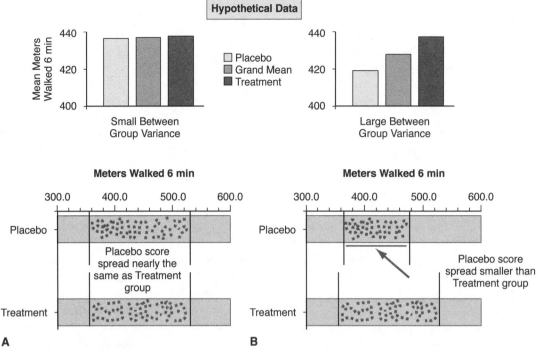

Figure 6-11 Hypothetical 6-minute-walk data analyzed under two different scenarios. (A) Small between-group variance. (B) Large between-group variance. Each dot in the dot plots represents a data point for one imaginary subject. Note that the within-group variance decreases overall primarily due to less variance within the placebo group (highlighted by the arrow).

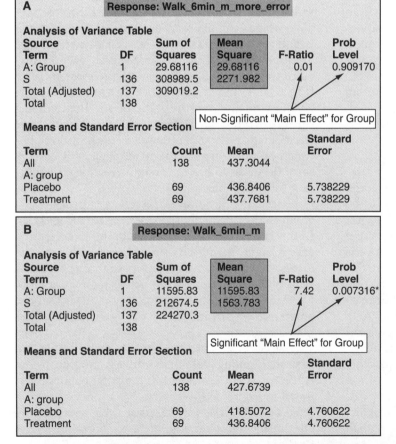

A

Response: Walk_6min_m_more_error

Analysis of Variance Table

Source Term	DF	Sum of Squares	Mean Square	F-Ratio	Prob Level
A: Group	1	29.68116	29.68116	0.01	0.909170
S	136	308989.5	2271.982		
Total (Adjusted)	137	309019.2			
Total	138				

Non-Significant "Main Effect" for Group

Means and Standard Error Section

Term	Count	Mean	Standard Error
All	138	437.3044	
A: group			
Placebo	69	436.8406	5.738229
Treatment	69	437.7681	5.738229

B

Response: Walk_6min_m

Analysis of Variance Table

Source Term	DF	Sum of Squares	Mean Square	F-Ratio	Prob Level
A: Group	1	11595.83	11595.83	7.42	0.007316*
S	136	212674.5	1563.783		
Total (Adjusted)	137	224270.3			
Total	138				

Significant "Main Effect" for Group

Means and Standard Error Section

Term	Count	Mean	Standard Error
All	138	427.6739	
A: group			
Placebo	69	418.5072	4.760622
Treatment	69	436.8406	4.760622

Figure 6-12 Example of a one-way ANOVA summary table generated from hypothetical 6-minute walk data with summary of mean walk distance in meters. Referring to the mean square terms, (A) summary of results with small between-group and larger within-group variances. (B) summary with large between-group and smaller within-group variances. "Response" in the heading of each panel refers to the dependent variable (in this case distance walked in 6 minutes). Output from NCSS.

"Group" factor in this example has two levels: Placebo and Treatment. There are 69 subjects in each group (number of observations = 138). The terms in the ANOVA summary table are defined as follows[o]:

- Source Term: the source of variance. A = between group variance, S = error variance. Note that if more than one factor is analyzed (for example, "Groups" followed from initial evaluation to discharge, then "Time" would be listed as "B: Time" under source and would hold two levels: initial and discharge evaluations. In addition, there would be an inter-action term "AB," which would show how group performance interacts or changes with time).
- Each source term that is not an error term is referred to as a "main effect." Thus, the *main effect* for "Group" in this example is statistically signifi-cant. It shows that the Placebo walk distance differs from the Treatment group walk distance. Inspection of the table of means indicates that the treatment group has longer (better) walking distance compared to Placebo (Fig. 6-12).[p]

  Degrees of freedom (DF). DF is a measure of the number of groups, subjects, or trials.

  DF for groups is $k - 1$, where k is the number of groups (hence, df = 2 – 1 = 1).

  DF for the error term is Observations – Group DF - 1, where Observations are the total number of measurements taken during the study.

  Total DF = number of subjects or observations.
- Sum of Squares: Sum of the squared deviations from either the grand mean or the individual group means (as occurs with the error term).
- Mean Square: Sum of squares divided by the respective DF.
- F ratio: Mean square between groups divided by Error MS (mean square within groups).

Figure 6-12A:

$$Group\ effect\ F\ ratio = \frac{Between\ Group\ Variance}{Within\ Group\ Variance}$$
$$= \frac{30}{2272} \cong 0.01,\ p > 0.05$$

Figure 6-12B:

$$Group\ effect\ F\ ratio = \frac{Between\ Group\ Variance}{Within\ Group\ Variance}$$
$$= \frac{11596}{1564} \cong 7.42,\ p < 0.05$$

[o]There may be slight differences among statistical software programs in reporting and labeling the ANOVA summary table.

[p]When an independent variable has more than two levels (e.g., placebo, treatment1, treatment2), then post-hoc testing is done to determine which pairwise comparisons within the factor are statistically different. Post-hoc testing is beyond the scope of this primer but additional in-formation on this topic can be found in Portney and Watkins.[34]

- Prob Level: The probability that the F ratio could occur simply by chance. Values less than 0.05 indicate a low chance probability and, therefore, results below this threshold are statistically signif-icant (indicated by the * in Fig. 6-12B) and likely due to the treatment intervention.
- By reviewing the DF in the ANOVA summary tables in Figure 6-12, the clinician knows that two different groups of patients were tested (df group + 1 = 2). Since 138 observations were made (df total = 138), then there must be 69 different patients per group (69 * 2 = 138).

Demonstration of One-Way Repeated Measures ANOVA

A repeated measures ANOVA ("RM-ANOVA") is a special type of ANOVA where *all* subjects are exposed to the treatments or clinicians assessing patient per-formance. In this type of ANOVA, the factor repre-senting "Patient" or "Subject" is always included. The analysis of the main effect for Patients or Subjects on the outcome measure of interest provides values for the calculation of the error term in the ANOVA, but the Patient main effect is not usually interpreted (it is assumed that patients differ from each other and the F ratio for the Patient main effect is ignored and is not considered a "factor" in the ANOVA).

Error terms in a RM-ANOVA are formed by an interaction of patients with each remaining factor in the analysis. Conceptually, the RM-ANOVA ac-counts for the fact that repeated measures on the same subjects are not independent data points. Thus, the error term in RM-ANOVA is typically smaller than in the basic ANOVA.[30] The maneuver of creating an error term based on repeated measures decreases the denominator of the F ratio (eq. 6-21) and results in a larger F statistic. Bigger F ratios have a better chance of reaching statistical significance.

In this demonstration, a hypothetical experiment involved 69 imaginary patients who were treated for gait disorders with yoga and then later received a walking program. The outcome measure (distance walked in 6 minutes) was evaluated after each treat-ment. The data for this hypothetical experiment and the design structure are shown in **Figure 6-13.**

The RM-ANOVA summary table from this demonstration is shown in **Figure 6-14.** By reviewing the DF, the clinician knows that 69 patients were tested (df Patient = 69 - 1 = 68), and a total of 138 observations (total DF) were made. There were two different treatments administered to this single group of patients (df Treatment = 2 – 1 = 1). This verifies that 69 patients were evaluated twice ($2 \times 69 = 138$). The significance of the Patient main effect is not rele-vant to the RM-ANOVA when the purpose of the

Patient	Treatment	Walk_6min_m
1	Yoga	402
1	Walking	471
2	Yoga	433
2	Walking	500
3	Yoga	417
3	Walking	499
4	Yoga	410
4	Walking	515
5	Yoga	466
5	Walking	452
6	Yoga	426
6	Walking	442
7	Yoga	439
7	Walking	458
8	Yoga	439

A

B

Figure 6-13 (A) Hypothetical data set up to generate a one-way repeated measures ANOVA using "Treatment" as the factor of interest. Fifteen of 138 rows are displayed here. The full data set is available on the bound-in disk (use "Ch6-Append_1-Way_RM-ANOVA" with either the NCSS or SPSS extension). Column headings show the labels of variables used in the analysis. (B) Study design showing "Treatment" main effect (differences among mean Yoga versus Walking treatments collapsed across patients). Note: the purpose of the RM-ANOVA in this case is to evaluate differences among treatments and uses the treatment main effect whereas the treatment effect is ignored when calculating ICC.

RM-ANOVA is to evaluate the difference between treatments (it is assumed that patients perform differently from each other).

The error term for a one-way RM-ANOVA is shown by the interaction between the "Patient" and "Treatment" factors (the "AB" term in Fig. 6-14). *In other words, the variance of each patient's score between trials.* The error term is the denominator of the F ratio that evaluates the treatment main effect.

$$Treatment\ F\ ratio = \frac{Between\ Group\ Variance}{Within\ Group\ Variance}$$
$$= \frac{11596}{1040} \cong 11.16,\ p < 0.05$$

In this case, the main effect for "Treatment" reached statistical significance (the F ratio occurs by chance in a null distribution less than 5% of the time). The report of means (**Fig. 6-14** bottom panel) shows that longer walk distance was achieved after the walking program compared to yoga (437 meters vs. 419 meters).

Understanding the Language of Repeated Measures (RM) ANOVA

The terms defining the components of ANOVA are different than the terms in a RM-ANOVA. In an ANOVA (without a repeated measure as a factor), the "between group" effect is any factor that compares separate groups of patients, such as the mean of patients in the treatment versus placebo groups. The "within group" effect compares patients' scores within a group, such as the spread of scores *within* the treatment and control groups.

For a RM-ANOVA, however, the terms "Between Subjects" and "Within Subjects" are used to determine differences between patients versus differences on a repeated measure, respectively. It is assumed that patients will differ from each other. The mean square

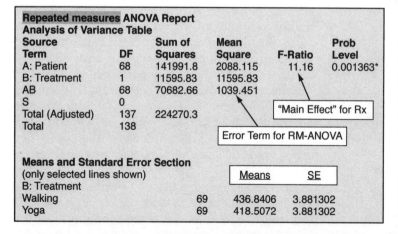

Repeated measures ANOVA Report					
Analysis of Variance Table					
Source Term	DF	Sum of Squares	Mean Square	F-Ratio	Prob Level
A: Patient	68	141991.8	2088.115	11.16	0.001363*
B: Treatment	1	11595.83	11595.83		
AB	68	70682.66	1039.451		
S	0				
Total (Adjusted)	137	224270.3			
Total	138				

"Main Effect" for Rx

Error Term for RM-ANOVA

Means and Standard Error Section			
(only selected lines shown)		Means	SE
B: Treatment			
Walking	69	436.8406	3.881302
Yoga	69	418.5072	3.881302

Figure 6-14 Example of a one-way repeated measures ANOVA summary table generated from hypothetical 6-minute walk data with summary of means (distance walked in 6 minutes in meters). Note that the error term under "Source" is "AB" (the interaction of Patient and Treatment factors. Although "Patient" is listed as a factor, it simply indicates subjects for calculation of the error term for the treatment main effect. The difference among patients, per se, is not the focus of the analysis and it is expected that patients will differ from each other on the outcome assessment. The mean square of this interaction is the denominator of the F ratio. Abbreviation: Rx = Treatment, SE = standard error of the mean.

Video Tutorial 6-5

Repeated Measures ANOVA for Evaluating Differences Between Two Treatments Using Statistical Software

Application:
• Illustrates how to use statistical software to produce a repeated measures ANOVA for evaluating the difference in walk distance scores between Yoga versus Walking treatments.

Demonstration Data:
• *Ch6-Append_1-Way_RM-ANOVA.**SO*** (for NCSS)
• *Ch6-Append_1-Way_RM-ANOVA.**Sav*** (for SPSS)

Steps:
1. Open the disk and navigate to this chapter.
2. Select Video Tutorial 6-5: Repeated Measures ANOVA Review.
3. View how to run the analysis using NCSS and SPSS statistical software.

Use of Software:
1. Verify that you have either NCSS or SPSS statistical software loaded on your computer.
2. Run the analysis illustrated in the video using the appropriate data set for the statistical software that you have installed.

---

for the Patient effect (patient mean square, or PMS), is generated in the RM-ANOVA summary table and is used in the calculation of reliability coefficients such as $ICC_{inter\ rater}$.

The clinician's attention is usually focused on the "Within Subjects" effect in a one-way RM-ANOVA. This effect describes the repeated measure. In other words, the factor that is repeated for all subjects in the study is the "Within Subjects" factor. For Figure 6-14, two forms of treatment (yoga and walking) were given to *all* patients. Therefore, "Treatment" is the "Within Subjects" factor. The F ratio that tests the significance of difference among treatment groups is based on a similar ratio format described for an ANOVA without repeated measures (that is, the variance in means between "groups" divided by the variance of scores within "groups"). *Groups in this case are the levels of the repeated measure: the treatment of yoga versus walking.*

$$\begin{aligned} \text{F ratio for Within} \\ \text{Subjects Effect} \end{aligned} = \frac{\text{Between "Group" Variance}}{\text{Within "Group" Variance}}$$

$$= \frac{\begin{aligned}\text{Variance of walk distance}\\\text{between Means of repeated}\\\text{Treatments}\end{aligned}}{\begin{aligned}\text{Variance walk distance}\\\text{within each treatment type}\end{aligned}}$$

The F ratio for the "Within Subjects" effect (read "Repeated Measure Effect" or "Treatment Effect") is statistically significant ($F_{1,68} = 11.16$, $p < 0.05$) and reveals that walk distance following the walking treatment is greater than following the yoga treatment (mean distance walked 437 vs. 419 m, respectively, Fig. 6-14).

Statistical Significance of Main Effects

In one-way ANOVAs (see Fig. 6-12) or one-way RM-ANOVAs (Fig. 6-14), the numerator and denominator of the F ratio each have statistical degrees of freedom. The notation of the F ratio usually includes the df for each part of the ratio. For example, in Figure 6-14, the F ratio calculated for the Treatment main effect with 1 df for treatment groups and 68 df for the repeated measures error term is:

$$F_{1,68} = 11.16$$

Statistical tables hold the values of F ratios (as well as other statistics) as if they were derived from a null distribution (see Chapter 13, "Statistical Tables—Critical Values F, $\alpha = 0.05$"). A null distribution of statistical values reflects statistics from a null result (no difference). This means, for example, that in a scenario where there is no Treatment effect (e.g., Yoga versus Walking interventions do not produce different walk distances), the statistical table will show the "critical" F ratio (for a given df pair) that occurs 5% of the time in a null distribution.[q]

Critical $F_{1,68} = 4.00$ (approximated from Fig. 6-15)

Statistical software programs automatically compare calculated statistics to critical values. However, the process used to select critical values for the F ratio in this example is illustrated in **Figure 6-15** to enhance the understanding of this procedure.

The 5% "critical point" in a null distribution is the point at which statisticians assign statistical significance. This critical point is called the alpha level (α). As F ratios increase, treatment effect increases and the probability of finding large F ratios in a null distribution decreases. Since the calculated F ratio is larger than the critical F ratio at $\alpha = 0.05$, then the calculated F ratio is statistically significant. In other words, the difference between yoga and walking treatments observed in the example (see Fig. 6-14) could have occurred by chance less than 5% of the time. This is true because statistical tables showing the distribution of F ratios in a null distribution (where there is no difference between groups) indicates that the *calculated F ratio* exceeds the *critical F ratio* in the table (Fig. 6-15). It

---

[q]Various statistical tables also hold critical values at other alpha levels in the null distributions (e.g., p = 0.01, or 1%).

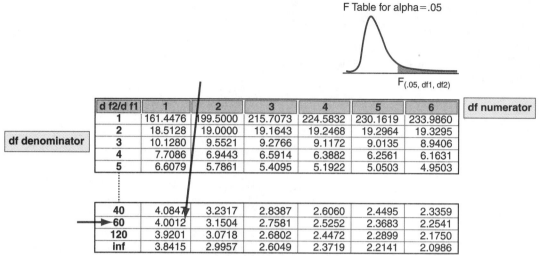

Figure 6-15 Excerpt from a statistical table showing the critical values of the F ratio at $\alpha = 0.05$. The approximate critical F ratio with df 1,68 is identified by the arrows. The full table appears in Chapter 13, "Statistical Tables." (Reprinted with permission from StatSoft, Inc. Electronic Statistics Textbook. StatSoft: Tulsa, OK, 2007. http://www.statsoft.com/textbook/stathome.html).

can be concluded that the difference between groups is likely to be caused by the intervention because in the null distribution, the observed difference (reflected in the F ratio) occurs rarely.

There is always the possibility that the determination of significant difference is incorrect. The probability of being incorrect is called Type I error, and in this example Type I error is 5%. This means that the determination of statistical significance carries a 5% error rate. Statisticians accept this error rate as reasonable when conducting research to establish a treatment effect. Many statistical programs provide the exact Type I error rate, and this value is the p value, or α.

$$\text{Type I Error} = p = \alpha \qquad \textbf{eq A6-22}$$

For example, in Figure 6-14, the Type I error for $F_{1,68} = 11.16$ is $p = 0.001$ (or less than 1%).

SUMMARY ON ANOVA BACKGROUND

- ANOVA is a procedure that partitions variance into between group (variance due to treatment) and within group (variance due to error).
- Repeated-measures ANOVA (RM-ANOVA) is a special case of ANOVA where the error term is influenced by the number of subjects (the "subject" or "patient" main effect).

- One-way ANOVA or one-way RM-ANOVA refers to a single independent variable under analysis (e.g., Group).
- The independent variable may have multiple levels (e.g., "Group" has two levels where there is Placebo versus Treatment "Group").
- For a given df, larger F ratios are less likely to occur in a null distribution than smaller F ratios.
- Assumptions underlying ANOVAs are commonly violated, but statistical software typically corrects for these violations.
- Information in the ANOVA summary tables is applied in different ways depending on the purpose of the study (consensus analysis versus testing significance of difference among groups or sessions).

The presentation of ANOVA in this appendix was focused on the contrast between the use of ANOVA for ICC versus ANOVA to evaluate differences among groups. When evaluating differences among groups or variables, ANOVAs can have multiple factors, each with multiple levels. For a broader discussion on this aspect of ANOVAs, the reader is referred to reference texts on statistical methodology.[34, 35]

PRACTICE

1. Two clinicians decided to test their level of consensus on measuring the severity of osteoarthritis from radiographic images of 35 patients with knee symptoms. The levels of severity were ranked "minimal," "moderate," and "severe." The contingency table is

		Clinician 1			
		Minimal	Moderate	Severe	Totals
Clinician 2	Minimal	10	3	2	15
	Moderate	5	5	1	11
	Severe	3	1	5	9
	Totals	18	9	8	35

   a. What is the proportion of observed agreements?
   b. What is the value of the statistic reflecting chance corrected agreement?
   c. What is the descriptive magnitude of kappa?

2. If the clinicians in question 1 decided to give credit for near misses (in other words, calculate a weighted kappa) using a quadratic weighting scheme, what would be the weighting constants for each cell below (assume minimal versus moderate and moderate versus severe ratings are penalized 1 point, whereas minimal versus severe ratings are penalized 2 points)?

		Clinician 1		
		Minimal	Moderate	Severe
Clinician 2	Minimal			
	Moderate			
	Severe			

3. a. What is the weighted kappa given the weighting constants in question 2?
   b. What is the descriptive magnitude of the weighted kappa?

4. Clinical experience indicated that there was little functional difference in patients who had radiographic ratings between "minimal" and "moderate" levels of involvement, so the clinicians decided to collapse the data into a 2×2 contingency table.
   a. What would the counts be in this new, smaller table?
   b. What is the new kappa and Po?
   c. What accounts for the discrepancy between kappa and Po?
   d. If kappa = 0.40 was the threshold for poor consensus, does the new kappa sufficiently exceed this threshold value?

5. A new scale to measure abnormal muscle tone was tested in a clinic. The grades for the scale were: slight increase in tone = 3, considerable increase in muscle tone = 2, and rigid limb = 1. A consensus measure was needed to determine if two practitioners would agree on patient evaluations. An ICC was preferred over a weighted kappa because the clinicians wanted to avoid implementing an arbitrary weighting scheme. The data for this practice question are on the bound-in disk for this chapter (**"Ch6-Practice ICC"** with either the NCSS or SPSS extension).
   a. What is the ICC reflecting the level of consensus between two clinicians not randomly selected (int**er** rater) who assessed tone on 27 randomly selected patients?
   b. Descriptively, what is the strength of this ICC?
   c. Given a patient's score of "2" on the muscle tone scale, what is the range of scores where the true value could be found within 95% of the time (with multiple theoretical replications of the study)?

REFERENCES

1. VanSwearingen JM, Brach JS. Validation of a treatment-based classification system for individuals with facial neuromotor disorders. Phy Ther 1998; 78: 678–689.
2. Currier LL, Froehlich PJ, Carow SD, et al. Development of a clinical prediction rule to identify patients with knee pain and clinical evidence of knee osteoarthritis who demonstrate a favorable short-term response to hip mobilization. Phys Ther 2007; 87:1106–1119.
3. Scheets PL, Sahrmann SA, Norton BJ. Use of movement system diagnoses in the management of patients with neuromuscular conditions: a multiple-patient case report. Phys Ther 2007; 87:654–669.
4. Wainner RS, Fritz JM, Irrgang JJ, et al. Development of a clinical prediction rule for the diagnosis of carpal tunnel syndrome. Arch Phys Med Rehabil 2005; 86:609–618.
5. Childs JD, Fritz JM, Flynn TW, et al. A clinical prediction rule to identify patients with low back pain most likely to benefit from spinal manipulation: a validation study. Ann Intern Med 2004; 141: 920–928.
6. Fritz JM, Delitto A, Erhard RE. Comparison of classification-based physical therapy with therapy based on clinical practice guidelines for patients with acute low back pain: a randomized clinical trial. Spine 2003; 28:1363–1372.
7. Ottenbacher K, Tomchek SD. Measurement in rehabilitation research: consistency versus consensus. Phys Med Rehabil Clin N Am 1993; 4:463–474.
8. Tooth LR, Ottenbacher KJ. The k statistic in rehabilitation research: an examination. Arch Phys Med Rehabil 2004; 85:1371–1376.
9. Sander AM, Seel RT, Kreutzer JS, et al. Agreement between persons with traumatic brain injury and their relatives regarding psychosocial outcome using the Community Integration Questionnaire. Arch Phys Med Rehabil 1997; 78:353–357.
10. Verheyden G, Nuyens G, Nieuwboer A, et al. Reliability and validity of trunk assessment for people with multiple sclerosis. Phys Ther 2006; 86:66–76.
11. Akinwuntan AE, De Weerdt W, Feys H, et al. The validity of a road test after stroke. Arch Phys Med Rehabil 2005; 86:421–426.
12. Razmjou H, Kramer JF, Yamada R. Intertester reliability of the McKenzie evaluation in assessing patients with mechanical low-back pain. J Orthop Sports Phys Ther 2000; 30:368–389.
13. Guggenmoos-Holzmnn I. The Meaning of kappa: probabilistic concepts of reliability and validity revisited. J Clin Epidemiol 1996; 49:775–782.
14. Sim J, Wright CC. The kappa statistic in reliability studies: use, interpretation, and sample size requirements. Phys Ther 2005; 85:257–268.
15. Watkins MW, Pacheco M. Interobserver agreement in behavioral research: importance and calculation. J Behav Educ 2000; 10:205–212.
16. Thompson WD, Walter SD. A reappraisal of the kappa coefficient. J Clin Epidemiol 1988; 41:949–958.
17. Cohen J. A coefficient of agreement for nominal scales. Educ Psychol Meas 1960; 20:37–46.
18. Landis JR, Koch GG. The measurement of observer agreement for categorical data. Biometrics 1977; 33:159–174.
19. Feinstein AR, Cicchetti DV. High agreement but low kappa, I. The problems of 2 paradoxes. J Clin Epidemiol 1990; 43:543–549.
20. Cicchetti DV, Feinstein AR. High agreement but low kappa II. Resolving the paradoxes. J Clin Epidemiol 1990; 43:551–558.
21. Riddle DL, Freburger JK. North American Orthopaedic Rehabilitation Research Network. Evaluation of the presence of sacroiliac joint region dysfunction using a combination of tests: a multicenter intertester reliability study. Phys Ther 2002; 82:772–781.
22. Verheyden G, Nieuwboer A, Mertin J, et al. The Trunk Impairment Scale: a new tool to measure motor impairment of the trunk after stroke. Clin Rehab 2004; 18:326–334.
23. Fleiss JL, Cohen J, Everitt BS. Large sample standard errors of kappa and weighted kappa. Psychol Bull, 1969; 72:323–327.
24. Hanley JA. Standard error of the kappa statistic. Psychol Bull 1987; 102:315–321.
25. Cohen J. Weighted kappa: nominal scale agreement with provision for scaled disagreement or partial credit. Psychol Bull 1968; 70:213–220.
26. Kraemer HC, Periyakoil VS, Noda A. Tutorial in biostatistics: Kappa coeffcients in medical research. Statistics in Medicine 2002; 21:2109–2129.
27. Soeken KL, Prescott PA. Issues in the use of kappa to estimate reliability. Med Care 1986; 24:733–741.
28. Fleiss JL. The Design and Analysis of Clinical Experiments. New York: Wiley, 1986.
29. Rae G. The equivalence of multiple rater kappa statistics and intraclass correlation coefficients. Educ Psychol Meas 1988; 48:367–374.
30. Portney LG, Watkins MP. Foundations of Clinical Research: Applications to Practice. Princeton: Prentice-Hall, 2000.
31. Hinze J. NCSS Help System. Kaysville, UT: NCSS, 2007.
32. Deyle GD, Henderson NE, Matekel RL, et al. Effectiveness of manual physical therapy and exercise in osteoarthritis of the knee: a randomized, controlled trial. Ann Intern Med 2000; 132:173–181.
33. Guyatt GH, Sullivan MJ, Thompson PJ, et al. The 6-minute walk: a new measure of exercise capacity in patients with chronic heart failure. Can Med Assoc J 1985; 132:919–923.
34. Portney LG, Watkins MP. Foundations of Clinical Research: Applications to Practice. Upper Saddle River, NJ: Prentice-Hall, 2009.
35. StatSoft Inc. Electronic Statistics Textbook. Tulsa, OK: StatSoft, 2007. http://www.statsoft.com/textbook/.

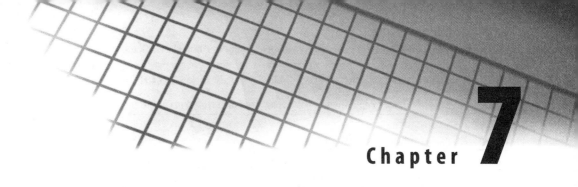

Chapter 7

Associations Among Clinical Variables

Clinical Question
• Is there an association among clinical variables (i.e., duration or type of treatment and outcome)?

Introduction

A leader of a rehabilitation team working in a hypothetical clinical setting sought to determine if a positive alliance between therapist and patient produced better therapeutic outcomes compared to situations where the patient and therapist did not have a good working relationship. Before initiating an in-clinic training program to address patient adherence to rehabilitation programs, she found a published review of literature reporting that strong patient-therapist alliances were associated with a pattern of positive outcomes, including treatment adherence, treatment satisfaction, and physical function.[1] Many of the research studies discussed in that review used some type of correlation coefficient to establish the extent of association between the strength of patient-therapist relationships and clinical outcomes. An understanding of correlation coefficients is necessary to critically review the literature and to serve as a basis for developing new patient adherence strategies.

The relationship between two variables, such as patient-therapist alliance and treatment adherence, are measured using correlation coefficients. Determining the extent of association between these and many other clinical variables serves several purposes:

• Measuring relationships that potentially guide clinical care;
• Providing a way to measure reliability (consistency of clinical measures across time);
• Providing a measure of criterion-related validity;
• Measuring the internal consistency of a clinical assessment tool.

Several additional examples of clinical literature using different types of correlation coefficients are summarized in **Table 7-1**.

Selecting the Appropriate Correlation Coefficient

The type of correlation coefficient that is selected to describe the extent of association depends upon the level of data being collected (review Chapter 6, Table 6-3) and the shape of the distribution of scores. Because two variables are involved in any "bivariate" correlation, there are many permutations related to the level of data each variable represents. For example, one variable may be continuous and not normally distributed while the second variable may be rank-ordered. Or, the first variable could be categorical while the second outcome is a normally distributed continuous variable. There are correlation coefficients that can accommodate many of these permutations.[6] However, for the purpose of this primer, the most commonly used correlation coefficients and the rules addressing their use are shown in **Table 7-2**.

General Principles Applied to Interpreting Correlation Coefficients

For all of the correlation coefficients outlined in Table 7-2, the magnitude of the coefficient indicates the strength of the association. The strength of

Table 7-1	Selected Examples of the Use of Correlations in Rehabilitation Research		
Authors	**Target Population**	**Type of Correlation Coefficient**	**Purpose of Measuring Association**
Lewis et al.[2]	Patients receiving home health services	Chi square	Association of selected patient characteristics with fall history
Sezer et al.[3]	Stroke	Spearman rank	Establish criterion-related validity of a hand function assessment
Vasconcelos et al.[4]	Post poliomyelitis syndrome	Pearson product moment	Association between scores on different clinical assessments of fatigue
Jensen et al.[5]	Neuromuscular disease and chronic pain	Cronbach's alpha	Determine internal consistency of FIM self-report assessment

Table 7-2	Commonly Used Correlation Coefficients and Rules for Their Use		
Rules for Use			
Correlation Coefficient	**Level of Data**	**Required Shape of the Distribution of Scores**	**Range**
Chi square[i] (χ^2 and r_{CV})	Association between two categorical variables[j]	Not applicable	−1 to +1
Spearman rank (r_s)	Association between: • two ordinal variables • one ordinal and one continuous variable • two non-normally distributed continuous variables	Not applicable	−1 to +1
Pearson product moment (r)	Association between two continuous and normally distributed variables	Normal distribution	−1 to +1
Cronbach's alpha	Association between scores on split-halves of a single clinical assessment tool of continuous, rank, or categorical data	Not applicable	0 to 1

[i]Conversion of χ^2 to a correlation coefficient is done using Cramer's V coefficient (r_{CV}). When the contingency table is 2×2, the correlation coefficient derived from χ^2 is called phi (φ).

[j]In some cases, rank-ordered data are used as categories that hold patient counts; for example, pain level is minimal, moderate, or severe. The cells in the contingency table, however, hold categorical data.

association does not imply cause and effect. With the exception of Cronbach's alpha, the correlation coefficients listed in Table 7-2 share several characteristics:

- The *descriptive significance* of the magnitude of the absolute value of the coefficient is judged arbitrarily. For the purpose of this primer, a "quarter system" is used:[a]

  | 0.75 to 1.00 | = Strong
  | 0.50 to 0.74 | = Moderate
  | 0.25 to 0.49 | = Weak
  | 0.00 to 0.24 | = Little to none

[a]Descriptive significance should include both direction and magnitude (e.g., "strong direct association," or "weak inverse association").

The sign of the coefficient indicates either a direct (+) or inverse (−) relationship (**Fig. 7-1**).

- *Statistical significance* is judged on a null hypothesis that the correlation coefficient equals 0 (H_0: $r = 0$). The alternative hypothesis is H_a: $r \neq 0$.

  If the coefficient has a probability of occurring in the null distribution of coefficients less than 5% ($p < 0.05$), then the correlation is judged to be statistically different from 0—in other words, "statistically significant."

  The critical values for determining statistical significance are found in Appendix B, Tables B-5 and B-6. Statistical software automatically calculates statistical significance in a process that is transparent to the user. Note that statistically significant correlation coefficients (those that differ from 0) do not necessarily indicate a strong relationship.

- The *percent of shared variance* is the coefficient squared and is called the coefficient of determination (eq. 7-1). Percent shared variance can range from 0% to 100%, with larger values indicating greater shared variance among the correlated variables. As the coefficient of determination increases:

    The "explained variance" increases (the variance of scores attributed or "explained" by the interaction of the two variables in the correlation).

    The unexplained variance decreases (variance due to other sources such as measurement error).

Coefficient of Determination = (Correlation Coefficient)²   **eq 7-1**

In conceptual terms, if the percent of shared variance is 40%, this means that 40% of the time as one variable changes, the other variable changes in a predictable manner (either in the same direction for positive correlations or in the opposite direction for negative correlations). This also means that 60% of the time as one variable changes the other variable changes in a **nonpredictable manner** (hence, "unexplained variance").

Interpretation of Correlation Coefficients: Overview

The correlation of hypothetical disability scores from initial evaluation to discharge in this example shows a Spearman rank coefficient (described in detail later) of $r_s = 0.45$ (Fig. 7-1A). According to the descriptive categories, a correlation of this sign and magnitude is "direct" and "weak," respectively. The coefficient of determination indicates that there is 20% shared variance (conceptually, as the initial disability scores increase, then the follow-up scores increase 20% of the time). This correlation coefficient is significantly different from 0 (so H_0: $r_s = 0$ is rejected) even though it is described as "weak."

The paradox between the statistical significance of a correlation coefficient and the descriptive magnitude is common.[7] This discrepancy occurs because the test of statistical significance is based on a low standard (r different from 0). Thus, many correlation coefficients will be significantly different from 0 without sufficient magnitude to explain the variance of scores. In order to provide a comprehensive

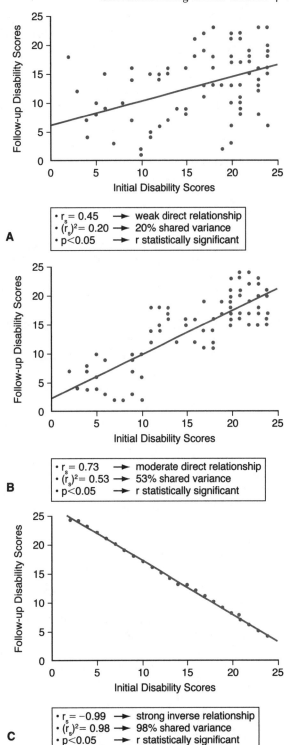

Figure 7-1 Bivariate scatter plots of hypothetical data demonstrating the three indices describing the association among two variables. For each panel, the first bullet is descriptive significance, the second bullet is the coefficient of determination, and the third bullet is statistical significance. Note that the correlation coefficients in all three panels are statistically different from $r_s = 0$. The least squares regression line (line of best fit) illustrates the direction of correlation; direct (+) vs. inverse (−).

assessment of correlation coefficients, it is recommended that researchers and clinicians report three indices of association (see Fig. 7-1):

1. Descriptive magnitude and sign
2. Coefficient of determination (r^2)
3. Results of hypothesis test (H_0: $r = 0$ vs. H_a: $r \neq 0$)

Chi Square (χ^2): Categorical Data

The chi square test of association (χ^2) answers the research question "Is there an association between categorical variables?" For example, Lewis et al.[2] examined the relationship between fall incidence and the type of medications used by clients receiving home care. A data set derived from their report is illustrated in **Figure 7-2**.

The primary requirement for using χ^2 is that the data entered into the contingency table are independent (e.g., not collected from repeated testing of the same patients).[8] The data in Lewis et al.[2] meet that criterion. Chi square is calculated by statistical software using the general formula[8]

$$\chi^2 = \sum \frac{(fo - fe)^2}{fe}$$ **eq 7-2**

where fo is the observed frequency for each cell[b], fe is the frequency expected by chance in each cell, and Σ is the sum from all of the cells in the contingency table.

The calculation of frequency counts expected by chance was described earlier for measuring consensus (refer to kappa, Chapter 6). In that case, only the cells on the agreement diagonal were of interest. Here, all cells in the contingency table contribute to the calculation of chi square. In order to view the background calculation of chi square in this example, a calculator developed using an Excel spreadsheet is provided on the bound-in disk. The output from the calculator is shown in **Figure 7-3**.

Yates Correction for Chi Square

Low sample size might lead to low expected frequencies. If the expected frequency in any cell is less than 1 and more than 20% of the cells have expected frequencies less than 5, then a Yates correction can be used to adjust (reduce) the size of chi square (Cochran,[9] cited by Portney and Watkins[10]). This adjustment is a conservative statistical procedure that

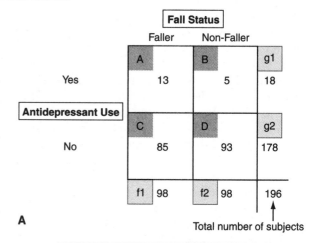

A

B

Figure 7-2 (A) Contingency table derived from Lewis et al.[2] (their Table 5) illustrating the medication status of patients classified as fallers vs. nonfallers; f1 and 2 = column totals, g1 and 2 = row totals. (B) Data set derived from the contingency table. Twenty-five of 196 rows of data are shown. The complete data set is available on the bound-in disk (open "Ch7_Chi_Square" with either the NCSS or SPSS extension). (Adapted from Lewis CL, Moutoux M, Slaughter M, Bailey SP. Characteristics of individuals who fell while receiving home health services. Phys Ther 2004; 84:23–32 with permission of the American Physical Therapy Association. This material is copyrighted and any further reproduction or distribution requires written permission from APTA.)

makes it more difficult to achieve statistical significance. The Yates correction subtracts 0.5 from the value of O - E before squaring. In Figure 7-3, both the Yates corrected chi square and the adjusted Cramer's V based on the Yates correction are illustrated in the result box

---

[b]Frequencies observed and expected by chance are defined with demonstrated calculations in Chapter 6.

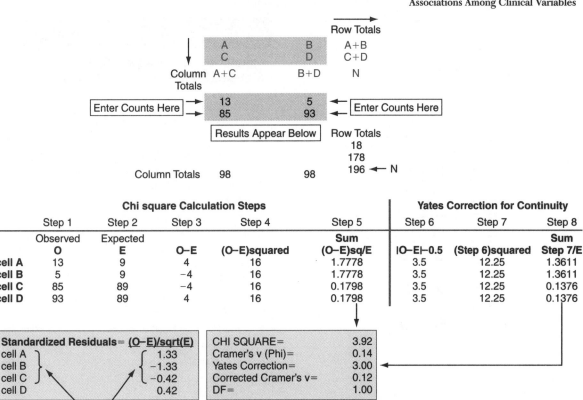

Figure 7-3 Steps for calculating χ^2 and Yates corrected χ^2 from a 2×2 table (shown in an Excel spreadsheet). O = observed frequencies, E = frequencies expected by chance, SQ = squared, sqrt = square root. The calculator is available on the bound-in disk ("P_Chi sq calculator").

at the bottom of the figure. While both types of chi square are shown, the practitioner must apply the Yates rule to determine if the Yates corrected chi square should be used instead of the unadjusted chi square.

Determining Statistical Significance of Chi Square

When association between two categorical variables is evaluated by chi square, statistical significance is influenced by the size of the contingency table. The critical chi square (e.g., the threshold for statistical significance) is determined by degrees of freedom (df). Larger contingency tables yield larger df. A simple drawing rule can be used to determine df for contingency tables of any size (refer to **Fig. 7-4** for selected examples). Drawing a line around *half of the perimeter* will leave some cells untouched. A count of those untouched cells is the df for that contingency table.

Once df are known, enter Table B-3 (Appendix B) to identify the critical chi square. In this demonstration (see Fig. 7-3), the table is 2×2 with df = 1. The critical chi square in Table B-3 is found at the intersection of the row with 1 df and the column with α (labeled "area" in the table) = 0.05. The critical value for the demonstration in Figure 7-3 is $\chi^2_{critical} = 3.84$. Since there is no cell with an expected frequency <1, Yates correction does not apply. Thus, the calculated χ^2 (3.92) is ≥ the critical value (3.84), and there is a statistically significant association between the variables in the study (antidepressant use and fall history). When the calculated χ^2 is < the critical value, then there is no significant association among the variables and the null hypothesis ($r_{cv} = 0$) cannot be rejected.

Standardized Residuals Identify Hot Spots

Standardized residuals provide a roadmap to the most important cells ("hot spots") in the contingency table.[c]

---

[c]The formula for calculating standardized residuals is shown in Figure 7-3.

Table Dimensions

2 x 2   df = 1

4 x 2   df = 3

4 x 4   df = 9

Figure 7-4 Determining for χ^2 contingency tables. A curved line is drawn through half of the perimeter as shown in each table. A count of the remaining cells is the df.

Video Tutorial 7-1

Calculating Chi Square and Related Statistics Using Statistical Software

Application:
• Illustrates how to use statistical software or an Excel spreadsheet to calculate chi square and related statistics that measure association between categorical variables.

Demonstration Data:
• *Ch7 Chi Square.**S0*** (for NCSS)
• *Ch7 Chi Square.**Sav*** (for SPSS)

Steps:
1. Open the disk and navigate to this chapter.
2. Select Video Tutorial 7-1: Association Among Clinical Variables: Chi Square.
3. View how to run the analysis using hardware.

Use of Software:
1. Verify that you have either NCSS or SPSS statistical software and Excel loaded on your computer.
2. Run the analysis illustrated in the video using the appropriate data set for the statistical software that you have installed.

The residuals are used only when χ^2 is statistically significant. The search for the largest positive and negative residuals is a post-hoc test (i.e., a test that *follows* the finding of statistical significance). The sign of these values allows the clinician to put words to the findings. For this example, the largest positive residual (see Fig. 7-3) is in Cell A, the count of fallers taking antidepressants. The positive sign indicates that *the count of people who were fallers taking antidepressants was significantly higher than would have occurred by chance.* The largest negative residual is in Cell B, the count of *non*fallers taking antidepressants (see Fig. 7-3). The negative sign indicates that the observed count in that cell is less than chance. In other words, *the count of people who were nonfallers taking antidepressants was significantly lower than would have occurred by chance.* Thus, the standardized residuals allow the practitioner to appreciate *how* medication status is related to falls.

Using Statistical Software to Calculate χ^2

If the user prefers statistical software, a cross-tabulation procedure is initiated to calculate χ^2. The output is shown in **Figure 7-5** (refer to video tutorial 7-1). Chi square is reported with statistical df and

the p value. The results are similar to the calculator using an Excel spreadsheet on the bound-in disk (see Fig. 7-3).

Converting χ^2 to a Correlation Coefficient

Chi square as calculated to this point is not comparable to other correlation coefficients where the range of possible values describing the extent of association is +1.00 (perfect direct association) to –1.00 (perfect inverse association). In order to place χ^2 in this format, it is necessary to convert the calculated χ^2 into a correlation coefficient using Cramer's V (denoted r_{CV} in this primer).[d]

$$r_{cv} = \sqrt{\frac{\chi^2}{N(q-1)}} \qquad \textbf{eq 7-3}$$

where χ^2 is the value of chi square, N is the total number of observations, and q is the number of rows or columns (whichever is smaller).

---

[d]Converting χ^2 to r_{CV} using the method shown will never be negative. Inspection of the cells on the A-D diagonal is necessary. When more cases occur on the A-D diagonal vs. the B-C diagonal, then the correlation is direct.

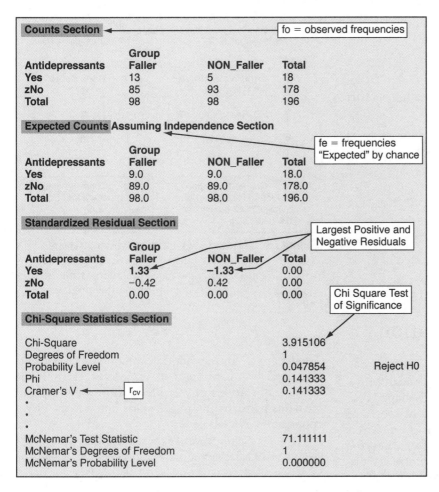

Figure 7-5 Chi square calculation and associated coefficients generated by statistical software analyzing the data set "Ch7_Chi Square." (Output from NCSS.) Output is truncated to highlight relevant results.

For the demonstration example:

$$r_{CV} = \sqrt{\frac{\chi^2}{N(q-1)}} = \sqrt{\frac{3.92}{196(2-1)}} = 0.14$$

The r_{CV} result agrees with that calculated in an Excel spreadsheet (see Fig. 7-3) and by statistical software (see Fig. 7-5).

Applying the three indices of association to the demonstration example:

- $r_{CV} = 0.14 \rightarrow$ little to no direct relationship
- $(r_{CV})^2 = 0.02 \rightarrow 2\%$ shared variance
- p <0.05 (refers to chi square test of significance) $\rightarrow r_{CV}$ is statistically different from 0

Using χ^2 With Dependent Data

In scenarios where data in a 2×2 contingency table are not independent (for example, test-retest assessment of the same patient sample), then McNemar's correction for χ^2 should be used in place of χ^2 for independent data. It is calculated as

$$\chi^2_{McNemar} = \frac{(b-c)^2}{b+c} \qquad \textbf{eq 7-4}$$

Where b and c correspond to actual counts in the respective cells of the contingency table.

$$\chi^2_{McNemar} = \frac{(b-c)^2}{b+c} = \frac{(5-85)^2}{5+85} = \frac{6400}{90} = 71.11$$

This result agrees with the McNemar statistic reported in Figures 7-3 and 7-5.[e]

Statistical software routinely reports the McNemar test in cross-tabulation analysis and it is up to the clinician to determine when it is appropriate to use this statistic. In the demonstration example, the data on antidepressants was acquired from two separate groups, so in this case the McNemar test results should be ignored. However, if the demonstration design was changed to reflect medication use pre- and post-balance training in the same subjects, then the McNemar adjustment would be the statistic that replaces χ^2 in the calculation of r_{CV}.

[e]When statistical software does not show the value of the McNemar adjustment, the clinician can easily calculate this adjustment using **equation 7-4**.

The results under this scenario would be:

$$r_{cv} = \sqrt{\frac{McNemar}{N(q-1)}} = \sqrt{\frac{71.11}{196(2-1)}} = 0.61$$

Applying the three indices of association to this test-retest alternate example:

Index	Result	Interpretation
Size and sign	$r_{CV} = 0.61$	→ moderate direct relationship
Coefficient of determination	$(r_{CV})^2 = 0.37$	→ 37% shared variance
Hypothesis test ($H_0: r_{CV} = 0$?)	$p < 0.05$	→ $r_{CV} \neq 0$

Parametric Versus Nonparametric Correlation Coefficients

Statistics that rely on the assumptions underlying a normal distribution of scores (i.e., a bell-shaped distribution with predictable percentages of scores at each standard deviation from the mean) are referred to as "parametric statistics." The use of z-scores, for example, relies on the assumption of a normal score distribution (see the appendix to Chapter 4). The use of parametric tests allows inferences beyond the sample at hand and can refer to the target *population* of patients being studied.[f] In this regard, the Pearson product moment correlation coefficient is a parametric test because it is used to evaluate normally distributed continuous scores.[11]

When statistics are designed to use non-normal data, they are referred to as "nonparametric" tests. Here, the Spearman rank correlation coefficient is selected as a common example of a statistic that does not depend on the assumptions linked to a normal distribution. Spearman correlation coefficients use the rank order of scores rather than the score itself and thus is a "distribution-free" statistic **(Fig. 7-6)**. By transforming scores to ranks, the assumptions of normality no

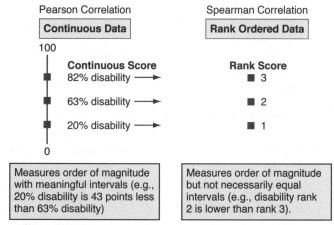

Figure 7-6 Illustration of continuous disability score and the corresponding rank scores as the type of data used by Pearson and Spearman correlation coefficients, respectively. Rank 1 assigned to smallest continuous value.

longer apply. Thus, when Spearman rank coefficients are used with continuous data, inferences are made about associations of variables within the sample of patients participating in the study and not the target population as a whole.

It is important to verify the assumption of normality prior to selecting a correlation coefficient because the type of statistic is one factor that will determine if the clinician can make inferences about the target population or limit the inferences to the immediate sample of patients.

Assumptions of Normality and Selection of Correlation Coefficients

A screening test for normality of the distribution of scores can be achieved by using statistical software **(Fig 7-7)**. When the assumption of normality is violated, researchers can attempt to transform the data to approximate a normal curve (refer to the next section) or use a correlation coefficient that does not depend on normality assumptions.

In demonstrating the application of correlation coefficients in this section, the demonstration data use hypothetical disability scores collected at the initial evaluation and then again at the time of discharge from the clinic. The question being answered in this demonstration: *"Is the level of disability of patients in my clinic at the time of discharge associated with the level of disability at the time of the initial evaluation?"* Many disability scores are considered

---

[f]Zeller and Levine[11] reported that the normality assumption underlying *r* is robust. In other words, they found that violation of the population normality assumption did not markedly alter the interpretation of *r*. For this primer, it is recommended that the Pearson product moment correlation coefficient be used when the data are normally distributed and continuous. In the case of a non-normal distribution of continuous data with a failed attempt to transform the data to a normal distribution, the use of Spearman correlation coefficients is recommended as the most conservative approach for the practitioner just beginning the clinical research process.

NCSS OUTPUT

Normality Tests Section									
	Skewness Test			**Kurtosis Test**			**Omnibus Test**		
Variable	**Value**	**Z**	**Prob**	**Value**	**Z**	**Prob**	**K2**	**Prob**	**Variable Normal?**
Initial_Disability	−0.61	−2.35	0.0190	2.08	−2.91	0.0036	13.96	0.0009	No
Followup_Disability	−0.11	−0.45	0.6498	2.10	−2.75	0.0060	7.76	0.0206	No

SPSS OUTPUT

Tests of Normality

	Kolmogorov-Smirnov[a]			Shapiro-Wilk		
	Statistic	df	Sig.	Statistic	df	Sig.
Initial_Disability	.190	88	.000	.899	88	.000
Followup_Disability	.076	88	.200*	.969	88	.035

a. Lilliefors Significance Correction
*. This is a lower bound of the true significance.

> Significant violation of normality when "sig" or p < 0.05. Decision: NOT NORMAL

Figure 7-7 Normality tests. Top: NCSS output uses D'Agostino normality tests for skewness, kurtosis as displayed. Bottom: SPSS uses Kolmogorov-Smirnov and Shapiro-Wilk tests for normality. In both cases, significant violation of normality is indicated by p < 0.05. Initial and follow-up hypothetical disability scores are used as the demonstration data. Higher scores = more disability. See file "Ch7_Spearman" on the bound-in disk for the complete data set.

continuous variables (e.g., 0%–100%, with higher scores indicating worse disability). In this example, a screening test for normality of hypothetical initial and follow-up disability scores revealed a non-normal distribution (see Fig. 7-7). Under these conditions (continuous data not normally distributed in at least one of the two variables under consideration), the Spearman rank correlation is an appropriate choice to measure the association of initial vs. follow-up disability scores.

• The determination of normality is made by statistical software. There are several tests of distribution shape listed in Figure 7-7 (tests for skewness and kurtosis). The types of skews tested are illustrated in **Figure 7-8.**
• There should be no skew in an ideal normal distribution of scores (e.g., the bell-shaped curve should be symmetrical with skew = 0). Normal curves should also show an optimal peak with no kurtosis.

The D'Agostino normality tests use a z-score to measure skew and kurtosis.[12] The omnibus test combines the assessment of skewness and kurtosis into a single index (referred to as the "K2" statistic). When

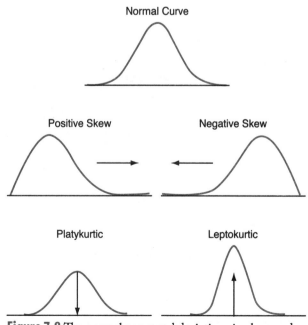

Figure 7-8 The normal curve and deviations in skew and kurtosis.

the z-score for any component of normality exceeds the critical z (±1.96 for a two-tailed test) or the probability of K2 is < 0.05, then the distribution fails the normality test. The Kolmogorov-Smirnov test is a nonparametric statistical test used to determine if two separate samples could have been drawn from populations with the same distributions (not relevant to this example where pre- and post-data came from the same subjects). Finally, the Shapiro-Wilk tests the hypothesis that the sample came from a normally distributed population. Note in Figure 7-7 that both the initial and follow-up disability scores fail at least one test of normality.

The correlation output from statistical software is shown in Figure 7-8. The output is in the form of a correlation matrix. These results correspond to the plot displayed in Figure 7-1A.

Determining Statistical Significance of Spearman Rank Correlation

The calculated r_s (0.45 in this example) is compared to a critical r_s, which is found in Appendix B, Table B-5. The critical r_s is found where the rows of the table ("n" or the number of paired observations) intersects with $\alpha = 0.05$ (either for a one- or two-tailed test). In the demonstration example, $n = 88$ and the two-tailed critical r_s at $\alpha = 0.05$ is 0.21. Because r_s calculated $(0.45) \geq r_s$ critical (0.21), the null hypothesis (H_0: $r_s = 0$) cannot be accepted and we defer to the alternative hypothesis (H_a: $r_s \neq 0$). The output from statistical software automatically calculates these results **(Fig. 7-9)**.

Interpretation of Spearman Rank Results

The interpretation of the Spearman rank correlation requires the three indices described earlier in the chapter:

Index	Result	Interpretation
Size and sign	$r_s = 0.45$	→ weak direct relationship
Coefficient of determination	$(r_s)^2 = 0.20$	→ 20% shared variance
Hypothesis test (H_0: $r_s = 0$?)	$p < 0.05$	→ $r_s \neq 0$

Thus, in this demonstration of imaginary patients, it is concluded that there is a weak relationship between levels of disability at discharge vs. at the time of the initial evaluation. Eighty percent of the variance of discharge disability scores cannot be explained by the variance of initial disability scores even though the correlation is significantly different from $r_s = 0$.

Criterion-Related Validity and Correlation Coefficients

Evidence for criterion-related validity[g] (also referred to as concurrent validity) is gathered by comparing the

[g]There are many different types of validity that are beyond the scope of this primer. Readers interested in an overview of the types of validity and the measures providing evidence for validity should refer to Sim and Arnell, Phys Ther 1993; 73 (2):102–115.

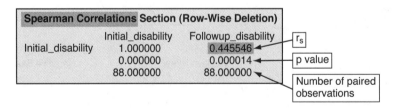

Figure 7-9 Output for Spearman rank correlation matrix; $r_s = 0.46$ (top panel: NCSS; bottom panel: SPSS). Sig = exact p value for level of significance. It is the probability of the correlation occurring by chance. The correlation coefficient is significantly different from 0 (p < 0.05).

results of a clinical assessment "with a measurable criterion that is accepted as a standard indicator of a concept or variable."[13, p.104]

For example, a new assessment tool that relied on timed measures of selected task performance (e.g., ascending stairs or moving from the floor to a standing position) was designed to measure mobility in elderly people.[14] Support for validity of this new tool, referred to as the Timed Movement Battery (TMB) Test, was obtained by correlating TMB results to well-known tools that are accepted as criterion standards for measuring mobility (the Timed Up & Go Test and the Berg Balance Test).[14] Strong correlations between the new measure of mobility and the established measures of mobility indicated that the new tool could serve as a valid measure of mobility.

Transforming Scores to Generalize Correlation Results to Target Populations

When continuous scores are analyzed for criterion-related validity, it is desirable to use parametric statistics if possible because of the ability to make inferences about the target population. For example, Verschuren et al.[15] developed shuttle run tests to measure aerobic power in children with cerebral palsy. These tests can be implemented in a clinical setting much easier than the criterion standard for measuring aerobic capacity (treadmill testing). The authors used peak oxygen uptake as one outcome measure (VO_2 measured in L/min). They found strong Pearson correlations between oxygen uptake among shuttle run tests and the criterion treadmill test, which supported the criterion-related validity of the new clinical tests.

For purposes of demonstration, an imaginary study with hypothetical data is provided to allow the reader to address the issue of transforming continuous data that might fail the tests of normality. This procedure is done so that a Pearson correlation coefficient can be used to support criterion-related validity. The data set for this demonstration is illustrated in **Figure 7-10**.

The first step in correlation analysis, as described earlier, is to determine if the data are normally distributed. **Figure 7-11** shows the results of the normality assessment and the hypothetical VO_2 variables failed the normality tests. At this juncture, a Pearson correlation coefficient is not optimal as a measure of association between the VO_2 measures for shuttle run vs. treadmill. The clinician can accept these results and use a Spearman rank correlation, or attempt to transform the scores to "reshape" the distribution.

Transforming the data so that the scores conform to a normal distribution is an acceptable procedure. There are several types of data transformations.[6] Here, a log transformation is applied (taking the log of the VO_2 scores). The transformed VO_2 scores now pass the *normality tests* (see Fig 7-11).

The correlation analysis proceeds with the transformed data. Output from statistical software using the Pearson product moment correlation coefficient is illustrated in **Figure 7-12**.

Determining Statistical Significance of Pearson Correlation

The calculated r (> 0.99 in this example) is compared to a critical r, which is found in Appendix B, Table B-6. The critical r is found where the rows of the table (df = $n - 1$) intersect with $\alpha = 0.05$ (either for a one- or two-tailed test). In the demonstration example, df = 8 - 1 = 7 and the two-tailed critical r at $\alpha = 0.05$ is 0.67. Since $r_{calculated}$ (0.99) $\geq r_{critical}$ (0.67), the null hypothesis ($H_0: r = 0$) cannot be accepted and we defer to the alternative hypothesis ($H_a: r \neq 0$). Statistical software automatically calculates the exact p value for the user.

Interpretation of Pearson Correlation Results

The interpretation of the Pearson correlation in this analysis of hypothetical data is:

Index	Result	Interpretation
Size and sign	$r = 0.99$	→ strong direct relationship
Coefficient of determination	$(r)^2 = 0.98$	→ 98% shared variance
Hypothesis test ($H_0: r = 0$?)	$p < 0.05$	→ $r \neq 0$

The conclusion to this demonstration using imaginary patients is that there is a strong direct relationship in peak aerobic capacity between the clinical test (shuttle run) and the criterion standard (treadmill testing). Thus, the imaginary data support the criterion-related validity of the clinical test.

Cronbach's Alpha

Cronbach's alpha is a statistic that measures the internal consistency of an evaluation tool. Internal consistency is a form of reliability that indicates if parts of the tool are correlated. The concept is that an assessment tool with high internal consistency should show high correlations when scores for each part of the split tool show a high association. The Cronbach alpha

Video Tutorial 7-2

Testing Normality and Selecting Correlation Coefficients Using Statistical Software

Application:
• Illustrates how to use statistical software to test the normality of the score distribution and to calculate Spearman rank order and Pearson product moment correlation coefficients.

Demonstration Data:
• *Ch7_Spearman.**S0*** (for NCSS)
• *Ch7_Spearman.**Sav*** (for SPSS)
• *Ch7_Pearson.**S0*** (for NCSS)
• *Ch7_Pearson.**Sav*** (for SPSS)

Steps:
1. Open the Essentials disk and navigate to this chapter.
2. Select Video Tutorial 7-2: Association Among Clinical Variables: Correlation.
3. View how to run the analysis using software.

Use of Software:
1. Verify that you have either NCSS or SPSS statistical software loaded on your computer.
2. Run the analysis illustrated in the video using the appropriate data set for the statistical software that you have installed.

should be thought of as a composite correlation of many iterations where the tool is split at different sections and then assessed with a correlation coefficient each time a split is made. Acceptable internal consistency is reflected by a Cronbach alpha 0.80 or above.[16] This coefficient is akin to a correlation coefficient but can only vary from 0 to 1.[6]

The Unified Parkinson's Disease Rating Scale (motor section, abbreviated UPDRSm) is selected to demonstrate the Cronbach alpha.[17] This assessment tool is comprised of 14 items each rated on a scale of 0 to 4. This 5-step severity gradation, with 0 representing absence of deficit and 4 representing maximum

Hypothetical Data

Subj	V02_ShuttleRun	V02_Treadmill	Log_V02_ShuttleRun	Log_V02_Treadmill
1	0.5	0.7	−0.3010299957	−0.15490196
2	1	1.2	0	0.07918124605
3	1.5	1.7	0.1760912591	0.2304489214
4	5	5.2	0.6989700043	0.7160033436
5	1	1.2	0	0.07918124605
6	1.5	1.7	0.1760912591	0.2304489214
7	0.2	0.4	−0.6989700043	−0.3979400087
8	0.3	0.5	−0.5228787453	−0.3010299957

Figure 7-10 Hypothetical data, set up for correlation analysis. Variables with VO_2 in the label are L/min. Those with "Log" in the label show the log of the respective VO_2 tests. Open the data set on the *Essentials CD* entitled "Ch7_Pearson" with either the NCSS or SPSS extension.

NCSS output

Normality Tests Section

Variable	Skewness Test Value	Z	Prob	Kurtosis Test Value	Z	Prob	Omnibus Test K2	Prob	Variable Normal?
V02_ShuttleRun	1.81	2.92	0.0035	5.03	2.63	0.0086	15.44	0.0004	No
V02_Treadmill	1.81	2.92	0.0035	5.03	2.63	0.0086	15.44	0.0004	No
Log_V02_ShuttleRun	0.15	0.25	0.8003	2.34	0.19	0.8532	0.10	0.9521	Yes
Log_V02_Treadmill	0.48	0.80	0.4210	2.61	0.55	0.5790	0.96	0.6202	Yes

SPSS output

Tests of normality

	Kolmogorov-Smirnov[a]			Shapiro-Wilk		
	Statistic	df	Sig.	Statistic	df	Sig.
V02_ShuttleRun	.343	8	.006	.714	8	.003
V02_Treadmill	.343	8	.006	.714	8	.003
Log_V02_ShuttleRun	.178	8	.200*	.962	8	.832
Log_V02_Treadmill	.190	8	.200*	.945	8	.662

No significant violation of normality (sig. or p>0.05)-NORMAL

Figure 7-11 Hypothetical shoulder aerobic capacity scores (VO_2) are used as a demonstration. Raw data (VO_2) do not pass the tests of normality, but log-transformed data are normally distributed for this imaginary patient sample.

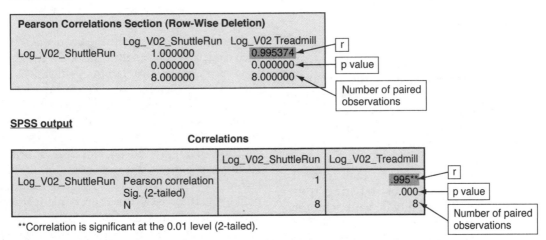

Figure 7-12 Output for Pearson product moment correlation matrix; $r = 0.99$ (top panel: NCSS; bottom panel: SPSS). Sig = exact p value for level of significance. It is the probability of the correlation occurring by chance. The correlation coefficient is significantly different from 0 (p < 0.05).

severity of that item, yields a composite score of 56 points.[18] Functions covered by the UPDRSm scale are illustrated in **Table 7-3**.

When Cronbach's alpha is calculated by statistical software in this demonstration, only a single coefficient is relevant. That single statistic is really a composite correlation. Conceptually, in the background, the UPDRSm is split—for example, at item 8 so that the score for items 1 through 6 (maximum score = 24) is correlated with the score for items 7 through 14 (maximum score = 32). This process is repeated many times with splits at different points (e.g., split at item 10, then split at item 3, and so forth randomly) until a composite (average) correlation coefficient is derived as the Cronbach alpha. For this demonstration, 105 imaginary patients with Parkinson's disease were evaluated using the UPDRSm. The data were recorded in the format shown in **Figure 7-13**.

The statistical output for the Cronbach analysis of the hypothetical data is 0.85[h] (Fig. 7-13B and C). Using the threshold of 0.80, the internal consistency of the UPDRSm was found to be acceptable in this demonstration analysis using imaginary patients.

Cronbach's alpha is typically used in research on the characteristics of clinical questionnaires and complements item analyses (such as factor or principal components analyses), which are beyond the scope of this primer. As a measure of internal consistency of a clinical assessment tool, the Cronbach statistic joins a battery of statistics that define the usefulness of the clinical evaluation along with floor/ceiling effects, the responsiveness of the tool (refer to Chapter 5), and meaningful clinical change (see Chapter 4).

Table 7-3	Components of the Unified Parkinson's Disease Rating Scale-Motor Section (UPDRSm)
Item	**Item Score Range**
1. Speech	0–4
2. Facial Mobility	0–4
3. Resting Tremor	0–4
4. Action Tremor	0–4
5. Rigidity	0–4
6. Finger Taps	0–4
7. Hand Movements	0–4
8. Rapid Alternating Movements	0–4
9. Leg agility	0–4
10. Rising from a chair	0–4
11. Posture	0–4
12. Gait	0–4
13. Postural Stability	0–4
14. Bradykinesia	0–4
Composite	0–56

Higher scores indicate more impairment. Refer to Goetz et al.[19] for implementation of the original scale and updates.[20]

[h]Standardized Cronbach's alpha is derived by subtracting the item means and dividing by the item standard deviations before calculating the alpha (Hinze, 2007).

Reliability: Consistency vs. Consensus

Reliability is repeatability. In the clinic, the use of reliable clinical assessment tools minimizes error (e.g., avoids measuring changes in the patient's score that are not related to the patient's functional status). The reliability of an assessment can be measured as consensus (agreement among raters, Chapter 6, or consistency among raters using correlation coefficients). Tooth and Ottenbacher emphasize the importance of distinguishing each form of reliability because the selection of statistical tests and the interpretation of reliability depend upon the intent to measure consensus vs. consistency.[21] For example, **Figure 7-14A** shows clinical assessment of shoulder abduction range of motion in degrees by two imaginary clinicians (in*ter* rater) who were not randomly selected. There is a high level of consistency between these clinicians as seen by the plot of scores assessed by clinician #1 vs. clinician #2 (Fig. 7-14B).

In this demonstration, the scores determined by each clinician are normally distributed and the Pearson product moment correlation coefficient is $r = 0.99$, showing near perfect consistency. As each clinician progressed from patient 1 to patient 4, the ROM scores increased. In other words, the clinicians' scores covaried almost perfectly with each other. Simple inspection of Figure 7-14A, however, shows that the ROM for patient #1, for example, is 5 degrees recorded by clinician #1 vs. 10 degrees recorded by clinician #2. These ROM measures do not agree. When agreement is assessed ($ICC_{inter\ rater\ fixed} = 0.73$), the measure of agreement is substantially lower than the measure of consistency. In contrast, **Figure 7-15** illustrates 100% precise agreement between the two clinical raters, but the data do not covary. This means

A

Subj_ID	X1_speech	X2_facial_expression	X3_tremor_at_rest
1	2	1	0
2	2	2	0
3	2	3	0
4	0	3	0
5	1	2	0
6	2	3	0
7	2	1	0
8	2	1	3
9	2	4	1
10	3	3	0
11	1	2	0
12	2	4	0
13	0	1	0
14	0	1	0
15	1	3	2
16	1	2	1
17	2	2	0
18	3	4	0
19	2	2	0
20	1	2	0
21	1	2	0
22	2	1	0
23	2	2	0
24	2	3	0
25	0	3	0
26	1	2	0

Hypothetical Data

B NCSS OUTPUT

	X1_speech	X2_facial_expression	X3_tremor_at_rest
X1_speech	1.000000	0.390016	0.023993...
X2_facial_expression	0.390016	1.000000	−0.062384...
X3_tremor_at_rest	0.023993	−0.062384	1.000000...
			(Correlations for UPDRSm
			test items 4-13 not shown)
X14_body_bradykinesia	0.128897	0.575575	0.043027...
Cronbachs Alpha = 0.845869		**Standardized Cronbachs Alpha = 0.836175**	

Figure 7-13 (A) Hypothetical data on UPDRSm, set up for Cronbach's alpha assessment. Only 26 rows (of 154 patients) and 3 test items (columns) holding the UPDRSm scores are shown. The complete data set is available on the bound-in disk. Open the file "Ch7_Cronbach Alpha" with either the NCSS or SPSS extension. (B) NCSS output for Cronbach's alpha appears at the bottom of a Pearson correlation matrix. (C) SPSS output simply reports Cronbach's alpha as "Alpha."

C SPSS OUTPUT

Reliability Statistics

Cronbach's Alpha	N of Items
.846	14

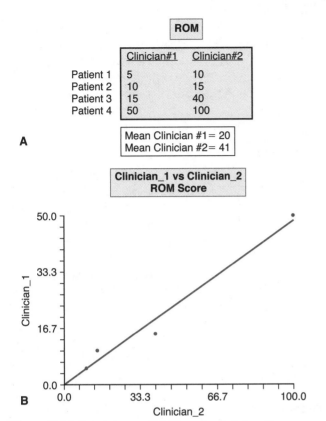

Figure 7-14 Consistency: (A) Hypothetical data from two clinicians evaluating shoulder abduction range of motion. (B) Scatter plot of the data from (A) showing a high level of consistency between clinicians ($r = 0.99$).

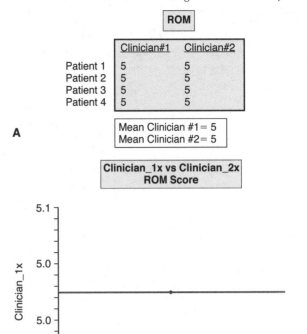

Figure 7-15 Agreement: (A) Hypothetical data from two clinicians evaluating shoulder abduction range of motion. (B) Scatter plot of the data in (A) showing no consistency between clinicians (r or $r_s = 0.00$).

that the correlation between clinicians #1 and #2 will be very low (r or $r_s = 0$; Fig. 7-15B).

The paradox between consistency and agreement is usually resolved by a clear research question coupled with statistics that match the type of data. When the research question relates to agreement, then percent agreement, kappa, weighted kappa, or an intraclass correlation coefficient are the statistics that should be considered (Chapter 6). If, however, the research question addresses consistency (covariance of scores), then χ^2 with Cramer's V, Spearman rank, or Pearson product moment correlation coefficients are more appropriate.

SUMMARY

Clinical application of correlation coefficients involves the assessment of association between rele-

vant clinical variables that may guide the care of the patient. Correlation analyses also help to establish reliability and the internal consistency of clinical assessment tools. The selection of a particular type of correlation coefficient depends upon the level of data, the normality of score distribution, and, in some cases, the dependency of data (e.g., whether the data are from the same patient tested twice or from different patients). Regardless of the correlation coefficient selected, three essential indices are used to interpret the meaning of correlation: the size and sign of the coefficient, the percent shared variance, and a statistical hypothesis test to determine if the degree of association is statistically different from 0.

PRACTICE

1. An imaginary clinical study of mobility enrolled patients randomly into a control and treatment group. The concern of the practitioners conducting the study was that the subjects might not have equivalent mobility deficits upon entering the study. They quantified mobility deficits by recording the type of assistive device used by each patient. The contingency table representing the counts is shown below:

Upon Entry to the Study		
Assist. Dev.	Control	Treatment
None	3	7
Crutches	2	9
Cane	12	5
Walker	10	13

Using the data set "Ch7_Practice 1" on the bound-in disk, evaluate the question "Is there an association between assistive devices and enrollment in the control or treatment groups at baseline?" Form your answers in terms of χ^2, df, and statistical significance. Also include size and sign of r_{CV}, coefficient of determination, and the results of the hypothesis test H_0: $r_{CV} = 0$. Then describe the results in words using standardized residuals as your guide.

2. If the contingency table in question 1 was collapsed into a 2×2 table, the data would be summarized as follows:

Upon Entry to the Study		
Assist. Dev.	Control	Treatment
No	3	7
Yes	24	27

Using the calculator developed in an Excel spreadsheet ("P_Chi sq calculator" on the bound-in disk), recalculate the results requested in question 1 and compare each set of findings.

3. An imaginary clinician was interested in the relationship between a timed mobility test (the Timed Up & Go Test in seconds—higher scores mean more impairment) and a functional balance measure (the Berg Balance Scale—higher scores mean less impairment). She tested 13 patients with stroke and collected the following data:

Patient	Berg	Timed_UP_GO
1	32	25
2	55	10
3	37	59
4	49	17
5	45	18
6	50	19
7	41	24
8	55	14
9	54	19
10	33	38
11	50	23
12	48	10
13	45	20

Using the data set "Ch7_Practice 2" on the bound-in disk, select the best statistic to evaluate the association between these two clinical measures and include a test of normality and the three essential indices for evaluating correlation coefficients. Be sure to describe in words what the correlation indicates.

4. If the test of normality was not conducted in question 3 and the clinician used a Pearson product moment correlation by mistake, would there be a difference in outcome in terms of the absolute value of the coefficient?

5. Is it possible to transform the Timed Up & Go data in "Ch7_Practice 2" into a normal-shaped distribution using a log transformation?

6. Using log transformations in the data set "Ch7_Practice 2", what is the best statistical method to measure association between the two clinical variables and what is the outcome?

REFERENCES

1. Hall AM, Ferreira PH, Maher CG, et al. The influence of the therapist-patient relationship on treatment outcome in physical rehabilitation: a systematic review. Phys Ther 2010; 90:1099–1110.

2. Lewis CL, Moutoux M, Slaughter M, et al. Characteristics of individuals who fell while receiving home health services. Phys Ther 2004; 84:23–32.

3. Sezer N, Yavuzer G, Sivrioglu K, et al. Clinimetric properties of the Duruoz Hand Index in patients with stroke. Arch Phys Med Rehabil 2007; 88:309–314.

4. Vasconcelos Jr OM, Prokhorenko OA, Kelley KF, et al. A comparison of fatigue scales in postpoliomyelitis syndrome. Arch Phys Med Rehabil 2006; 87:1213–1217.

5. Jensen MP, Abresch RT, Carter GT. The reliability and validity of a self-report version of the FIM instrument in persons with neuromuscular disease and chronic pain. Arch Phys Med Rehabil 2005; 86: 116–122.

6. Portney LG, Watkins MP. Foundations of Clinical Research: Applications to Practice. Princeton: Prentice-Hall, 2000.

7. Di Fabio RP. Significance of relationships. J Orthop Sports Phys Ther 1999; 29:572–573.

8. Ottenbacher K. The chi-square test: its use in rehabilitation research. Arch Phys Med Rehabil 1995; 76:678–681.

9. Cochrane WG. Some methods for strengthening the common χ^2 test. Biometrics 1954; 10:417–451.

10. Portney LG, Watkins MP. Foundations of Clinical Research: Applications to Practice. Upper Saddle River, NJ: Prentice-Hall, 2009.

11. Zeller RA, Levine ZH. The effects of violating the normality assumption underlying r. Sociol Meth & Res 1974; 2:511–519.

12. D'Agostino RB, Ralph B., Belanger A, et al. A suggestion for using powerful and informative tests of normality. Amer Stat 1990; 44:316–321.

13. Sim J, Amell P. Measurement validity in physical therapy research. Phys Ther 1993; 73:102–115.

14. Creel GL, Light KE, Thigpen MT. Concurrent and construct validity of scores on the Timed Movement Battery. Phys Ther 2001; 81:789–798.

15. Verschuren O, Takken T, Ketelaar M, et al. Reliability and validity of data for 2 newly developed shuttle run tests in children with cerebral palsy. Phys Ther 2006; 86:1107–1117.

16. Carmines EG, Zeller RA. Reliability and Validity Assessment, Vol. 17. Beverly Hills, CA: SAGE, 1979.

17. Cubo E, Stebbins GT, Golbe LI, et al. Application of the Unified Parkinson's Disease Rating Scale in progressive supranuclear palsy: factor analysis of the motor scale. Movement Disorders 2000; 15:276–279.

18. Richards M, Marder K, Cote L, et al. Interrater reliability of the Unified Parkinson's Disease Rating Scale Motor Examination. Movement Disorders 1994; 9:89–91.

19. Goetz CG, Stebbins GT, Chmura TA, et al. Teaching tape for the motor section of the Unified Parkinson's Disease Rating Scale. Movement Disorders 1995; 10:263–266.

20. Goetz CG, Fahn S, Martinez-Martin P, et al. Movement Disorder Society-sponsored revision of the Unified Parkinson's Disease Rating Scale (MDS-UPDRS): process, format, and clinimetric testing plan. Movement Disorders 2007; 22:41–47.

21. Tooth LR, Ottenbacher KJ. The k Statistic in rehabilitation research: an examination. Arch Phys Med Rehabil 2004; 85:1371–1376.

Prediction of Clinical Outcome

Clinical Questions
• What is the outcome that patients and caregivers can expect from treatment?
• What is the patient's prognosis?

Introduction

Frequently in clinical practice the patient or caregiver will ask, "What can I expect from the treatment that you provide?" or "What is my prognosis in terms of rehabilitation outcome?" The experience of the practitioner will play a key role in making judgments about clinical outcome. However, clinical experience can be supplemented with evidence-based literature that addresses prediction of outcome in similar target populations. Practitioners may wish to know how patient status at the initial evaluation will influence the likelihood of a good rehabilitation outcome. Which cognitive and behavioral deficits influence return to work for people with traumatic brain injury?"[1] What are the clinical profiles that influence functional independence following rehabilitation for people with stroke?[2] For people with hip fractures, what clinical features following surgery have value for predicting ambulation independence?[3]

Good predictive models not only help practitioners inform patients and caregivers about the patient's prognosis but in some cases (e.g., traumatic brain injury) can guide care or redirect "… the use of certain therapeutic interventions in those predicted to have a good outcome and reduce their use in those predicted to have a poor outcome."[4(p.425)]

What Is a Prediction Model?

The term *model* simply means an equation. For selected models predicting outcome following traumatic brain injury, the patient intake scores on the variables of interest (*predictors* or *independent variables*) are entered into the equation to yield either a *predicted* outcome (e.g., the amount of care the patient might need at the time of treatment completion),[5] the predicted risk that the patients will be severely disabled,[4] or a predicted maximum likelihood that the patient will be classified in a certain group (a dichotomous outcome such as *return to work or not*).[1]

Two commonly used methods to develop prediction models in rehabilitation are linear regression and logistic regression analyses (**Fig. 8-1**). These procedures have the common goal of predicting patient outcome or classification to guide care, but the type of predicted outcome differs for each method. Linear regression models predict outcome for continuous variables (e.g., disability scores, functional independence measures, strength, or cognitive scores). Logistic regression, in contrast, predicts a dichotomous outcome (e.g., independent in self-care versus not independent, return to work versus unable to return to work) for the appropriate target population.

The ultimate goal is to apply a prediction model in a clinical setting for *new* patients who were not part of the original model development. If the prediction model is strong, then accurate predictions of outcome will result. However, if the model is weak, it might not be useful in a clinical environment.

This chapter provides essential information for practitioners seeking to understand the fundamental

Study Design: Predicting Outcomes with Regression Analysis

Figure 8-1 Common design and statistical procedures to predict outcome. *Note: there are forms of logistic regression that can be used with polytomous data, but this procedure (referred to as multinomial logistic regression) is beyond the scope of this text.

Patient true status is known

Patients in the study are assessed:
- Variables recorded that will be *used in the future* as
- Outcome measures
- Predictors

Model (equation) developed for prediction of Outcome

Simple Regression—single predictor
Multiple Regression—multiple predictors

Linear Regression

Predicts Continuous Outcome*

Logistic Regression

Predicts Dichotomous Outcome

Model is tested

Patients in the study are re-evaluated using the model to determine how well predicted outcome agrees with actual outcome.

Alternatively, the model is applied to a new group of patients in the target population for validation of prediction.

concepts underlying the development of prediction models and the use of prediction models in clinical practice.

Linear Prediction Models: Validity

When linear regression is used to predict outcome, there are three statistical issues that clinical researchers should address to ensure that the prediction model yields a valid estimate of outcome:

1. *Absence of redundancy (multicollinearity).* The term *multicollinearity* refers to associations among the predictors in the model. For example, if age and strength are correlated, then only one of these variables can be used to predict dependence level following rehabilitation. In other words, if multicollinearity is present, the prediction model will be biased because some of the predictors are redundant. When multicollinearity is discovered, the variable contributing most to the redundancy of the prediction is removed and the regression analysis is repeated (the exact procedure is described later in this chapter).

2. *Slope of the overall regression line different from 0.* In multiple regression, the line of best fit through the data is multidimensional and difficult to illustrate. However, it is conceptually similar to the line of best fit in simple regression (single predictor variable versus a single outcome measure yielding a straight prediction line). A statistical procedure called *ANOVA on regression* will determine if the slope of the overall regression line statistically differs from 0 (null hypothesis H_0: slope = 0). The slope of the prediction line represents the amount of error in the prediction. Slopes approaching ±1.00 have less prediction error than lower slopes. The reason for this

phenomenon is related to the magnitude of residuals surrounding the prediction line (described later).

A prediction line slope different from 0 does not necessarily indicate a strong model. On the other hand, if the slope of the regression line is not different from 0, then it cannot be considered a strong predictive model. The impact of a low slope on prediction of outcome is shown in **Figure 8-2**. The variables plotted are hypothetical disability scores (higher scores = more self-perceived disability).

Residuals and Prediction Line Slope: Comparing Predicted Versus Actual Outcomes

An analysis of "residuals" can be helpful as a descriptive tool for visualizing the discrepancies between actual versus predicted values. A residual in the context of prediction models is defined as the difference between an actual outcome versus a predicted outcome:[a,b]

$$\text{Residual} = \text{Actual Outcome} - \text{Predicted Outcome} \quad \textbf{eq 8-1}$$

For example, if initial disability scores were used to predict disability scores following rehabilitation in a simple linear regression analysis, inspection of a scatter plot might look like the plot in **Figure 8-3A**. In this

[a]In **Chapter 7,** the post hoc analysis used residuals to evaluate the cells contributing the most to the association between 2 categorical variables. In that context, the residual analysis identified cells with counts greater than (+) or less than (-) the counts expected by chance.

[b]In **Chapter 7,** the post-hoc analysis used residuals to evaluate the cells contributing the most to the association between two categorical variables. In that context, the residual analysis identified cells with counts greater than (+) or less than (–) the counts expected by chance.

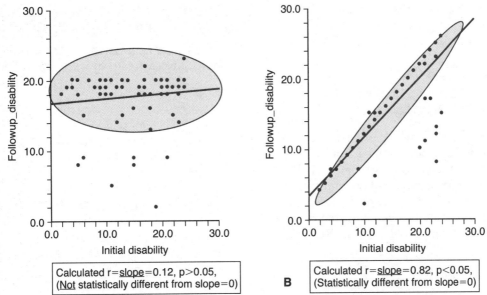

Calculated r=<u>slope</u>=0.12, p>0.05,
(<u>Not</u> statistically different from slope=0)

A

Calculated r=<u>slope</u>=0.82, p<0.05,
(Statistically different from slope=0)

B

Figure 8-2 Hypothetical data demonstrating the slope of the line of best fit generated from a linear regression analysis. (A) As the initial disability score increases along the *x*-axis, there is little change in the follow-up disability score (*y*-axis). The slope of the prediction model is nearly flat, and the prediction of disability level following rehabilitation is poor. Shaded area illustrates some of the *unexplained* variance between initial and final disability scores. (B) As the initial disability score increases along the *x*-axis, the follow-up scores on the *y*-axis also rise and the slope of the prediction model is relatively large and significantly different from 0. This prediction model appears to provide a good prediction of outcome following rehabilitation. Shaded area illustrates *explained* variance.

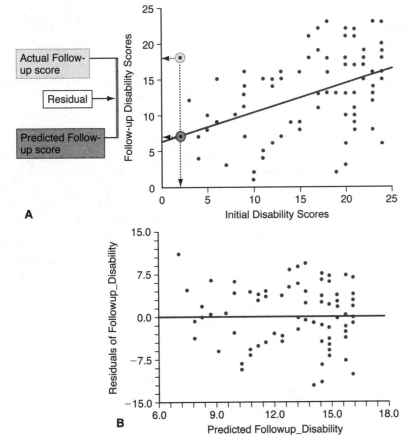

Figure 8-3 (A) Scatter plot and simple linear regression with line of best fit (least squares regression line). Highest circled point isolates a hypothetical patient's data point discussed in the text. The residual is the difference between actual and predicted disability scores. (B) Plot of residuals for each imaginary patient in this demonstration.

analysis, both the patient's *actual* outcome and *predicted* outcome are known. The predicted value is found on the prediction line for any observed value on the *x*-axis.

The prediction model for this scatter plot is:

Predicted Discharge Disability =
(.41* Initial_Disability) + 6.28

Thus, an imaginary patient who participated in the hypothetical study had an actual initial disability score = 2 and an actual follow-up disability score = 18. The residual analysis generates a predicted outcome when inserting the actual initial score in the prediction equation. The predicted outcome is then compared to the actual outcome using equation 8-1 (see Fig. 8-3A).

Patient's actual initial score = 2
Patient's actual outcome score = 18

Using the prediction model, the patient's predicted outcome is:

(.41* **2**) + 6.28 = **7**
Residual = Actual Outcome – Predicted
Outcome = 18 – 7 = **11**

Statistical software generates plots of residuals for all patients in the study (**Fig. 8-3B**). Ideally, the residuals should be 0. Residuals with large departures from 0 indicate a poor correspondence between actual and predicted outcomes.

The sum of the squared residuals is a measure of error. Larger values indicate a greater scatter of points (more error) surrounding the prediction line (see Fig. 8-2). The "line of best fit" minimizes the sum of the squares of the residuals. Thus, the line of best fit is called the "least squares regression line" or the "prediction line."

3. R^2. The coefficient of determination when multiple predictors are used to predict an outcome is a multiple R^2. Here, the capital R^2 refers to the amount of shared variance between *all* predictors and the predicted variable. This value is interpreted as the percent shared ("explained") variance between the predictors and the outcome score. Usually, a large R^2 reflects a strong predictive capacity of the model because there is substantial "explained variance"; that is, as the predictors change there is a consistent change in the value of the outcome measure, thus "explained variance." Note that r^2 (lowercase) was described in Chapter 7 as the percent of explained variance between just two variables without intent to predict one variable from the other.

Video Tutorial 8-1

Multiple Linear Regression and Correction for Multicollinearity Using Statistical Software

Application:
- Illustrates how to use statistical software to calculate a multiple linear regression and correct the analysis for excessive multicollinearity in a hypothetical data set with imaginary patients.

Demonstration Data:
- *Ch8-Multiple linear regression.**S0*** (for NCSS)
- *Ch8-Multiple linear regression.**Sav*** (for SPSS)

Steps:
1. Open the disk and navigate to this chapter.
2. Select Video Tutorial 8-1: Prediction of Clinical Outcome: Linear Regression.
3. View how to run the analysis using software.

Software:
1. Verify that you have either NCSS or SPSS statistical software loaded on your computer.
2. Run the analysis illustrated in the video using the appropriate data set for the statistical software that you have installed.

Linear Prediction Equations

All linear regression models assume that changes in the outcome measure vary with changes in the predictors of outcome in a linear fashion. Also, for the prediction models covered in this text, there is always only 1 *dependent* (predicted) variable. Simple linear regression means that there is a single predictor variable, whereas multiple linear regression will have multiple predic**tors** or independent variables. The form of a simple linear regression model is the equation for a straight line (see **eq 8-2**), and the form of a multiple linear regression prediction model is a variant of the equation for a straight line (see **eq 8-3**):

$$\hat{y} = mx + b \qquad \textbf{eq 8-2}$$
$$\hat{y} = m_1x_1 + m_2x_2 + \cdots + b \qquad \textbf{eq 8-3}$$

where $\hat{y}$ is a predicted continuous variable, x is a predictor variable, m is the slope for the corresponding predictor variable, and b is the y intercept of the linear regression line. As the patient's prognosis can rarely be predicted accurately with a single predictor, multiple linear regression typically serves as a better prediction model.

Demonstration: Predicting Clinical Outcomes Using Multiple Linear Regression

Previous literature has shown that factors including age, severity of physical disease, and duration of disease affect ability to drive.[6] This demonstration is a hypothetical study to create a prediction model for braking reaction time (the outcome measure) for imaginary people with Parkinson's disease. The predictor variables in this example are disease severity as assessed by the Hoehn and Yahr Scale[7,8] (only three of five stages included: stage 1 = unilateral disease, stage 2 = bilateral disease without postural instability, stage 3 = postural instability), age, Parkinson's disease duration (in years), and the duration of taking anti-Parkinson's medications (also in years). The data set for this demonstration is shown in **Figure 8-4**.

When developing a linear prediction equation it is necessary to know the values of both the dependent and independent variables (recorded in Fig. 8-4). Braking time in seconds is measured using a driving simulator such as that used in an actual study.[6] For the purpose of this primer, the development of a prediction equation is achieved in three steps.

Step 1: Assess Redundancy of Predictors (Multicollinearity)

The concept of prediction is based on the assumption that each independent variable provides unique information about the outcome. If independent variables are related to each other, then multicollinearity exists. Multicollinearity must be corrected before a prediction equation is derived. In statistical software, the regression analysis is run first to determine the extent of multicollinearity **(Fig. 8-5)**.

Hoehn-Yahr stages

1. Unilateral involvement only usually with minimal or no functional disability
2. Bilateral or midline involvement without impairment of balance
3. Bilateral disease: mild to moderate disability with impaired postural reflexes; physically independent
4. Severely disabling disease; still able to walk or stand unassisted
5. Confinement to bed or wheelchair unless aided

A

Patient_num	Hoehn_Yahr_Stage	Age	Brake_RT_s	PD_duration_yrs	PD_meds_duration_yrs
103	3	83	0.59	8.6	7.6
104	3	49	0.65	4.2	3.2
105	1	67	0.97	8.6	7.6
106	1	76	0.29	9.3	8.3
107	2	63	0.74	10.7	9.7
108	2	90	0.41	10.2	9.2
109	2	85	1.31	10.4	9.4
110	2	61	0.23	4.5	3.5
111	2	88	0.93	5.7	4.7
112	2	85	0.53	11.3	10.3
113	2	87	1.06	5.3	4.3
114	2	83	1.33	6.3	5.3
115	2	54	0.24	11.1	10.1
116	2	83	0.62	11.4	10.4
117	2	78	1.1	6.9	5.9
118	2	88	0.29	6.8	5.8
119	2	74	0.63	10	9
120	3	58	0.24	12.8	11.8
121	3	78	1.19	11.6	10.6
122	3	63	0.2	6.9	5.9
123	3	58	0.41	5.3	4.3
124	3	79	1.17	9.8	8.8
125	3	67	0.86	8	7
126	3	68	1.49	12.1	11.1
127	3	78	1.24	4.4	3.4

B

Figure 8-4 (A) Hoehn-Yahr stages for determining severity of Parkinson's disease. Adapted from Goetz CG, Poewe W, Rascol O, et al., Movement Disorder Society Task Force Report on the Hoehn and Yahr Staging Scale: Status and Recommendations. Movement Disorders Vol. 19, No. 9, 2004, pp. 1020-1028 with permission from John Wiley and Sons copyright 2004. (B) Hypothetical data, set up for multiple linear regression to predict brake reaction time in people with Parkinson's disease. Only 25 of 154 rows are displayed. The full data set is available on the bound-in disk (open "Ch8-Multiple linear regression" with either the NCSS or SPSS extension). Abbreviations: PD = Parkinson's disease, s = seconds. Hoehn-Yahr stage is a disease severity score.

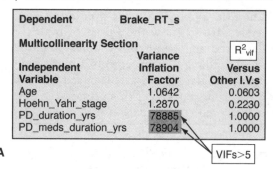

A

B

Figure 8-5 Assessment of multicollinearity. (A) Two predictors of brake reaction time (arrows) have high correlations with the remaining predictor variables or with each other. (B) Elimination of duration on medication removes multicollinearity (all VIFs now <5). Refer to "Ch8-Multiple linear regression" data set on the bound-in disk. Output from NCSS v2007. Abbreviations: VIF = variance inflation factor, IVs = Independent variables, PD = Parkinson's disease. Irrelevant portions of the output not shown. (Brake_RT_s = brake reaction time in seconds)

When *predictor variables* are correlated with each other, they "share variance." *It should be emphasized that the focus here is strictly on the predictor side of the model.* If multicollinearity is present, then redundancy in the prediction model is corrected by eliminating the most offending predictor first and then rerunning the regression analysis. The offending variable is identified by a variance inflation factor (VIF) ≥5 (eq 8-4). When any predictor has a VIF ≥5, then that variable should be removed from the model. If more than one predictor has VIF ≥5, then the variable with the largest VIF should be removed first to determine if a single predictor elimination will correct multicollinearity. If elimination of the predictor with the largest VIF does not correct multicollinearity, then there is a systematic removal of single (one-at-a-time) remaining predictors that have VIF ≥5 until multicollinearity is reduced to an acceptable level (VIF <5 for every predictor).

$$VIF = \frac{1}{1 - R_{vif}^2}$$ **eq 8-4**

where R_{vif}^2 is the shared variance of a selected predictor variable "regressed" on (in other words, correlated with) the remaining predictor variables.[9]

For example, the $R_{vif}^2 = 0.22$ for the Hoehn-Yahr disease severity score (**Fig. 8-5A**). This indicates that the selected predictor variable accounts for 22% of the variation of the remaining predictors in the model. The VIF for this R_{vif}^2 is 1.28 (**eq 8-4**). This means that the predictor has a low correlation with other predictors (VIF <5) in the model and should be retained in the analysis.

However, the hypothetical demonstration shown in Figure 8-5A indicates that two other potential clinical predictors of brake reaction time during driving simulation have VIFs ≥5: the duration of Parkinson's disease in years and the duration of taking medications for Parkinson's disease (abbreviated "PD_duration_yrs" and "PD_meds_duration_yrs," respectively). The VIF for the duration of taking medicine for PD has the highest VIF and is removed first. Rerunning the regression analysis shows that all remaining VIFs for the predictors are now below 5 (**Fig. 8-5B**). This allows the practitioner to continue to the next step in the analysis.

Step 2: Determine If Slope of the "Line of Best Fit" Differs From 0

The test of the slope of the line of best fit against a reference of slope = 0 is akin to testing the magnitude of a correlation coefficient against a reference of r or $r_s = 0$ (Chapter 7). Here, ANOVA on regression partitions the total variance of scores into *variance that is explained by the model* (mean square for the "model" term—the numerator of the F ratio) *and variance unexplained by the model* (error mean square—the denominator of the F ratio).[10]

$$F\ ratio\ regression = \frac{Mean\ Square\ Explained}{Mean\ Square\ Error}$$

eq 8-5

Using **equation 8-5,** the F ratio testing the slope of the prediction line is

$F_{3,150}$ on regression = 0.29/0.07 = 4.41, p <0.05

where the subscripts $F_{3,150}$ are the df for the model (number of predictors) and the error term, respectively.

In conversational terms, the F ratio on regression means that when the **predicted** variable changes in concert with the **predictors,** then the variance is "explained" by the predictors. Changes in the predictors that are *not* associated with changes in the predicted score are referred to as "unexplained variance" or error. The goal is to have a relatively large amount of explained variance (F ratio numerator) and a relatively small unexplained variance (F ratio denominator). The df for the model term reflects the number of predictor variables.[10] In this demonstration, the multiple regression analysis using three variables to predict brake reaction time has a slope that differs from 0 (**Fig. 8-6,**

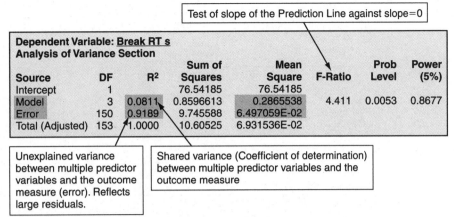

Test of slope of the Prediction Line against slope=0

Dependent Variable: <u>Break RT s</u>
Analysis of Variance Section

Source	DF	R^2	Sum of Squares	Mean Square	F-Ratio	Prob Level	Power (5%)
Intercept	1		76.54185	76.54185			
Model	3	0.0811	0.8596613	0.2865538	4.411	0.0053	0.8677
Error	150	0.9189	9.745588	6.497059E-02			
Total (Adjusted)	153	1.0000	10.60525	6.931536E-02			

Unexplained variance between multiple predictor variables and the outcome measure (error). Reflects large residuals.

Shared variance (Coefficient of determination) between multiple predictor variables and the outcome measure

Figure 8-6 ANOVA on regression: Test of the slope of a multiple regression line against slope = 0 using an F ratio. The mean square components for calculation of the F ratio are highlighted. Analysis generated from the data set on the bound-in disk ("Ch8-Multiple linear regression") shows that the line of best fit predicting brake reaction time ("Brake_RT_s") has a slope significantly different from 0 ($F_{3,150}$ = 4.41, p <0.05). The coefficient of determination for the entire model (R^2) is 0.08 = 8%. The df for "model" reflects the number of predictors.

$F_{df\ numerator,\ df\ denominator}$; $F_{3,150}$ = 4.41, p <0.05). However, as noted earlier, a prediction line slope that differs from 0 does not necessarily mean that the prediction model is strong.

Step 3: Determine the Extent of Shared ("Explained") Variance

In this demonstration, R^2 = 0.08 (see Fig. 8-6). This means that age, severity of disease, and duration of disease covary with driving brake reaction time only 8% of the time. The results of this demonstration analysis of hypothetical data emphasize the phenomenon that a statistically significant model (just like a statistically significant bivariate correlation coefficient) can differ from a reference slope of 0 but not reflect substantial explained variance among predictor variables and the predicted outcome. The amount of shared variance (R^2) will assist the clinician in making determinations about the strength of the prediction model. Unfortunately, there is no widely accepted rule for how much explained variance must be present to yield a good prediction model. Clinical judgment regarding unique characteristics of the patient and his or her circumstances is necessary to apply any prediction rule in a clinical setting.

Are Some Predictor Variables More Important Than Others?

A statistically significant prediction model even with a substantial R^2 does not mean that all predictors contribute equally to the prediction of outcome. Each predictor variable ideally contributes something to the overall slope of the multiple regression line of best fit (a regression coefficient; **Fig. 8-7**). However, some predictor variables contribute more to the slope (and thus the prediction of outcome) than other variables.

Figure 8-7 shows the prediction equation and identifies the significant predictor variables. In this demonstration, the patient's age and severity of disease (Hoehn and Yahr stage) are statistically significant predictors of brake reaction time measured in seconds, whereas the duration of disease is not. The significant predictors have regression coefficients, or "slopelets" (slope contributions to the overall line of best fit), that differ from 0. The significance of each slopelet is evaluated with a t-score (described later). Each predictor variable has a slopelet that combines with other predictor variables to create the overall prediction line. So when the slopelet for a given predictor variable is statistically significant, it simply means that the contribution of that variable to the overall slope of the prediction line is >0.

Clinical researchers seeking to identify the best predictors in the model can either:

• focus on the *t-scores*. The t-score in this case is a type of a z-score. The t-score is formed by the ratio

$$t\ score\ regression = \frac{slope\ coefficient - 0}{SE\ slope\ coefficient} \quad \textbf{eq 8-6}$$

where the slope coefficient is labeled as B or b(i) in the statistical software output (see Fig. 8-7), and SE is the standard error of the slope coefficient (refer to Chapter 4 Appendix for review of standard error).

Note that **equation 8-6** answers the question: Is the contribution of this predictor to the slope of the overall prediction line greater than 0? In this demonstration, age has the highest t-score absolute value that is statistically significant at a probability of p <0.05 (|t| = 2.56, p = 0.01; the intercept p value is ignored).

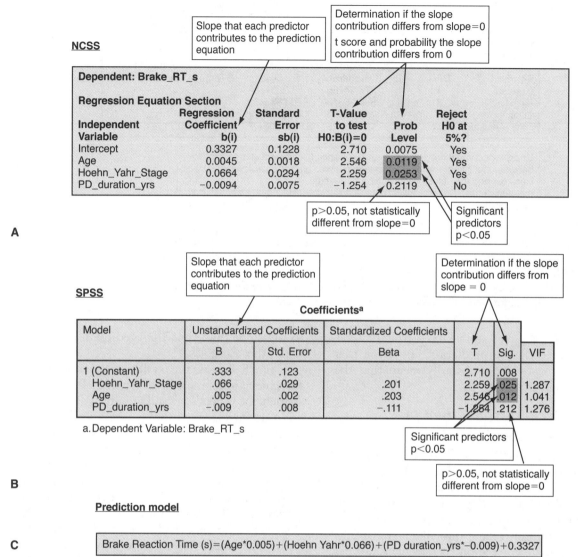

Figure 8-7 Analysis of the contribution of each predictor to the prediction model in a multiple linear regression analysis. (A) NCSS output. (B) SPSS output. (C) Prediction model derived from statistical output. Abbreviations: Brake_RT_s = brake reaction time in seconds, PD = Parkinson's disease, B or b(i) = regression coefficient (slope contribution to the prediction line), t = t-test on slope contribution to prediction line, "Sig" = significance level or probability of occurring by chance, VIF = variance inflation factor, constant = Y intercept of the prediction line.

The sign of the t-score represents the direction of the association (+ for direct and − for inverse). In contrast, the duration of Parkinson's disease in years is not a statistically significant predictor of brake time because the contribution to the overall prediction line is no better than 0 ($|t| = 1.254$, $p = 0.2119$).[c] Since each predictor has different units, the magnitude of the

slope contribution (Fig. 8-7, "b(i)" in NCSS or the column of numbers under "B-Unstandardized Coefficients" in SPSS) in raw form cannot be used to compare the value of each predictor in the overall model. Some statistical programs report beta weights, which are standardized coefficients (Fig. 8-7B). The magnitude of beta weights shows the relative importance of the predictors contributing to the overall slope of the prediction line. In this example, age is a statistically significant predictor ($p < 0.05$) and has the largest beta weight (0.203 under the "beta" column; Fig. 8-7B).

The practice of identifying the most important predictors in a prediction model that passes the

[c]Statistical df for the t ratio on regression slope contribution of each predictor is $n - 1$. In this demonstration, there are 154 subjects, so $n - 1 = 153$. Enter the critical t table in Appendix B **(Table B-2)** and the critical t for a two-tailed test at $p = 0.05$ is ±1.96. Since n is large, this critical value is the same as a critical z for a two-tailed test at $p = 0.05$.

multicollinearity test and the test of prediction line slope >0 in the ANOVA on regression adds depth and detail to the regression analysis. Evaluation of the contributions of individual predictors to the model may be of help when trying to derive the best minimal set of predictors, for instance, when trying to reduce the number of clinical tests given to the patient. However, in practice, the prediction model is used in its entirety to render a prediction of outcome. In other words, *all* variables that are contained in the prediction model, once it passes the multicollinearity and regression ANOVA tests, are included in the prediction of outcome regardless of the amount of their individual contributions to the slope of the prediction line. It is left to the clinical researcher to trim and retest a new model for multicollinearity and the regression line slope if a model with fewer predictors is desired (see also the section "Selection of the Best Predictors").

Making the Prediction

The value of a good prediction model when used to supplement clinical practice is the ability to make reasonable predictions of outcome given the status of the patient at the time of the initial evaluation. For example, the demonstration data set yields a prediction model that has the form:

Prediction of Brake Reaction Time Using Hypothetical Data[d]

$$\hat{y} = m_1x_1 + m_2x_2 + \cdots + b$$
$$= 4.54085618267474\text{E-03*Age+}$$
$$6.64306193675109\text{E-02*Hoehn\_Yahr\_Stage+}$$
$$-9.42193098804128\text{E-03*PD\_duration\_yrs+}$$
$$0.332702300495548$$

where $\hat{y}$ = predicted brake reaction time, m = slope contribution of each variable, and b is the y intercept.

A new imaginary patient enters the clinic who is 76 years of age. He was diagnosed with Parkinson's disease 8 years ago and is at stage 2 on the Hoehn and Yahr Severity Scale. What is his predicted brake reaction time in seconds?

Predicted Brake Reaction time[e] =
4.54085618267474 E-03*(76 years)+
6.64306193675109E-02*(2 points)+
−9.42193098804128E-03*(8 years) +
0.332702300495548

[d]Numbers reported in statistical software have a high degree of precision. The values following 2 decimal places are shaded to focus the reader on a manageable number. When using the prediction model generated from statistical software, it is recommended to copy and paste the equation into an Excel spreadsheet for processing. Note that the model is reported with coefficients in exponent form. This alters the appearance of the equation but not the content.
[e]When performing the calculations, only the numbers are entered (e.g., 76 instead of "76 years").

Predicted Brake Reaction time = 0.74 seconds

Note that the prediction equation is generated by statistical software and can be copied and then pasted into an Excel spreadsheet. The predictor values for the new patient are entered in place of the variable names, and the calculation yields the brake reaction time that is predicted for this patient (0.74 sec).

Is the Prediction From Linear Regression Useful?

In the demonstration of multiple linear regression to predict brake reaction time in imaginary people with Parkinson's disease, we know the following:

- Multicollinearity has been addressed by removing the offending "correlated" variable.
- Slope of the model (the prediction equation or line of best fit) is different from slope = 0.
- Multiple $R^2 = 8\%$.
- A new imaginary patient's age, disease severity, and disease duration can be entered into the equation to predict brake time in seconds.

Thus, while the overall prediction equation is free from a preponderance of multicollinearity and has a slope that differs from 0, the amount of explained variance between predictors and the dependent measure is very low. This means that the prediction might not be accurate because as the values for each independent variable change, there is not a strong correspondence to changes in the dependent variable (brake reaction time).

Selection of Best Minimal Set of Predictors Using Linear Prediction Models

Regression analysis can be used as a tool to select the minimal set of best predictors for any outcome of interest. The rehabilitation literature describes many different approaches to variable selection, including forward and backward stepwise procedures (selected procedures covered in Chapter 9). While these procedures are popular and widely used, the max R_2 procedure is considered a superior alternative (also called "all possible regressions").[9] When 15 or fewer predictor variables are evaluated simultaneously, this procedure identifies the best model with the fewest predictors (e.g., the model where R_2 stabilizes and the addition of predictors does not improve predictive capacity). Variable selection using prediction models is addressed in Chapter 9. The focus of the current chapter is on the interpretation of regression models given a set of variables without regard to the variable selection procedure.

Once predictors are selected for the linear model, t-scores can be used to identify the most important predictors within the set (Fig. 8-7).

Logistic Regression: Overview Predicting Dichotomous Clinical Outcomes

Logistic regression generates a prediction model that is conceptually similar to prediction models generated by linear regression (see Fig. 8-1), except that the prediction

- focuses on a dichotomous outcome (e.g., target condition likely present or not)
- yields a prediction of risk using odds ratios (e.g., what is the risk that a patient with a certain set of signs and symptoms will actually have the target condition?).

Identifying the target and reference conditions in the data set is typically done using the codes 0 = Reference condition and 1 = Target condition. However, words can also be designated as Reference (e.g., develop disability = "No") versus Target (develop disability = "Yes"). The logistic regression equation is designed to predict the probability that the patient belongs to the target group.

The format of the prediction equation from *simple* logistic regression is similar to simple linear regression (**Fig. 8-8**). Both simple models use one predictor. In simple logistic regression, however, the outcome variable is the natural log of the predicted odds ratio (also called a logit).

The generic format of the *multiple* logistic model is analogous to the multiple regression prediction equation (**Fig. 8-9**). Both multiple models use multiple independent variables to predict a single outcome measure. As noted earlier, the outcome for linear regression models is usually a continuous variable, whereas the outcome for logistic regression is a dichotomous outcome.

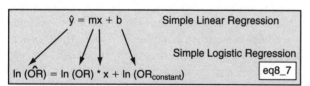

Figure 8-8 Analogy of simple linear (top) and logistic regression equations (bottom). Abbreviations: OR = odds ratio, x = predictor score, $\hat{y}$ = continuous outcome measure, m = slope coefficient, b = y intercept for the linear regression prediction line, ln $(\hat{OR})$ = logit, ln = natural logarithm. The constant in logistic regression is analogous to b, but logistic regression has no line of best fit (predictions are dichotomous and not made on a continuous line).

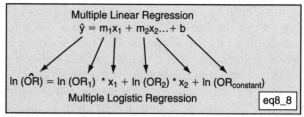

Figure 8-9 Generic formats for multiple linear regression (top) and multiple logistic regression equations (bottom). Abbreviations: see Figure 8-8.

Multiple Versus Simple Logistic Regression

The essential features of multiple logistic regression are the same as simple logistic regression. Both statistical procedures:

- generate a single predicted dichotomous outcome (dependent variable)
- distinguish between a *target* condition (e.g., return to work) and a *reference* condition (e.g., unable to return to work)[f]
- utilize the logit (the natural logarithm of the predicted odds ratio) as the outcome of the prediction equation
- have the decision rule that when predicted probability (the logit converted to a probability) is >50%, the patient is classified as likely to have the target condition or be assigned to the target group.

The primary differences between multiple and simple logistic regression analyses are

- multiple logistic procedures use more than one predictor (independent) variable
- the odds ratios generated by statistical software are "adjusted" or controlled for the remaining predictors in the multiple logistic model.

The statistic central to predicting the probability that a patient will be in the target versus reference group in logistic regression is based on the odds ratio (OR).

What Is an Odds Ratio?

An odds ratio is a statistic that measures risk.[g] For example, the risk of physical disability in people with

---

[f]Note that designation of the target and reference conditions is at the discretion of the practitioner. Once each condition is identified, the model predicts the target condition.

[g]Odds ratios are usually intended to determine the odds of contracting disease in exposed versus unexposed persons in retrospective case-control experimental designs (Motulsky 1995). ORs are also used as a measure of effect size between two treatment conditions (Sim et al. 1995).

sarcopenia (loss of muscle mass) compared with those with normal skeletal mass indices was reported to be 3.03 (95% CI; 1.21-7.61).[11] This means that people with sarcopenia are 3 times more likely to have a disability compared to those who do not have sarcopenia.

The 95% confidence interval indicates the range of odds ratios that could occur with theoretical replication of the study using different patients, thus accounting for sampling error. When the number 1 occurs in the 95% CI for an odds ratio, that ratio is *not* a significant predictor of risk. The rationale for discounting ORs with 1 in the CI is that the true value of the OR could be 1 as the study is replicated. In other words, a person with sarcopenia could simply be only 1 time more likely to have the target condition (in this case, disability) compared to those without sarcopenia, regardless of the magnitude of the point estimate. If an OR could be 1, then a finding of the OR adds nothing to risk prediction.

Odds ratios can be calculated from a 2×2 contingency table or by using simple logistic regression. When a contingency table is used, the OR is calculated by

$$Odds\,Ratio = \frac{AD}{BC} \qquad \textbf{eq 8-9}$$

where the letters A through D correspond to the standard cell labels for a 2×2 contingency table (Chapter 2, Fig. 2-1).

Using hypothetical data with imaginary patients, a 2 × 2 contingency table for calculating the point estimate for risk of developing a disability in a patient with sarcopenia is illustrated in **Figure 8-10A**. The calculation of the 95% CI for an OR is most conveniently done using statistical software **(Fig. 8-10B)**.

When there is a single predictor of the target condition (e.g., presence of sarcopenia predicting occurrence of disability), then the odds ratio is *unadjusted*. This means that no other factors are considered in the risk estimate and hence the OR is *not adjusted* for any additional clinical or demographic variables.

What Is an Adjusted *Odds Ratio?*

Just as with an unadjusted odds ratio, the adjusted odds ratio is an estimate of risk. When multiple predictors are included in a logistic prediction model, an odds ratio is generated for each predictor. These odds ratios, however, are adjusted so that the risk estimate is corrected for every remaining predictor in the model. For example, consider age and a baseline upper extremity function score entered as predictors of feeding ability (adequate versus not adequate). The odds ratio for the predictor variable "baseline upper extremity function" is corrected for age of the patient. In other words, the odds ratio for upper extremity function reflects the risk of having inadequate feeding behaviors *when age is held constant*. A convenient way to remember the meaning of the adjusted odds ratio in this example is to think of patients who have the same age before determining the odds ratio for baseline upper extremity function as a predictor of feeding ability. This process extends to age as the remaining variable in the model so that the odds ratio for age is corrected for baseline upper extremity function.

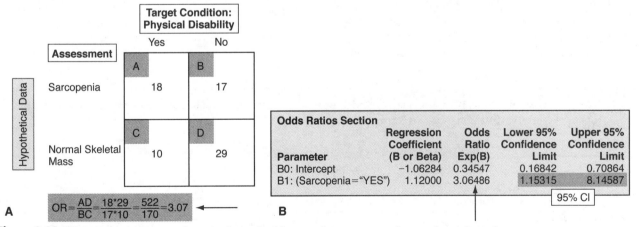

Figure 8-10 (A) Hand calculation of an unadjusted odds ratio (point estimate) using hypothetical data from imaginary patients. (B) Statistical software output that includes both the point estimate for the unadjusted odds ratio and the 95% CI. The parameter "intercept" is used in the model as a constant. The regression coefficient is the natural log of the odds ratio. Arrows highlight the OR point estimate for each method of calculation. Abbreviations: OR = odds ratio. Data set with imaginary patient outcomes is on the bound-in disk entitled "Ch8-Simple Logistic Regression." Modified from NCSS v2007.

Adjusted odds ratios are typically larger than unadjusted odds ratios because the unadjusted values reflect the control of at least one additional predictor variable. If age is added to the demonstration data set shown in Figure 8-10A, it can be seen that the adjusted odds ratio for sarcopenia's influence on the prediction of disability is reduced (from an *unadjusted* R = 3.07 to an *adjusted* OR = 2.77; Table 8-1).

Demonstration: Simple Logistic Regression

In this demonstration there are 74 imaginary patients who received an initial evaluation for sarcopenia and disability in terms of physical function. The distribution of imaginary patients into categories of presence and absence of sarcopenia as well as disability is shown in Figure 8-10A.

Logistic regression requires a precise definition of the target and reference condition. In this demonstration, the target condition is "disability = yes" and the reference condition is "disability = no." This means that the logistic prediction model will determine the probability that a patient will develop disability given the presence or absence of the predictor variable (sarcopenia). The predictor is coded 1 = sarcopenia and 0 = no sarcopenia.

Making the Prediction of Dichotomous Outcome

The simple logistic prediction model for this demonstration is

Predicting disability for imaginary patients with and without saropenia model for predicting disability = YES (target condition)

$$\ln(\hat{OR}) = \ln(OR) * x + \ln(OR_{constant})$$
$$1.12000224758764*(1) + (-1.06284383375115)$$
$$\text{Sarcopenia code} = 1 = \text{"Condition Present"}$$
$$\Downarrow$$
$$= 1.12000224758764*(1) + (-1.06284383375115)$$
$$= 0.057$$

Conversion of the predicted natural log of the OR to predicted odds:

$$\text{Predicted Odds} = e^{(logit)} \qquad \textbf{eq 8-10}$$

where the term "e" is the base of the natural logarithm.[h]

In this demonstration the predicted odds for developing a disability with sarcopenia is

$$\text{Predicted odds} = e^{\hat{x}} = e^{0.057} = 1.06$$

The large number of shaded digits following the decimal point is needed to enhance the accuracy of prediction. In order to make a "dichotomous" prediction, it is necessary to convert the predicted OR into a probability:

$$\text{Probability} = \frac{odds}{odds + 1} \qquad \textbf{eq 8-11}$$

The conversion of predicted odds to probability in the sarcopenia example is

$$\text{Probability} = \frac{1.06}{1.06 + 1} = 0.51 \; or \; 51\%$$

---

[h]On a scientific calculator, the key e^x is the base of the natural logarithm. Enter 0.057 as the logit in this example and press e^x; this will yield the predicted odds of 1.06. For spreadsheet applications, enter the function "Exp(logit)" into a blank cell without quotes. In this demonstration =Exp(0.057) will also yield the predicted odds.

Table 8-1	**Comparison of Unadjusted (A) vs. Age-Adjusted (B) Odds Ratio for Sarcopenia as a Risk Factor Contributing to Disability in Hypothetical Data With Imaginary Patients (Highlighted)**

ODDS RATIOS SECTION (REFERENCE GROUP: DISABILITY = NO)					
	Parameter	Regression Coefficient (B or Beta)	Odds Ratio Exp(B)	Lower 95% Confidence Limit	Upper 95% Confidence Limit
(A) *UNADJUSTED* →	B1: (Sarcopenia = "YES")	1.1218	**3.07**	1.15502	8.16304
	B1: Age	−0.05151	0.94980	0.87143	1.03522
(B) *ADJUSTED* →	B2: (Sarcopenia = "YES")	1.02006	**2.77**	1.02433	7.50879

NCSS output edited to show comparison of odds ratios. To reproduce this comparison, use the data set "Ch8-Adjusted OR" on the bound-in disk with either the NCSS or SPSS extension. Two runs are required; first with only sarcopenia as a predictor of disability as in Fig. 8-10B, and then with age added in the model as a continuous predictor variable.

The cut-point for dichotomous prediction is 50%. For a given patient, once his or her specific predictor information is placed in the predictor equation (e.g., the presence "1" or absence "0" of sarcopenia), then the outcome probability >50% means that the patient is best classified as "at risk" for the target condition (disability). If the resulting probability from the logistic model is <50%, then this predicts a likelihood that the patient will be in the "reference" group (in this example, the reference group is "no disability").

The outcome probability generated by the logistic regression model after conversion to a probability in this demonstration is 52%, so it is likely that this imaginary patient *with sarcopenia* is classified at risk for disability.

In the case where a different imaginary patient *did not* have sarcopenia, the logistic model is applied using "0" in place of "No" to show no sarcopenia.

Sarcopenia code = 0 = "Not present"
$$\Downarrow$$
$$= 1.12000224758764*(0) + (-1.06284383375115)$$
$$= -1.06$$

Conversion of the predicted natural log of the OR to predicted odds:

$$\widehat{\text{Predicted Odds}} = e^x = e^{-1.06} = 0.35$$

Conversion of predicted odds to probability:

$$\text{Probability} = \frac{0.35}{0.35 + 1} = 0.26 \text{ } or \text{ } 26\%$$

Using the 50% rule, the model predicts that this patient *without sarcopenia* does not likely belong to the target group because the predicted probability of having the target condition is less than 50%.

Goodness-of-Fit: Is the Dichotomous Prediction Useful?

Studies developing prediction models enroll and then assess patients so that the actual status of each patient is known before the study proceeds (see Fig. 8-1). The clinical value of the logistic prediction equation is based on the strength of agreement between the actual versus predicted classifications of the patients. Thus, the amount of agreement between actual and predicted outcome will determine if the model derived from the logistic analysis is a good prediction model.

At the beginning of the hypothetical study for this demonstration (Fig. 8-10A), note that the classification from clinical evaluations is not perfect. There are 17 imaginary patients who have sarcopenia but

without disability (Cell B). In addition there are 10 imaginary patients who have normal skeletal muscle mass but who also show disability (Cell C). Given this imperfection in the observed relationship between sarcopenia and the presence of disability, the question at this juncture is "how well do the *actual* observations of patient disability compare with their *predicted disability* status?"

In order to determine how good the model is for correctly predicting outcome, statistical software places the information from each patient in the study into the prediction equation, *one patient at a time*. The prediction for each patient, based on the 50% rule is recorded. Then the *actual* classification of the patient (has the target condition or not) is compared against the *predicted* classification **(Table 8-2)**. There is no widely accepted magnitude for percent agreement when judging goodness of fit. Practitioners, therefore, need to consider the statistical output in the context of the clinical problem that is addressed by the model.

Video Tutorial 8-2

Simple Logistic Regression Using Statistical Software

Application:
• Illustrates how to use statistical software to run a simple logistic regression analysis on a data set with imaginary patient outcomes, make a prediction of patient classification using the logistic model generated from that analysis, and also evaluate "goodness of fit" (how well the predicted patient classification corresponds to the actual classification of the patient).

Demonstration Data:
• *Ch8-Simple Logistic regression.***S0** (for NCSS)
• *Ch8-Simple Logistic regression.***Sav** (for SPSS)

Steps:
1. Open the *Essentials* disk and navigate to this chapter.
2. Select Video Tutorial 8-2: Prediction of Clinical Outcome: Logistic Regression.
3. First view how to run the analysis using statistical software. Then view the use of the logistic model to predict patient classification in Excel. Please note video demonstrates multiple logistic regression.

Software:
1. Verify that you have either NCSS or SPSS statistical software loaded on your computer and Excel.
2. Run the analysis illustrated in the video using the appropriate data set for the statistical software that you have installed.

Table 8-2	Goodness-of-Fit Contingency Table Using Hypothetical Data to Compare Actual Presence of the Target Condition From Clinical Evaluation vs. the Predicted Status of Target Condition When the Logistic Model Is Applied

CLASSIFICATION TABLE FOR OBSERVED ("ACTUAL") VS. PREDICTED ("ESTIMATED") PRESENCE OF DISABILITY

Hypothetical Data

		Predicted Outcome		
	Actual	NO Disability	YES Disability	Total
Clinical Evaluation	NO Disability	29	17	46
	YES Disability	10	18	28
	Total	39	35	74

Percent correctly classified = 63.5%

Data from Figure 8-10A. Highlighted cells indicate agreement between actual and predicted disability status. Output modified from NCSS v2007.

Multiple Logistic Regression: Multiple Predictors of Dichotomous Outcome

Earlier it was noted that the patient's prognosis can rarely be predicted with a single predictor variable in any regression analysis. The clinical reality that multiple factors influence outcomes of care or the classification of patients into categories that guide care will require that many factors are simultaneously considered in any prediction model. When multiple variables are used as predictors of a single dichotomous outcome, a multiple logistic regression analysis is used. For example, Benedictus et al.[1] studied people with traumatic brain injury and evaluated the influence of cognitive and behavioral impairment on return to work. Multiple logistic regression was used as part of their analyses because the predicted outcome measure was dichotomous (return to work "yes" or "no").[i] Predictors of outcome included a modified version of the Glasgow coma scale[12] and four scales designed to separately measure physical, cognitive, behavioral, and social sequelae for patients with different levels of injury severity.

Demonstration of Multiple Logistic Regression

In this demonstration, imaginary patients with traumatic brain injuries were evaluated to determine if selected independent variables could accurately predict return to work ("RTW"). In this example, the reference condition is 0 = unable to return to work, whereas the target condition was 1 = return to work. The predictor variables were

- Glasgow Coma Score (GCS; **Table 8-3,** lower scores indicate worse severity);
- Average Physical_Score (0-4, with 4 being non-impaired performance on selected activities of daily living);
- Average Cognitive_Score (0-4 with 4 being non-impaired cognition in terms of memory and visual discrimination).

The output in **Table 8-4A** shows that the Glasgow Coma Score is the only statistically significant predictor of assignment to the target group (those imaginary patients likely to return to work; "RTW") because the number 1 does not appear in the 95% confidence interval. When all variables are taken together to predict RTW, **Table 8-4B** shows that 72.4% of the cases are correctly classified by the logistic prediction model. The prediction equation generated by statistical software for this demonstration is

Estimated Logistic Regression Model(s)

Model For RTW = YES
(−.072701825794601*Cognitive_Score) + (.316095226692772*GCS) +

Table 8-3	Glasgow Coma Scale	
Behavior	**Response**	**Score**
Eye opening	Spontaneous	4
	To speech	3
	To pain	2
	None	1
Verbal response	Oriented	5
	Confused conversation	4
	Words (inappropriate)	3
	Sounds (incomprehensible)	2
	None	1
Best motor response	Obey commands	6
	Localize pain	5
	Flexion - Normal	4
	Flexion - Abnormal	3
	Extend	2
	None	1
Total Coma Score Range		3/15 - 15/15

Adapted from The Lancet, Vol. number 23;1(8017), Jennett B, Teasdale G. Aspects of coma after severe head injury. Pages 878-81. Copyright (1977), with permission from Elsevier.

[i]"No" indicated return to work at a lower level or not at all.

| Table 8-4 | **(A) Adjusted Odds Ratios from a Multiple Logistic Regression Using Hypothetical Data on Imaginary Patients With Traumatic Brain Injury.** Glasgow coma score (GCS) is a significant predictor of return to work (highlighted). (B) Goodness-of-fit using all variables in the model. |

(A) ODDS RATIOS SECTION (REFERENCE GROUP: RTW = NO)

Parameter	Regression Coefficient (B or Beta)	Odds Ratio Exp(B)	Lower 95% Confidence Limit	Upper 95% Confidence Limit
B0: Intercept	−2.60436	0.07395	0.00986	0.55453
B1: Ave_Cognitive_Score	−0.07270	0.92988	0.60202	1.43630
B2: GCS	0.31610	1.37176	1.10565	1.70192
B3: Ave_Physical_Score	−0.17967	0.83555	0.50006	1.39611

(B) CLASSIFICATION TABLE

		Predicted Outcome		
	Actual RTW	NO	YES	Total
Clinical Evaluation	NO	26	15	41
	YES	9	37	46
	Total	35	52	87
	Percent correctly classified = 72.4%			

Output edited to add clarity to labels. Abbreviations: RTW = return to work. Reference condition RTW = no.
Prediction model predicts target group, which is RTW = yes.

$$(-.179670577605 * \text{Physical\_Score}) +$$
$$(-2.60435937758944)$$

This equation predicts the likelihood that a patient will return to work given his or her scores on each predictor variable. For example, if the patient in question has:
Average Cognitive score = 2,
Glasgow Coma Score = 8,
Average Physical Score = 1,
then the probability that this patient will be in the target group is 0.40, or 40%:

$$= (-.07 * 2) + (.31 * 8) + (-.17 * 1) + (-2.60)$$

Logit	−0.40
predicted odds	0.67
predicted probability	**0.40** ← or 40%

This means that a patient with the clinical profile outlined above is only 40% likely to return to work and thus is classified as "unable to return to work."

Are Some Predictors of Dichotomous Outcome More Important Than Others?

The determination of which variables are most important in the logistic prediction model is based on a Wald test. This test evaluates the contribution of each predictor to the overall prediction equation and is a type of z-score (similar to the t-score evaluation of H_0: slope = 0 for multiple *linear* regression; see Fig. 8-7). The most significant predictor has the highest absolute value for Wald score **(Table 8-5)**; in this case, the Glasgow Coma Score (GCS) Wald = |2.87|. The probability that the GCS makes a contribution to the dichotomous prediction that *equals 0* is very unlikely at p = 0.004 and is considered the only predictor in the equation that adequately predicts a patient's likelihood to return to work (RTW).

Video Tutorial 8-2

***Multiple Logistic Regression* Using Statistical Software**

Application:
• Illustrates how to use statistical software to run a multiple logistic regression analysis on a data set with imaginary patient outcomes, make a prediction of patient classification using the logistic model generated from that analysis, and also evaluate "goodness of fit" (how well the predicted patient classification corresponds to the actual classification of the patient).

Demonstration Data:
• *Ch8-Multiple Logistic regression.**S0*** (for NCSS)
• *Ch8-Multiple Logistic regression.**Sav*** (for SPSS)

Continued

Steps:

1. Open the *Essentials* disk and navigate to this chapter.
2. Select Video Tutorial 8-2: Prediction of Clinical Outcome: Logistic Regression.
3. First view how to run the analysis using statistical software. The view the use of the logistic model to predict patient classification in Excel. Video also demonstrates simple logistic regression.

Software:

1. Verify that you have either NCSS or SPSS statistical software loaded on your computer and Excel.
2. Run the analysis illustrated in the video using the appropriate data set for the statistical software that you have installed.

Logistic Prediction Models: Validity

For logistic regression, multicollinearity can be assessed with a correlation matrix (Pearson product moment or Spearman rank; see Chapter 7). Predictor variables that show fair to excellent correlations with each other and also have low Wald scores that show nonsignificant contributions to the prediction model should be considered for elimination. With regard to evaluating the "slope" of the prediction equation against a reference of 0, conceptually, there is no linear prediction line because the prediction in logistic regression is dichotomous, not continuous. The use of R^2 (the proportion of variation in the outcome variable accounted for by the independent variables) is not recommended for logistic regression because of ambiguity of interpretation when adapted to logistic prediction models.[9] An alternative to this test for those uninitiated in statistics is to evaluate goodness-of-fit using the percent of patients accurately classified by the logistic model (see Table 8-2).

SUMMARY

- Regression analysis is used to predict patient outcome from patient classification.
- Linear regression predicts continuous outcome measures.
- Logistic regression predicts the probability that a given patient either has or does not have the target condition (a dichotomous outcome).
- In both cases (logistic or linear regression), the outcome or predicted variable is the dependent variable, whereas the predictor variables are the independent variables.
- When there is a single predictor, the procedures are referred to a *simple* logistic or linear regression.
- When there are multiple predictors, the procedures involve *multiple* logistic or linear regression.
- There is only one dependent (predicted) variable in linear and logistic regression covered in this text.
- Logistic regression uses a prediction equation where:
  - the patient's unique profile (e.g., his or her performance scores on various clinical assessments) is entered into the prediction equation (one patient at a time) to predict outcome.
  - the prediction results in the natural logarithm of the odds ratio (called a logit) that is converted to a probability score.
- Probabilities >0.50, or 50%, indicate that the patient is likely to have the target condition.
- Predicted diagnosis is compared to actual diagnosis to determine how well the prediction equation fits the outcome for each patient (goodness-of-fit).

Table 8-5	**Identifying Significant Predictors in the Logistic Regression Model Using the Wald Score (z Value) Calculated by Dividing the Regression Coefficient by the Standard Error of the Coefficient.** Note that the GCS has the highest absolute value of the Wald score that is also statistically significant with p <0.05 (highlighted).

PARAMETER SIGNIFICANCE TESTS SECTION (REFERENCE GROUP: RTW = NO)					
Parameter	Regression Coefficient (B or Beta)	Standard Error	Wald z Value (Beta = 0)	Wald Prob. Level	Odds Ratio Exp(B)
B0: Intercept	−2.60436	1.02794	−2.534	0.01129	0.07395
B1: AVE_Cognitive_Score	−0.07270	0.22183	−0.328	0.74311	0.92988
B2: AVE_Physical_Score	−0.17967	0.26192	−0.686	0.49274	0.83555
B3: GCS	0.31610	0.11003	2.873	0.00407	1.37176

Abbreviations: RTW = return to work. GCS = Glasgow Coma Scale.

PRACTICE

1. In a study by Buatois et al.,[13] they reported a risk model for recurrent falls in a population of community-dwelling elderly people. A portion of that model appears in **Table 8-6.** From the information given in this truncated table, calculate the probability of recurrent falls for each variable assuming each row in the table is treated as a simple logistic model with target group (recurrent fallers) = 1 and reference group (nonrecurrent fallers) = 0 .

Probability of Recurrent Falls

History of falling (coded 1) _____

Living alone (coded 1) _____

Medications ≥ (coded 1) _____

Sex female (coded 1) _____

2. Referring to Table 8-6, now assume that the model shown is the result of a multiple logistic regression. For a patient who does not have a history of falling (code = 0), but who is male (code = 0) and is living with someone (code = 0) and taking more than 4 medications (code = 1), what is the probability that this patient will be a recurrent faller?

3. Ng et al.[2] retrospectively evaluated the clinical characteristics influencing rehabilitation outcome in people with posterior cerebral artery stroke. The authors used multiple regression analysis to predict changes in functional independence from admission to discharge (the total FIM change score)[j] following rehabilitation. The variables that appeared in their prediction model are shown in **Table 8-7.** Which independent variables were found to be statistically significant predictors of the change in total FIM scores from initial evaluation to discharge from a rehabilitation program? (The constant or *y* intercept of the prediction line is not considered an independent variable.)

4. The minimal clinically important difference in the total FIM score from initial evaluation to discharge from rehabilitation has been reported as 22 points.[14] With regard to Table 8-7, assuming that a patient was coded 0 for female, that length of stay is days in rehabilitation, and that no interrupted stay (e.g., no temporary transfer to acute care) was coded 0:

   a. what would the predicted FIM change score be for an imaginary female who suffered from a stroke who also spent 10 days in a rehabilitation facility with *no* interrupted stay and with an admission total FIM total = 60?

   b. does the predicted change score reach the threshold for meaningful clinical change?

   c. if the patient's profile changed on only one variable (interrupted stay coded 1), what would be the revised predicted FIM change score?

Table 8-6	Risk Model for the Prediction of Recurrent Falls by Multiple Logistic Regression			
Variable	**Regression Coefficient (Standard Error)**	**P**	**Odds Ratio**	**95% Confidence Interval**
History of falls (yes)	1.55 (0.24)	< .0001	4.72	(3.00-7.43)
Living alone (yes)	0.56 (0.24)	.021	1.75	(1.08-2.82)
Medications (≥ 4 drugs per day)	0.51 (0.23)	.025	1.66	(1.06-2.60)
Sex (female)	0.48 (0.25)	.052	1.62	(0.99-2.65)
Intercept	−3.46 (0.24)			

Reprinted from Buatois S, Perret-Guillaume C, Gueguen R, et al. A simple clinical scale to stratify risk of recurrent falls in community-dwelling adults aged 65 years and older. Phys Ther 2010; 90:550-560, with permission of the American Physical Therapy Association. This material is copyrighted, and any further reproduction or distribution requires written permission from APTA.

[j]FIM is the Functional Independence Measure consisting of 13 motor and 5 cognitive items. Each item is scored 1 = total assistance needed through 7 = complete independence. Score range is 18-126, with higher scores showing less dependence on others.

Table 8-7	Multiple Linear Regression Analysis Model on the Change in FIM Score			
Variable	B+	SE	t+	P
Constant	3.585	14.829	0.242	.810
Sex	7.402	2.633	2.811	.006
LOS in rehabilitation	0.279	0.089	3.148	.002
Total admission FIM score	0.855	0.273	3.129	.002
Total admission FIM score (squared)	−0.007	0.002	−3.307	.001
Interrupted stay	−12.683	4.452	−2.849	.006

Reprinted from Ng YS, Stein J, Salles SS, Black-Schaffer RM. Clinical characteristics and rehabilitation outcomes of patients with posterior cerebral artery stroke. Arch Phys Med Rehabil 2005; 86:2138-43, with permission from Elsevier. Abbreviations: B = unstandardized slope coefficient, SE = standard error for the slope coefficient, t = t-score on the slope contribution of each variable (H_0: slope = 0), P = probability.

5. Duke and Keating[3] studied people with hip fractures in order to develop a predictive model for determining prognosis for independence of transfers and ambulation 2 weeks following corrective surgery. The results of one of their logistic prediction models are shown in **Table 8-8.**

Functional independence 2 weeks postsurgery was predicted using:

Logit = −2.7411 + 3.6889 (distance walked dichotomized) − 2.0422 (supine-to-sit)

where distance walked was coded either "1" for <2 m or "2" ≥2 m supine-to-sit was rated as "1" (maximal assist or worse) or "2" (moderate assist or better), and Logit is the natural log of the predicted odds ratio for ambulation independence.

A caregiver wants to know the prognosis of his or her relative who received surgry for a hip fracture

a. for an imaginary patient evaluated 2 days following surgery who was not able to walk more than 2 m but was able to move from supine to sit with moderate assistance, what was the probability that this patient would be independent 2 weeks following surgery?

b. if the patient in 5a was able to walk >2 m as well as move with moderate assistance from supine to sit, what would be the revised prediction of functional independence at 2 weeks postsurgery?

Table 8-8	Logistic Regression Analysis of Mobility 2 Days Following Surgery for People With Hip Fractures. The predictors of independence in transfers and ambulation 2 weeks following the surgery.				
Variable	OR	95% CI	P	Classification Accuracy (%)	
Transfer supine to sitting (0-2, 3-6)	0.13	.02-.93	.04	86	
Distance walked (<2 m, >2 m)	40.00	4.12-398.47	.00		

Reprinted from Arch Phys Med Rehabil 2002; 83, Duke RG, Keating JL. An investigation of factors predictive of independence in transfers and ambulation after hip fracture. Pp. 158-64 copyright 2002 with permission from Elsevier.

Transfer from supine to sitting was measured using a 7-point Iowa Level of Assistance Scale (higher scores = more independent).

REFERENCES

1. Benedictus MR, Spikman JM, van der Naalt J. Cognitive and behavioral impairment in traumatic brain injury related to outcome and return to work. Arch Phys Med Rehabil 2010; 91:1436-1441.

2. Ng YS, Stein J, Salles SS, et al. Clinical characteristics and rehabilitation outcomes of patients with posterior cerebral artery stroke. Arch Phys Med Rehabil 2005; 86:2138-2143.

3. Duke RG, Keating JL. An investigation of factors predictive of independence in transfers and ambulation after hip fracture. Arch Phys Med Rehabil 2002; 83:158-164.

4. MRC CRASH Trial Collaborators, Perel P, Arango M, Clayton T, et al. Predicting outcome after traumatic brain injury: practical prognostic models based on large cohort of international patients. Brit Med J 2008; 336:425-429.

5. Black K, Zafonte R, Mills S, et al. Sitting balance following brain injury: does it predict outcome? Brain Injury 2000; 14:141-152.

6. Singh R, Pentland B, Hunter J, et al. Parkinson's disease and driving ability. J Neurol Neurosurg Psychiatry 2007; 78:363-366.

7. Goetz CG, Poewe W, Rascol O, et al. Movement Disorder Society Task Force Report on the Hoehn and Yahr Staging Scale: Status and Recommendations. Movement Disorders 2004; 19:1020-1028.

8. Hoehn M, Yahr M. Parkinsonism: onset, progression and mortality. Neurology 1967; 17:1049-1055.

9. Hinze J. NCSS Help System. Kaysville, UT: NCSS, 2007.

10. Portney LG, Watkins MP. Foundations of Clinical Research: Applications to Practice. Princeton, NJ: Prentice-Hall, 2000.

11. Chien M-Y, Kuo H-K, Wu Y-T. Sarcopenia, cardiopulmonary fitness, and physical disability in community-dwelling elderly people. Phys Ther 2010; 90:1277-1287.

12. Jennett B, Teasdale G. Aspects of coma after severe head injury. Lancet 1977; Apr 23; 1(8017):878-881.

13. Buatois S, Perret-Guillaume C, Gueguen R, et al. A simple clinical scale to stratify risk of recurrent falls in community-dwelling adults aged 65 years and older. Phys Ther 2010; 90:550-560.

14. Beninato M, Gill-Body KM, Salles S, et al. Determination of the minimal clinically important difference in the FIM instrument in patients with stroke. Arch Phys Med Rehabil 2006; 87:32-39.

Chapter 9

Identifying Responders to Rehabilitation Interventions

Clinical Questions
- What is a clinical decision rule?
- Can clinical decision rules be used to classify patients in a manner that guides care?
- Is there a way to identify people who are likely to respond to a particular type of rehabilitation treatment ("responders")?

Introduction

Beattie and Nelson[1] describe clinical prediction rules (CPRs) as a way to combine relevant clinical findings to calculate the numeric probability of the presence of a specific disorder or likelihood of a clinical outcome. Since most of the clinically important information is incorporated into the CPR score, clinical efficiency and diagnostic accuracy can be improved from the use of a validated CPR.[2]

Common uses of CPRs are to assist practitioners in

- *Making a diagnosis,*
- *Developing a prognosis,* or
- *Classifying patients* into categories that are intended to guide care.[1,3-6]

In Chapter 3, the validity of a single diagnostic test was evaluated using sensitivity, specificity, and likelihood ratios. Diagnostic certainty was measured in terms of posttest probabilities. In practice, clinicians often rely on a battery of tests rather than a single clinical test to determine if the patient has a particular diagnosis, prognosis, or classification. CPRs address the potential inaccuracy of using a single diagnostic measure by incorporating multiple tests or clinical observations that guide clinical decision making.

Prediction Rule Versus Decision Rule

Recently, a distinction has been made between a *prediction* rule and a *decision* rule.[1,6]

A clinical prediction rule provides a score that represents the probability of outcome.[6] As such, prediction rules do not dictate a specific clinical intervention. Clinical decision rules (CDRs), however, are directive and explicitly recommend a precise plan of action.

The contrast between a prediction rule and a decision rule is illustrated by comparing the rule for determining the probability of deep venous thrombosis[7-9] and the Ottawa Ankle Rule.[10] The rule for deep vein thrombosis provides a score with a risk rating of "low," "moderate," or "high" risk for the target condition.[8] These classifications serve as an adjunct to clinical decision making without mandating how the patient should be followed or what subsequent interventions are necessary. The value of this CPR is that additional testing may not be necessary for patients diagnosed as low risk on the rule (in combination with a negative blood test), thus reducing cost and patient test-time burden.[11] For rehabilitation professionals, this CPR increases the awareness of risk factors for thrombosis and helps clinicians determine the urgency for patient referral where management of a potential clot can be pursued.[2] Thus, clinical judgment is enhanced with use of the rule, but the rule itself does not require a particular intervention. The Ottawa Ankle rule,[10] however, directs the clinician to a specific intervention (e.g., to acquire x-rays of the ankle and foot) depending upon the pain/tenderness profile of the injured client. When a CPR guides the care of the patient, it is called a CDR.

In rehabilitation practice, CPRs are designed to predict the presence of pathology (e.g., carpal tunnel syndrome)[12] or, through regression analyses, the prognosis of the patient (Chapter 8). The probability of a *diagnosis* or prognosis generated from a CPR is based on a set of clinical signs and symptoms with the greatest predictive value. In these situations, identifying the "responders" to a particular type of treatment is not relevant. When a CDR is used, however, the focus turns to *patient classification* based on a clinical profile that predicts the likelihood that a patient will respond to treatment (classified as a "responder") in a way that is distinct from nonresponders to therapy.[3,13-18]

Reilly et al.[6] indicate that decision rules can be derived from prediction rules. The process of validating a clinical decision (intervention), however, entails the support of efficacy studies (randomized controlled trials) and systematic reviews that confirm the value of the intervention.[3] Discussion about the merits of specific decision rules is beyond the scope of this primer, because debates about clinical practice standards require a specialty and practice-specific context. The fundamental aspects and statistical concepts used to develop CDRs to guide the care of the patient, however, will be addressed here.

The Need for Clinical Rules: One Size Does Not Fit All

Practitioners will often find contradictory or ambiguous results in the literature regarding the efficacy of rehabilitation interventions. One potential reason for equivocal findings of treatment efficacy is the lack of patient classification into relevant subgroups based on clinical signs and symptoms.[13,16,19,20] When the same treatment is applied to all patients who have stroke or all patients who have back pain, for example, specific patient profiles are ignored, and those who respond to treatment may be lost in the average of those who do not respond. Several clinical researchers have argued for patient classification systems so that specific treatments can be tailored to patients with a specific clinical profile (see, for example, Scheets et al.,[20] Fritz et al.,[19] Maluf et al.,[21] Alonso-Blanco et al.,[13] and Cleland et al.[15]). The goal is to use clinical rules to place the patient in a certain category of intervention that will guide the development of a treatment program. As noted in Chapter 6, misclassification (or no classification) of the patient might reduce efficacy of care,[14,19] but this assumption has not yet been systematically validated for many classification schemes.

Steps in Developing CDRs: Overview

There are three steps to developing a CDR (**Fig. 9-1**).[3] First, the clinician identifies a comprehensive set of factors that have predictive value. These factors might include certain aspects of health history, performance on selected clinical assessment tools at the time of initial evaluation, or the patient's expectations of outcome.[1]

Before the rule can be used in the clinic, it must be validated by testing its accuracy in different clinical environments where it is used by clinicians with a range of experience.[5] There are four levels of validation (**Table 9-1**). Level 1 is the strongest validation, whereas level 4 is the weakest. The validation process at the strongest level (level 1) addresses the question: Does the rule change clinician behavior or improve patient outcome?

Deriving Clinical Rules With the Highest Predictive Value

Deriving a minimal set of the best clinical predictors is important because evaluating every historical item

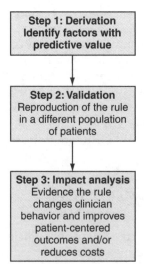

Figure 9-1 Steps in the development of a clinical prediction rule. These steps may also be applied to the development of CDRs. Step 1 is highlighted as the focus of this chapter. (Adapted from Childs JD, Cleland JA. Development and application of clinical prediction rules to improve decision making in physical therapist practice. Phys Ther 2006; 86: 122–131, with permission of the American Physical Therapy Association. This material is copyrighted, and any further reproduction or distribution requires written permission from APTA.)

Table 9-1	Levels of Validation for CPRs		
Level of Validation	**What Was Done to Validate?**	**Appropriate Use of Clinical Decision Rule**	**Strength of Validation**
4	Derived but not validated or validated only in retrospective databases, or by statistical techniques	Rules that need further evaluation before they can be applied clinically	*Weak*
3	Validated in only 1 narrow prospective sample	Rules that clinicians may consider using with caution and only if patients in the study are similar to those in the clinician's clinical setting	
2	Demonstrated accuracy in either 1 large prospective study including a broad spectrum of patients and clinicians or validated in several smaller settings that differ from one another	Rules that can be used in various settings with confidence in their accuracy	
1	At least 1 prospective validation in a different population and 1 impact analysis, demonstrating change in clinician behavior with beneficial consequences	Rules that can be used in a wide variety of settings with confidence that they can change clinician behavior and improve patient outcomes	*Strong*

Adapted from McGinn T, Wyer P, Wisnivesky J, Devereaux PJ, Stiell I, Richardson S, Guyatt G. Chapter 17.4. Clinical prediction rules. Table 17.4-1. In: Guyatt G, Rennie D, Meade MO, Cook DJ, eds. Users' Guides to the Medical Literature: A Manual for Evidence-Based Clinical Practice. 2nd ed. New York: McGraw-Hill, 2008.

and performing every possible physical exam is inefficient and could lead to inaccurate results.[22] The process begins by identifying the broadest set of potentially relevant clinical attributes.

- *Comprehensive Pool of Predictors* **(Fig. 9-2A):** Extensive clinician input is required to ensure that all important predictors are included at the beginning of the derivation process.[5] Reliability for each variable must be established before considering any potential measure for inclusion in the rule. If agreement about the patient's functional level among therapists is poor when a particular clinical test is applied, then the possibility of misclassifying the patient is magnified due to random error (factors not related to patient status, such as skill or experience of the clinician; see Chapter 6).
- *Cursory Evaluation of Predictive Capacity* **(Fig. 9-2B):** Authors differ on how they evaluate the predictive capacity of clinical measures. In some cases, likelihood ratios have been calculated for each potential predictor. The goal in using this procedure is to determine if the magnitude of the point estimate reaches a predetermined threshold for meaningful effects on posttest probabilities (i.e., +LRs >2; –LRs <0.5).[12] Others have used the finding of statistically significant associations

between the clinical measure and a criterion standard for response or lack of response to therapy.[17] Simple (univariate) logistic regression can also be used to determine the size and significance of unadjusted odds ratios to estimate the risk of having the target condition when each variable is assessed independently of the remaining variables in the pool (see Chapter 8).[23] At this stage, subjective evaluation of the predictive capacity for variable inclusion in the rule uses relatively liberal criteria (e.g., p values larger than 0.05). The use of confidence intervals will further assist clinicians who wish to modify the prediction rule based on selecting variables with statistically significant contributions to prediction of outcome.[23]

- *Narrow the Field of Predictors* **(Fig. 9-2C):** The comprehensive pool of variables is trimmed to yield a subset of factors with substantial predictive value. The final stage of variable trimming to derive the prediction rule can be accomplished with multiple logistic regression.[12,17,22,23] This statistical procedure was described in Chapter 8 as a method of predicting dichotomous clinical outcomes, but it is also commonly used during the development of prediction rules as a "variable reduction technique."[22]

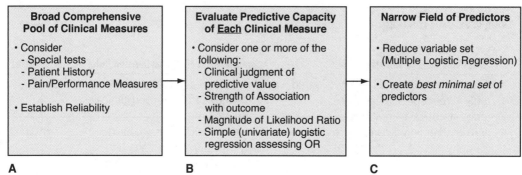

Figure 9-2 Steps in deriving clinical rules with the best minimal set of clinical predictors.
Abbreviations: OR = odds ratio

Identifying Responders Using CDRs

There are many examples of CDRs that are designed to identify responders to some type of rehabilitation intervention.[13,17,23,24] (See Childs et al.[3] for additional review.) The goal is to establish a clinical profile that the clinician can use following the initial evaluation to select an effective intervention strategy. Patients with a "responder" profile are predisposed to a high likelihood of successful outcome when a specific treatment is rendered. For example, Flynn et al.[17] developed a CDR that identifies patients with nonradicular low-back pain who have a high likelihood of improvement following spinal manipulation. They reported five variables that formed a clinical decision rule for patients with low-back pain who are likely to respond favorably to spinal manipulation (**Table 9-2**).

Patients in this target population need not be positive on all of the five variables in the rule. However, the likelihood that a particular patient will respond favorably to the intervention increases with the number of items included in the rule (**Table 9-3**). For example, if a patient enters the clinic at the initial evaluation and is positive on at least any three components of the rule, then that patient has a 68% probability of successful outcome following spinal manipulation. This probability is actually the post-test probability given a prevalence of 45% (see Chapter 3 for review of post-test probability and prevalence).

At the level of at least three positive traits, there is a sensitivity of 94% and a specificity of 64%. Sensitivity in this context is the number of patients responding to therapy according to the rule (Cell A) divided by the total number of "responders" identified by the criterion standard (Cells A + C; **Fig. 9-3**). Specificity for this level of traits present is the number of nonresponders identified by the rule (Cell D) divided by the number of nonresponders identified by the

Table 9-2	Clinical Decision Rule Developed by Flynn et al. for Identifying Patients with Nonradicular Low-Back Pain Who Are Likely to Respond to Spinal Manipulation[17]

Clinical Decision Rule	Target Population	Criterion for Success
1. Duration of symptoms <16 days	People with nonradicular low back pain with an initial Oswestry Disability Score at least 30%	>50% improvement in self-perceived disability
2. Fear Avoidance Beliefs Questionnaire Work subscale score <19		
3. At least one hip with >35° of internal rotation range of motion		
4. Hypomobility in the lumbar spine		
5. No symptoms distal to the knee		

Flynn T, Fritz J, Whitman J, Wainner R, Magel J, Rendeiro D, Butler B, Garber M, Allison S. A clinical prediction rule for classifying patients with low back pain who demonstrate short-term improvement with spinal manipulation. Spine 2002; 27:2835–2843.

criterion standard (Cells B + D). In this example, the responder criterion standard was a person who had >50% improvement in the Oswestry Disability Score (scale illustrated in Chapter 5, Fig. 5-3).

Likelihood ratios are calculated in the same manner as illustrated in Chapter 3. Large positive likelihood ratios without a "1" in the 95% CI indicate that being positive on a given number of traits in the rule will improve "diagnostic certainty" or, in this case, the certainty that the patient will be a "responder" to the intervention. Note the substantial jump in certainty between the +LR for at least three versus four traits

Table 9-3	Number of Predictors Present and Probability of Successful Outcome in a Clinical Prediction Rule for Patients with Nonradicular Low-Back Pain				
No. of Predictor Variables Present	Sensitivity	Specificity	Positive Likelihood Ratio	Probability of Success* (%)
5	0.19 (0.09, 0.35)	1.00 (0.91, 1.00)	infinite (2.02, infinite)	—
4+	0.63 (0.45, 0.77)	0.97 (0.87, 1.0)	24.38 (4.63, 139.41)	95
3+	0.94 (0.80, 0.98)	0.64 (0.48, 0.77)	2.61 (1.78, 4.15)	68
2+	1.00 (0.89, 1.0)	0.15 (0.07, 0.30)	1.18 (1.09, 1.42)	49
1+	1.00 (0.89, 1.0)	0.03 (0.005, 0.13)	1.03 (1.01, 1.15)	46

*The probability of success is calculated using the positive likelihood ratio and assumes a pretest probability of success of 45%. Accuracy statistics with 95% confidence intervals for individual variables for predicting success.

Reprinted from Flynn T, Fritz J, Whitman J, Wainner R, Magel J, Rendeiro D, Butler B, Garber M, Allison S. A clinical prediction rule for classifying patients with low back pain who demonstrate short-term improvement with spinal manipulation. Spine 2002; 27:2835–2843 with permission from Wolters Kluwer Publisher.

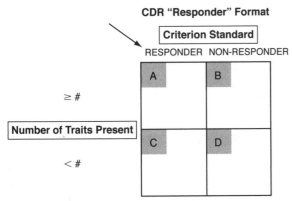

Figure 9-3 Visualization of a contingency table to evaluate sensitivity, specificity, and likelihood ratios for studies designed to identify responders to rehabilitation interventions. CDR = clinical decision rule; # = number of traits present (e.g., ≥3 and <3).

present in the rule (+LRs 2.61 vs. 24.38, respectively; see Table 9-3).

Demonstration of Clinical Decision Rule Derivation

A hypothetical clinical decision rule is derived in this demonstration to identify responders to a standardized exercise program. This exercise protocol is designed to improve function for imaginary people with osteoarthritis. Following a literature review to confirm reliability, the broad assessment of our imaginary patients included the variables shown in **Table 9-4**.[a]

Data for the imaginary patients with knee and hip osteoarthritis have been created artificially and have no link to any real study. Seventy-one imaginary patients were evaluated as a sample of convenience. All imaginary patients received the same exercise program. Some imaginary patients responded to exercise while others did not ("nonresponders" in the Group column in Fig. 9-4). The outcome measure for response to the exercise intervention in this demonstration was the total score on the Western Ontario and McMaster Universities Osteoarthritis Index (WOMAC).[31] This tool measures stiffness, pain, and physical function and is a condition-specific assessment for people with osteoarthritis.[31] The WOMAC total score was measured at the initial evaluation and again after 1 month of the standard exercise program. Lower scores represent improvement. If an imaginary patient achieved a 20% improvement on this index, then the patient was considered to be a "responder."[b]

A portion of the hypothetical data set is illustrated in **Figure 9-4**. Data are coded as condition present (1) or absent (0). For example, imaginary patient #1:

• Is classified as a non-responder (showed less than 20% improvement in the WOMAC total score from initial to follow-up)
• Has a Borg exertion score greater than 12 at the initial evaluation
• Has joint narrowing in the knee or hip joint space on x-ray at the initial evaluation

[a]In clinical practice the broad scope of potential predictor variables will likely include many variables. Only five clinical variables are shown here due to space limitations.

[b]The WOMAC scores are not shown in the demonstration data set. When subtraction of initial versus follow-up WOMAC total score showed ≥20% improvement in the hypothetical data, the label "responder" was entered into the Group column in Figure 9-4.

Table 9-4	Demonstration of Potential Predictor Variables for Responders to a Hypothetical Standardized Exercise Program		
Demonstration Variable	**Manner Used in Demo**	**Where to Read More About the Actual Clinical Test**
WOMAC	Criterion Standard Responder ≥20% improvement	Roos et al.[25]
Potential Predictor Variables:		
1. Borg Perceived Exertion Scale	Scores less than 12 indicate lower exertion levels during exercise	Borg[26]
2. Radiographic evidence of joint space narrowing	Imaging reveals narrowing or not	Wolfe and Lane[27]
3. Age greater than 45 years	Dichotomous (yes or no)	—
4. Assistive device used	Dichotomous (yes or no)	—
5. Pain (derived from VAS)	Dichotomous (high or low)	—
6. Gait variability	Dichotomous (yes or no)	Huang et al.[28], VanSwearingen[29]
7. Hip motion asymmetry on medial rotation	Dichotomous (yes or no)	Flynn et al.[17]
8. Mini-Mental State Examination Score	Scores less than 24 indicate cognitive impairment	Folstein et al.[30]

Here condition = Borg score less than 12.
1=present; 0=not present (so not present means Borg score is >12)

Here condition = Age>45 years
1=yes; 0=no (so no means less than 45 years old)

Patient_num	Group	Group_coded	Borg_Exertion_Scale_LT12	Joint_Space_Narrowing	Age_GT_45yrs	Assit_Device	Pain	Gait_Variability	Hip_motion_asym	Mini_Mental_GT-24
1	NON_Responder	0	0	1	0	0	0	0	0	1
2	NON_Responder	0	0	1	1	0	0	0	0	0
3	NON_Responder	0	0	1	0	1	0	0	0	0
4	NON_Responder	0	0	1	0	1	0	0	0	0
5	NON_Responder	0	0	1	0	0	1	0	0	0
6	NON_Responder	0	1	1	0	0	0	0	0	0
7	NON_Responder	0	0	1	1	1	0	0	0	0
8	NON_Responder	0	0	1	1	1	0	0	0	0
9	NON_Responder	0	0	0	1	1	0	0	0	0
10	NON_Responder	0	0	0	1	1	0	0	0	0
11	NON_Responder	0	0	0	1	1	0	0	0	0
12	NON_Responder	0	0	0	0	1	1	0	0	0
13	NON_Responder	0	0	0	0	1	1	0	0	0
14	NON_Responder	0	0	0	0	1	1	0	0	0
15	NON_Responder	0	1	0	0	1	0	0	0	0
16	NON_Responder	0	1	0	0	0	1	0	0	0
17	NON_Responder	0	1	0	0	0	1	0	0	0
18	Responder	1	1	0	0	0	1	0	0	0
19	NON_Responder	0	0	1	1	0	0	0	0	0
20	NON_Responder	0	0	1	1	0	0	0	0	0
21	NON_Responder	0	0	1	0	1	0	0	0	0
22	NON_Responder	0	0	1	1	0	0	0	0	0
23	NON_Responder	0	0	1	0	1	0	0	0	0
24	NON_Responder	0	0	1	0	0	1	0	0	0
25	Responder	1	0	1	0	0	1	0	0	0

Figure 9-4 Hypothetical data, set up to demonstrate the statistical process that derives a clinical decision rule. Column headings show the labels of variables used in the analysis. Only a portion of the data set is shown here. The complete data set is found on the bound-in disk ("Ch 9-Clinical Decision Rule" with either the NCSS or SPSS extension). Codes 0 = condition absent; 1 = condition present.

- Is less than 45 years of age[c]
- Does not use an assistive device for walking
- Has a low pain score
- Does not have gait variability
- Does not have hip medical rotation asymmetry
- Has a Mini Mental State Examination Score less than 24 (impaired).

[c]In order to dichotomize a continuous variable for inclusion in the data set, a ROC analysis can be used. Refer to Chapter 4.

Predictive Capacity of Each Clinical Measure: Simple Logistic Regression

Univariate logistic regression has been selected here to determine the predictive capacity of *each* variable that is considered for inclusion in the rule. The Wald z test is used to determine if each potential predictor, standing alone, is a statistically significant predictor of patients likely to respond to the exercise program (see **Chapter 8** for a review of the Wald statistic). The Wald statistic (**equation 9-1**) in logistic regression is calculated as

$$Wald\ z\ test\ score = \left(\frac{Coefficient}{SE\ Coefficient} \right) \quad \textbf{eq 9-1}$$

where coefficient ("B") is the natural log of the odds ratio (akin to the slope in a linear regression model) and SE is the standard error of B. The Wald z probability approximates a normal distribution[32] and can be estimated using Table B-1 (Appendix B). For example, a Wald z score of 2.87 covers 0.4979 of the area from 0 to z in Table B-1 and thus has a probability occurring by chance of (0.5 – 0.4979), or 0.002 at each tail of the normal curve.

The critical p value for this stage of rule derivation is set at p <0.10 instead of the standard p value of 0.05. This is done to loosen the threshold for variable inclusion in the rule and tends to allow a broader list of predictor variables for consideration. Using the critical p <0.10, variables are identified as candidate to be evaluated in the next stage of variable reduction (**Table 9-5**). Note that the only variable not passing the univariate test as a significant predictor of responders at the stage of the variable elimination process is age.

Narrow the Field of Predictors: Multiple Logistic Regression

All remaining variables are now entered into a multiple logistic regression to determine if the model has the best minimal set of predictors. The multiple logistic regression described in Chapter 8 was used strictly to generate a prediction equation without regard to the selection of the best predictors. Here, a variable selection routine will be added to the multiple logistic analysis that will yield the best minimal subset of predictor variables for the decision rule.

There is a change in both the magnitude and statistical significance of odds ratios when making the transition from a univariate logistic analysis (which produces an unadjusted odds ratio) to a multivariate logistic analysis (which creates adjusted odds ratios). This happens because each variable in the multivariate analysis is evaluated with respect to all of the other variables in that analysis. In other words, the multivariate analysis looks at the group of variables entered and adds or removes variables to find the best subgroup.

There are many ways to add or remove variables in the final stage of decision-rule formation. Some authors narrow the field of predictors using "backward steps."[13] This method starts with all variables from the previous stage (e.g., see Table 9-5 with age removed) and then removes variables one at a time to determine which subgroup has the best predictive capacity. Another option is to start with no variables and add one at a time until the best subgroup of variables is identified ("forward steps").[17,33] In order to avoid removing a reasonable predictor variable in either case, the critical p value for variable removal from the model is typically larger than 0.05.

In this demonstration analysis, a *forward stepwise procedure* was coupled with the multiple logistic regression to narrow the field of predictors to a final optimal set of the fewest variables (**Fig. 9-5**). The

---

Table 9-5	**Separate Univariate Logistic Regression Analysis Used to Analyze Each Potential Predictor Variable for Predicting Responders to a Hypothetical Standardized ExerciseProgram in an Imaginary Sample of Patients with Osteoarthritis.**

Critical p value for inclusion in the rule at this stage is p <0.10. The variable age (highlighted) does not meet the p value threshold for inclusion in the rule.

Potential Predictor Variable	Wald Test Value	Wald Probability Level**	Unadjusted Odds Ratio
Borg Exertion Score	2.87	0.004	4.30
Joint space narrowing	1.69	0.090	2.49
Age	0.85	0.396*	1.53
Assistive device	2.63	0.009	4.63
Pain	3.23	0.001	5.71
Gait variability	4.51	0.000	15.66
Hip motion asymmetry	4.60	0.000	26.40
Mini-Mental State Examination Score	4.65	0.000	16.50

*Variable has p >0.10 and will be excluded from the pool.
**Two-tailed probabilities

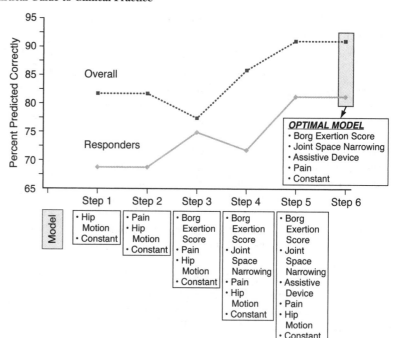

Figure 9-5 Goodness-of-fit (percent of correctly identified patients overall and responders) as predictor variables are added and removed. Modified from SPSS v18. Note: The constant, akin to the y intercept in linear regression, is included in each model.

statistical output will show which variables have nonsignificant Wald test scores. The Wald p values will identify nonsignificant predictors in our responders. These "nonsignificant" variables are systematically eliminated one-by-one in a "*stepwise*" fashion, either by rerunning the analysis without the predictor that is *most nonsignificant* (having the largest Wald p value greater than the designated critical p value), or automatically by statistical software, depending upon the particular software package that is used. In this demonstration, variables needed to have a Wald p value of ≤ 0.05 to enter the model and ≥ 0.10 to be removed from the model.[d] The iterative stepwise process continues until all variables included in the final model are statistically significant predictors of responders. A significant predictor in this phase of the variable elimination process is based on the adjusted and liberal p value <0.10. This means that in order to remove a potential predictor variable from the model, the p value for that variable must be >0.10 (Table 9-5). This process allows researchers to be very "inclusive" and keep potentially important predictors by using a high threshold for elimination from the model.

Goodness-of-Fit and the Optimal Clinical Decision Rule

The concept of finding the best minimal set of responder predictors can be visualized by noting the percent of correctly classified patients as variables are entered or removed from the model (see Fig. 9-5). At the start of this iterative process seven variables were considered (all predictor variables in the demonstration data set except for age). Gait variability and the Mini Mental State Examination Score were never entered into the model (both variables had Wald scores with p values >0.05). Now, with five remaining variables, the forward stepwise procedure evolves as illustrated in Figure 9-5.

At step 1, only hip motion asymmetry is entered. This model correctly predicts only 69% of responders and only 82% of patients overall (responders + nonresponders). As variables are added to the model at step 2 (Pain), step 3 (Borg Exertion Score), step 4 (Joint Space Narrowing), and step 5 (Assistive Device), the percent of patients correctly classified increases. At step 6, however, hip motion asymmetry was removed from the model. Since the percent correct classification in steps 5 and 6 is the same and the model at step 6 has fewer variables than the model at step 5, then step 6 produces the optimal *minimal* set of predictors of responders to the hypothetical exercise program (Fig. 9-5).

[d]Advanced statistical procedures use a measure called the **log**-likelihood to guide the selection of an optimal prediction model. Log-likelihoods transform very small likelihoods into large negative numbers that are more convenient for processing. A detailed discussion of this procedure is beyond the scope of this text.

Applying a CDR in the Clinic

Logistic regression equations are sometimes cumbersome to use in a clinical setting because the output of the logistic model must be converted to a probability of having the target condition (see Chapter 8). When a patient is evaluated, counting presence or absence of a specified number of predictive signs and symptoms may be more useful for determining the probability that the patient will respond to a particular type of rehabilitation. For example, Flynn et al.[17] calculated the probability of successful rehabilitation outcome by using the number of predictor variables present rather than weighting the importance of each predictor variable (see Table 9-3).

In the demonstration example, deriving a hypothetical CDR for exercise responders in a sample of imaginary patients with osteoarthritis, a four-variable model (not counting the constant) was derived (see Fig. 9-5). The number of positive traits in the CDR is counted for each patient. A ROC analysis is performed on each level of positive traits **(Table 9-7)**. The ROC analysis for this demonstration reveals that imaginary patients having at least three positive signs on the rule will have a 96% probability of responding to the rehabilitation intervention. The probability for success drops markedly when only two signs are present (51%).

Is The Rule Strong Enough to Justify Further Validation?

The question facing clinicians at this point relates to the value of the prediction rule. Do the magnitudes of the likelihood ratios justify further validation of the CPR? Fagan's Nomogram[34] can be used to estimate the post-test probability of an accurate CTS diagnosis by entering the positive likelihood ratio and assuming a pretest probability of success of 45% (review Chapter 3

for definition and calculation). **Figure 9-6** shows the amount of improvement in predicting a response to therapy that is realized by applying the rule at each number of positive signs. Note that in this demonstration exercise with hypothetical data, the post-test probabilities improve responder prediction accuracy about 51% in the best-case scenario (from 45% pretest probability to 96% post-test probability when three or more predictors are present).

If these data were real, it would be reasonable to conclude that the CDR for a standardized exercise program is highly predictive for responders to therapy. These results would justify further study to validate the CDR for use in clinical practice (see Fig. 9-1).

Limitations Addressing Validity of CDRs

The process of using unweighted predictors to identify responders differs from a logistic regression model because each predictor in logistic regression has an assigned weight. In other words, even when all predictors in the model are significant predictors for identifying responders to the intervention, some predictors may be better than others. For example, the Wald test score for the Borg exertion measure is slightly larger than the Wald score for joint space narrowing, even though both variables are significant predictors **(Table 9-6)**. If the logistic regression equation were used to predict "responders" to rehabilitation, then each variable has an assigned weight ("slope") that contributes to the prediction (see equation 8-8). When posttest probabilities are generated from the number of variables present, however (see Table 9-7, Fig. 9-6), the presence or absence of each variable carries the same weight as other variables. When three variables from a four-variable model are present at the patient's initial evaluation, for

Table 9-6	**Final Variables for Decision Rule Using Multiple Logistic Regression and a Forward Stepwise Procedure.** (Wald p <0.05 to enter and p ≥0.10 to remove from the model.) Column with Wald p values is highlighted. Note all final variables in the model have p values p <0.10. Output modified from SPSS v18. Abbreviations: B = natural log of the adjusted odds ratio, SE = standard error of B, Wald = z-score test of significance of each predictor, df = degrees of freedom, sig = p value.

MULTIPLE LOGISTIC REGRESSION						
	B	**S.E.**	**Wald***	**df**	**Sig.**	**Adjusted Odds Ratio**
Borg_Exertion_Scale_LT12	5.494	1.480	13.785	1	.000	243.246
Joint_Space_Narrowing	4.548	1.341	11.501	1	.001	94.438
Assist_Device	4.431	1.282	11.945	1	.001	83.993
Pain	5.887	1.614	13.300	1	.000	360.187
Constant	−11.954	2.776	18.544	1	.000	.000

*Wald values in SPSS are z-scores squared and are calculated using

$$Wald\ z\ test\ score = \left(\frac{Coefficient}{SE\ Coefficient}\right)^2$$

Table 9-7	The Probability of Success (Identifying a Responder to the Hypothetical Exercise Program) Derived From a ROC Analysis				
No. Predictor Variables Present	Sensitivity (95% CI)	Specificity (95% CI)	+Likelihood Ratio (95% CI)	−Likelihood Ratio (95% CI)	Posttest Probability*
4	0.25 (0.13–0.42)	1.00 (0.91–1.00)	Infinite	0.75 (0.61-0.92)	—
3+	0.81 (0.65–0.91)	0.97 (0.87–1.00)	31.69 (4.55–220.91)	0.19 (0.09-0.40)	96%
2+	1.00 (0.89–1.00)	0.21 (0.11–0.36)	1.26 (1.07–1.48)	0.00 (—)	51%
1+	1.00 (1.00–1.00)	0.00 (0.00–0.09)	1.00 (1.00–1.00)	Infinite	45%

*Based on a pretest probability of 45% and the +LR.

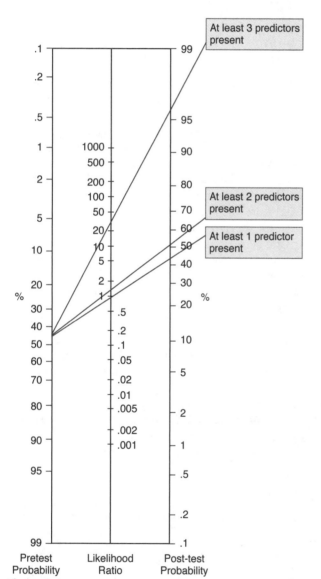

Figure 9-6 Fagan's nomogram[34] used to estimate posttest probabilities for each level of the clinical decision rule derived from hypothetical data in the demonstration exercise. (Reprinted and adapted with permission from Fagan TJ. Letter: Nomogram for Bayes's theorem. N Engl J Med 1975; 293:257. Copyright 1975 Massachusetts Medical Society. All rights reserved.)

example, this could mean that *any combination* of three variables would lead to a posttest probability of 96% in the demonstration (see Table 9-7).

Some CDR studies give the same treatment to all patients and evaluate the status of each patient on the rule.[13,15-17] This design identifies patients positive on the rule who are "responders." However, it does not necessarily demonstrate that the treatment is effective because the treatment was not a variable in the study. Hancock et al.[35] suggest that treatment efficacy must be evaluated along with status on the rule (allowing examination of the rule status × treatment interaction). Otherwise, if all patients receive the same treatment, it might be difficult to conclude that "responders" do better than "nonresponders" because of the *treatment*. Validation studies using randomized controlled trials (e.g., Childs et al.[14]) may alleviate this concern. Fitzgerald[36] presents options that would support either a one-study approach (a design that includes a rule status × treatment interaction) vs. a two-study approach (a study of rule status first following by a randomized controlled trial to validate the rule) to derivation of the decision rule. Others caution against the use of single-arm trials (rule status as the only factor) because this design detects measures of good prognosis regardless of the treatment.[36-38]

"Overfitting" can also influence CDR validity during the derivation process.[39] The problem of "overfitting occurs when too many predictor variables are used with too few participants."[39(p.643)] A guide for the minimum number of subjects per predictor variable in logistic regression is $n = 10$.[40] Thus, if the derivation of a CDR produces eight potential predictor variables, then the study would need 80 patients to support the validity of the logistic regression model that derived the CDR. One possible solution to overfitting is to select a pool of variables with some plausible relationship to the response to rehabilitation.[41]

SUMMARY

- CDRs are best used as an adjunct to assist clinicians in making decisions about treatment.
- Three steps are needed to develop a valid CDR: derivation of the rule, validation, and impact analysis. This primer has focused on derivation of the rule.

• The process of rule derivation involves the narrowing of a broad field of clinical variables to arrive at the best minimal set of predictor variables (see Fig. 9-2).

• Several factors may influence the validity of the CDR derivation, including the design of the study (single- vs. double-arm clinical trial) and overfitting the logistic regression model that derives the rule.

PRACTICE

1. Use the data set on the bound-in disk "Ch 9-Clinical Decision Rule" to generate a logistic prediction equation using the four best predictors of responders to exercise in Table 9-6.
   a. Show that prediction model.
   b. What is the probability of being a responder if the patient at initial evaluation has the following traits:
   Borg_Exertion_Scale_LT12—no
   Joint_Space_Narrowing—yes
   Assist_Device—yes
   Pain—yes
   c. Using a nomogram, a prevalence of 45%, and a +LR = 31.69 (see Table 9-7), what is the level of certainty that the hypothetical exercise program will result in a positive outcome?

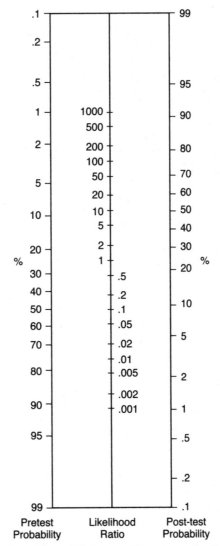

(Reprinted and adapted with permission from Fagan TJ. Letter: Nomogram for Bayes's theorem. N Engl J Med 1975; 293:257. Copyright 1975 Massachusetts Medical Society. All rights reserved.)

d. Comparing the answers to question 1b and 1c, does the use of multiple logistic regression in this case have a substantially different outcome compared to the "unweighted" analysis using number of traits present for the clinical decision rule?

2. Explain the difference between odds ratios generated by simple (univariate) vs. multivariate logistic regression.

3. Which statistical procedure translates the clinical decision rule into probabilities based on the number of traits present?

4. Use the data set *Ch9-Clinical Decision Rule* on the bound-in disk.
   a. Generate a ROC analysis of two variables present for the hypothetical CDR shown in Table 9-7.
   b. Then use the appropriate p calculator to generate sensitivity, specificity, and +LR point estimates and 95% CIs.
   c. What is the posttest probability of exercise success when a patient has at least two traits present on the rule?

5. Wald z-scores approximate z values for a normal distribution and are thus interpreted as z-scores. What is the probability that a Wald score = 0.85 occurs by chance in a two-tailed normal distribution?
   a. if an independent variable were evaluated as a potential predictor variable and had a Wald z = 0.85, would this variable be considered a statistically significant predictor?

REFERENCES

1. Beattie P, Nelson R. Clinical prediction rules: What are they and what do they tell us? Austral J Physiother 2006; 52:157–163.
2. Riddle DL, Wells PS. Diagnosis of lower-extremity deep vein thrombosis in outpatients. Phys Ther 2004; 84:729–735.
3. Childs JD, Cleland JA. Development and application of clinical prediction rules to improve decision making in physical therapist practice. Phys Ther 2006; 86:122–131.
4. Laupacis A, Sekar N, Stiell IG. Clinical prediction rules. A review and suggested modifications of methodological standards. JAMA 1997; 277:488–494.
5. McGinn TG, Guyatt GH, Wyer PC, et al. Users' guides to the medical literature: XXII: How to use articles about clinical decision rules. Evidence-Based Medicine Working Group. JAMA 2000; 284:79–84.
6. Reilly BM, Evans AT. Translating clinical research into clinical practice: impact of using prediction rules to make decisions. Ann Intern Med 2006; 144:201–209.
7. Riddle DL, Hoppener MR, Kraaijenhagen RA, et al. Preliminary validation of clinical assessment for deep vein thrombosis in orthopaedic outpatients. Clin Orthop Relat Res 2005; 432:252–257.
8. Wells PS, Anderson DR, Bormanis J, et al. Value of assessment of pretest probability of deep venous thrombosis in clinical management. Lancet 1997; 350:1795–1798.
9. Wells PS, Hirsh J, Anderson DR, et al. Accuracy of clinical assessment of deep-vein thrombosis. Lancet 1995; 345:1326–1330.
10. Stiell IG, McKnight RD, Greenberg GH, et al. Implementation of the Ottawa Ankle Rules. JAMA 1994; 271:827–832.
11. Wells PS, Anderson DR, Rodger M, et al. Evaluation of D-dimer in the diagnosis of suspected deep-vein thrombosis. N Engl J Med 2003; 349:1227–1235.
12. Wainner RS, Fritz JM, Irrgang JJ, et al. Development of a clinical prediction rule for the diagnosis of carpal tunnel syndrome. Arch Phys Med Rehabil 2005; 86:609–618.
13. Alonso-Blanco C, Fernández-de-las-Peñas C, Cleland JA. Preliminary clinical prediction rule for identifying patients with ankylosing spondylitis who are likely to respond to an exercise program. Am J Phys Med Rehabil 2009; 88:445–454.
14. Childs JD, Fritz JM, Flynn TW, et al. A clinical prediction rule to identify patients with low back pain most likely to benefit from spinal manipulation: A validation study. Ann Intern Med 2004; 141:920–928.
15. Cleland JA, Childs JD, Fritz JM, et al. Development of a clinical prediction rule for guiding treatment of a subgroup of patients with neck pain: Use of thoracic spine manipulation, exercise, and patient education. Phys Ther 2007; 87:9–23.
16. Currier LL, Froehlich PJ, Carow SD, et al. Development of a clinical prediction rule to identify patients with knee pain and clinical evidence of knee osteoarthritis who demonstrate a favorable short-term response to hip mobilization. Phys Ther 2007; 87:1106–1119.
17. Flynn T, Fritz J, Whitman J, et al. A clinical prediction rule for classifying patients with low back pain who demonstrate short-term improvement with spinal manipulation. Spine 2002; 27:2835–2843.
18. Stanton TR, Hancock MJ, Maher CG, et al. Critical appraisal of clinical prediction rules that aim to optimize treatment selection for musculoskeletal conditions. Phys Ther 2010; 90:843–854.
19. Fritz JM, Delitto A, Erhard RE. Comparison of classification-based physical therapy with therapy based on clinical practice guidelines for patients with acute low back pain: a randomized clinical trial. Spine 2003; 28:1363–1372.
20. Scheets PL, Sahrmann SA, Norton BJ. Use of movement system diagnoses in the management

of patients with neuromuscular conditions: a multiple-patient case report. Phys Ther 2007; 87: 654–669.

21. Maluf KS, Sahrmann SA, Van Dillen LR. Use of a classification system to guide nonsurgical management of a patient with chronic low back pain. Phys Ther 2000; 80:1097–1111.

22. Holleman DR, Simel DL. Quantitative assessments from the clinical examination: How should clinicians integrate the numerous results? J Gen Intern Med. 1997; 12:165–171.

23. Kuijpers T, van der Windt DAWM, Boeke AJP, et al. Clinical prediction rules for the prognosis of shoulder pain in general practice. Pain 2006; 120:276–285.

24. Iverson CA, Sutlive TG, Crowell MS, et al. Lumbopelvic manipulation for the treatment of patients with patellofemoral pain syndrome: Development of a clinical prediction rule. J Orthop Sports Phys Ther 2008; 38:297–309.

25. Roos EM, Klassbo K, Lohmander LS. WOMAC Osteoarthritis Index: reliability, validity, and responsiveness in patients with arthroscopically assessed osteoarthritis. Scand J Rehabil Med 1999; 28: 210–215.

26. Borg G. Perceived exertion as an indicator of somatic stress. Scand J Rehabil Med 1970; 2:92–98.

27. Wolfe F, Lane NE. The longterm outcome of osteoarthritis: rates and predictors of joint space narrowing in symptomatic patients with knee osteoarthritis. J Rheumatol 2002; 29:139–146.

28. Huang WNW, VanSwearingen JM, Brach JS. Gait variability in older adults: Observational rating validated by comparison with a computerized walkway gold standard. Phys Ther 2008; 88:1146–1153.

29. VanSwearingen JM, Paschal KA, Bonino P, et al. The modified Gait Abnormality Rating Scale for recognizing the risk of recurrent falls in community-dwelling elderly adults. Phys Ther 1996; 76(9):994–1002.

30. Folstein MF, Folstein SE, McHugh PR. Mini-mental state: A practical method for grading the cognitive state of patients for the clinician. J Psych Res1975; 12:189–198.

31. Martin DP, Engelberg R, Agel J, et al. Comparison of the musculoskeletal function assessment questionnaire with the short form-36, the Western Ontario and McMaster Universities Osteoarthritis Index, and the sickness impact profile health-status measures. J Bone Joint Surg [Am] 1997; 79:1323–1335.

32. Hinze J. NCSS Help System. Kaysville, UT: NCSS, 2007.

33. Hicks GE, Fritz JM, Delitto A, et al. Preliminary development of a clinical prediction rule for determining which patients with low back pain will respond to a stabilization exercise program. Arch Phys Med Rehabil 2005; 86:1753–1762.

34. Fagan TJ. Letter: Nomogram for Bayes's theorem. N Engl J Med 1975; 293:257.

35. Hancock M, Herbert RD, Maher CG. A guide to interpretation of studies investigating subgroups of responders to physical therapy interventions. Phys Ther 2009; 89:698–704.

36. Fitzgerald GK. Commentary (Stanton TR, Hancock MJ, Maher CG, et al. Critical appraisal of clinical prediction rules that aim to optimize treatment selection for musculoskeletal conditions. Phys Ther. 2010; 90:843–854). Phys Ther 2010; 90:856–858.

37. Maher CG. Letter (Childs JD, Cleland JA. Development and application of clinical prediction rules to improve decision making in physical therapist practice. Phys Ther 2006; 86:122–131). Phys Ther 2006; 86:759.

38. Stanton TR, Hancock MJ, Maher CG, et al. Author response (Stanton TR, Hancock MJ, Maher CG, et al. Critical appraisal of clinical prediction rules that aim to optimize treatment selection for musculoskeletal conditions. Phys Ther. 2010; 90:843–854. Phys Ther 2010; 90:856–858). Phys Ther 2010; 90:858–859.

39. Cibulka MT, Harrell FE. Letter ("Some factors predict successful short-term outcomes..." Mintken PE, Cleland JA, Carpenter KJ, et al. Phys Ther. 2010; 90:26–42). Phys Ther 2010; 90:643–644.

40. Peduzzi P, Concato J, Kemper E, et al. A simulation study of the number of events per variable in logistic regression analysis. J Clin Epidemiol 1996; 49: 1373–1379.

41. Hancock MJ. Commentary on (Cleland JA, Mintken PE, Carpenter K, et al. Examination of a clinical prediction rule to identify patients with neck pain likely to benefit from thoracic spine thrust manipulation and a general cervical range of motion exercise: multi-center randomized clinical trial. Phys Ther. 2010; 90:1239–1250). Phys Ther 2010; 90: 1250–1252.

Assessment of Outcome Over Time

Clinical Question
• How can I assess outcomes over time for a group of patients in my clinic?

Types of Patient Outcome Measures

Generic, disease-specific, and patient-specific assessments of rehabilitation outcome are used or have been recommended for use in many clinical settings (**Table 10-1**).[1,2] Disease-specific assessments are uniquely designed to determine the level of function for patients within a specific diagnostic category. For example, the Jebsen-Taylor hand function test[3] is intended for use with patients who have upper-extremity and hand disorders. This test evaluates a range of hand functions, including feeding, writing, and picking up small objects. Examples of other disease-specific outcome measures are outlined in Table 10-1.

In contrast to disease-specific assessments, a generic outcome assessment is designed to measure broad aspects of behavior that are common to any patient. The Short-Form 36 (SF-36) is an example of a generic health-related assessment that evaluates both physical and mental health of clients regardless of diagnosis.[4] In this generic assessment, the patient will answer questions like "does your health limit you in lifting or carrying groceries?"[4]

When the type of outcome is "patient-specific," the assessment of rehabilitation effectiveness is established through a collaborative process between the therapist and client.[1] A key feature of this method of outcome assessment is to simply ask patients at the initial evaluation to identify which areas of function they hope to improve over the course of rehabilitation. Patient-specific outcome is usually measured by patient self-assessment following the completion of treatment.

Why Manage Outcome Assessment?

The primary reasons for collecting and analyzing clinic-centered patient outcomes are quality-of-care monitoring, ongoing quality improvement, and reimbursement.[11,12] Third-party payors require documentation of patient function when the patient is evaluated, treated, and then reevaluated.[13] To qualify for cap exceptions to avoid specified limits in reimbursement, the Centers for Medicare & Medicaid Services (CMS) has mandated that the clinician must document all conditions and complexities that might affect treatment.[13] One way to satisfy this requirement is to use predetermined outcome assessments for patients entering the clinic.[8]

Selecting valid and reliable outcome measures for use in the clinic and collecting patient outcomes over time facilitate the assessment of changes in patient performance (**Fig. 10-1**). The psychometric characteristics of various outcome measures reported in the literature should be assessed by the practitioner when selecting the most appropriate tool for a particular clinical environment. These characteristics include diagnostic validity (Chapter 3), meaningful clinical change (Chapter 4), responsiveness of the tool (Chapter 5), level of consensus or reliability (Chapter 6), criterion-related validity (Chapter 7), and the feasibility or burden on the patient when applying the assessment.

The collection of outcomes data has been shown to be feasible for routine clinical practice.[14] Various recording forms have been advocated to systematically record important patient information (see, for example, Horn and Gassaway,[15] Guccione et al.,[8] or Granger et al.[10]).

Table 10-1	Examples of Clinical Outcome Measures		
Outcome Measure	**Description**		**Examples**
Disease-specific	Measures status related to a particular disorder (e.g., hand dysfunction, stroke, back pain)		Jebsen-Taylor hand function test[3] Unified Parkinson's Disease Rating Scale (UPDRS)[5] Fugl-Meyer Sensory Motor Assessment (stroke) [6] Roland-Morris Disability Scale (low back dysfunction) [7]
Generic	Measures health outcome regardless of diagnosis		OPTIMAL (Outpatient Physical Therapy Improvement in Movement Assessment Log)[8] Short-Form 36 (SF-36)[4] Sickness Impact Profile[9] Functional Independence Measure[10]
Patient-specific	Measures goals set by the patient (e.g., increase walking endurance)		Set by the patient and the clinician[1]

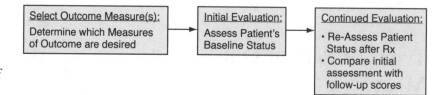

Figure 10-1 The fundamental practice of outcome assessment.

After collecting measures of outcome, practitioners can perform simple analyses of trends that provide a "clinic-centered" index to determine if groups of patients who receive treatment at a local facility show meaningful improvement following rehabilitation.

Assessing Clinical Outcomes for Groups of Patients

When all patients who enter a clinic receive the same assessment protocol, then assessment of outcome for that particular group of patients is done by comparing the initial score vs. reevaluation scores (Fig. 10-1). For example, all patients entering a rehabilitation clinic with a diagnosis of Parkinson's disease might be evaluated with the Unified Parkinson's Disease Rating Scale.[5] All patients with back pain might be assessed using the Roland-Morris Disability Questionnaire,[7] and all patients with stroke evaluated with a Star Cancellation Test for visual neglect.[16]

As an alternative to these disease-specific assessments, the clinic administrator might prefer a generic assessment for initial vs. follow-up comparisons of function. The benefit of selecting a generic assessment is that the same tool can be used to assess every patient entering the clinic regardless of diagnosis. This feature greatly simplifies an in-clinic outcome assessment.

One tool recommended by the Centers for Medicare & Medicaid Services is the Outpatient Physical Therapy Improvement in Movement Assessment Log (OPTIMAL).[8,13] This generic self-assessment tool measures difficulty and self-confidence in performing 21 movements that a patient needs to accomplish in order to do various functional tasks **(Fig. 10-2)**.[8] Each item is scored from 1 (able to do without any difficulty) to 5 (unable to do). A sum of the 21 items gives a composite score that can vary from 21 (best performance) to 105 (worse performance).[a] The OPTIMAL test first inquires about difficulty performing tasks and then queries patients about their level of confidence in performing each task (1 = fully confident in ability to perform task, 5 = not confident in ability to perform).

Demonstration Exercise: Patient Outcome Assessment

In this demonstration exercise, a hypothetical rehabilitation clinic uses the OPTIMAL tool for six consecutive imaginary patients entering the clinic.

[a]The most current version of this tool is available at the American Physical Therapy web link: www.apta.org/AM/Template.cfm?Section=Research&CONTENTID=36589&TEMPLATE=/CM/ContentDisplay.cfm.

Optimal Instrument

Difficulty–Baseline

Instructions: Please circle the level of difficulty you have for each activity today.	Able to do without any difficulty	Able to do with little difficulty	Able to do with moderate difficulty	Able to do with much difficulty	Unable to do	Not applicable
1. Lying flat	1	2	3	4	5	9
2. Rolling over	1	2	3	4	5	9
3. Moving–lying to sitting	1	2	3	4	5	9
4. Sitting	1	2	3	4	5	9
5. Squatting	1	2	3	4	5	9
6. Bending/stooping	1	2	3	4	5	9
7. Balancing	1	2	3	4	5	9
8. Kneeling	1	2	3	4	5	9
9. Walking–short distance	1	2	3	4	5	9
10. Walking–long distance	1	2	3	4	5	9
11. Walking–outdoors	1	2	3	4	5	9
12. Climbing stairs	1	2	3	4	5	9
13. Hopping	1	2	3	4	5	9
14. Jumping	1	2	3	4	5	9
15. Running	1	2	3	4	5	9
16. Pushing	1	2	3	4	5	9
17. Pulling	1	2	3	4	5	9
18. Reaching	1	2	3	4	5	9
19. Grasping	1	2	3	4	5	9
20. Lifting	1	2	3	4	5	9
21. Carrying	1	2	3	4	5	9

22. Thinking about *all* of the activities you would like to do, please mark an "X" at the point on the line that best describes your *overall* level of difficulty with these activities today.

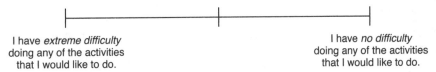

I have *extreme difficulty* doing any of the activities that I would like to do.　　　　　I have *no difficulty* doing any of the activities that I would like to do.

23. From the above list, choose the 3 activities you would most like to be able to do without any difficulty (for example, if you would most like to be able to *climb stairs, kneel* and *hop* without any difficulty, you would choose: 1. _12_ 2. _8_ 3. _13_)

1. ____ 2. ____ 3. ____

Figure 10-2 Outpatient Physical Therapy Improvement in Movement Assessment Log (OPTIMAL). Only the task difficulty assessment is shown. (Reprinted from http://www.apta.org/AM/Template.cfm?Section=Research&CONTENTID=36589&TEMPLATE=/CM/ContentDisplay.cfm with permission of the American Physical Therapy Association. This material is copyrighted and any further reproduction or distribution is prohibited.)

The tool is scored at initial evaluation and then again at the time of a follow-up assessment. The OPTIMAL outcome scores generated from this imaginary study are shown in **Table 10-2**. Note that only the task difficulty is addressed in this data set. If clinicians were to conduct the test in a real clinical environment, then both the task difficulty and the patient's level of confidence in performing each task would be rated.[8]

Questions 1–21 in the OPTIMAL tool are labeled in the data set **(Fig. 10-3)** as either baseline (BL) or discharge (DC) along with the question number (e.g., BL_Q1 indicates baseline evaluation,

OPTIMAL question 1). Questions that are not applicable to a particular patient are left blank.[b] This means that the number of questions completed by each patient will probably be different. For example, at baseline, patient #1 completed all 21 questions on task difficulty, whereas patient #2 completed only 18 (see the variable column "BL_Count_cells," Fig. 10-3 top panel).

[b]OPTIMAL questions 22 and 23 evaluate global status measured on a scale that differs from task difficulty and were not evaluated in the demonstration exercise.

| Table 10-2 | Paired Scores (% Difficulty of Task Performance Measured by the OPTIMAL Tool) for Imaginary Patients With Shoulder and Back Dysfunction Derived From the Raw Data in Table 10-2. Positive *difference scores* indicate improvement at discharge (more % disability minus less % disability = positive change score). |

		SHOULDER DYSFUNCTION		
Patient Number	% Difficulty Score at Initial Evaluation	% Difficulty Score at Discharge	Difference Score (Initial – Discharge)	Performance Better (+) or Worse (−)?
3	74	25	+49	Better
4	71	20	+51	Better
6	71	32	+39	Better
	Mean = 72 SD = 1.73	Mean = 26 SD = 6.03	Mean = 46 SD = 6.43	

		BACK DYSFUNCTION		
Patient Number	% Difficulty Score at Initial Evaluation	% Difficulty Score at Discharge	Difference Score (Initial – Discharge)	Performance Better (+) or Worse (−)?
1	77	26	+51	Better
2	23	21	+2	Better
5	67	20	+47	Better
	Mean = 56 SD = 28.73	Mean = 23 SD = 3.22	Mean = 33 SD = 27.21	

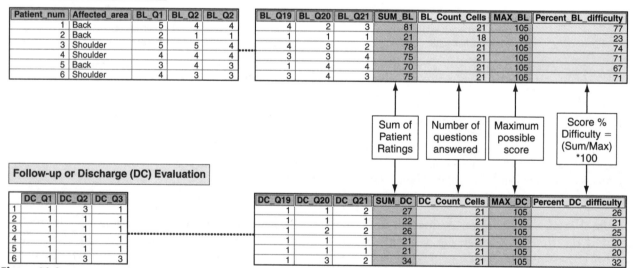

Initial Baseline (BL) Evaluation

Patient_num	Affected_area	BL_Q1	BL_Q2	BL_Q2		BL_Q19	BL_Q20	BL_Q21	SUM_BL	BL_Count_Cells	MAX_BL	Percent_BL_difficulty
1	Back	5	4	4		4	2	3	81	21	105	77
2	Back	2	1	1		1	1	1	21	18	90	23
3	Shoulder	5	5	4		4	3	2	78	21	105	74
4	Shoulder	4	4	4		3	3	4	75	21	105	71
5	Back	3	4	3		1	4	4	70	21	105	67
6	Shoulder	4	3	3		3	4	3	75	21	105	71

Sum of Patient Ratings → SUM

Number of questions answered → Count_Cells

Maximum possible score → MAX

Score % Difficulty = (Sum/Max) *100 → Percent_difficulty

Follow-up or Discharge (DC) Evaluation

	DC_Q1	DC_Q2	DC_Q3		DC_Q19	DC_Q20	DC_Q21	SUM_DC	DC_Count_Cells	MAX_DC	Percent_DC_difficulty
1	1	3	1		1	1	2	27	21	105	26
2	1	1	1		1	1	1	22	21	105	21
3	1	1	1		1	2	2	26	21	105	25
4	1	1	1		1	1	1	21	21	105	20
5	1	1	1		1	1	1	21	21	105	20
6	1	3	3		1	3	2	34	21	105	32

Figure 10-3 Data set showing OPTIMAL outcomes at baseline ("BL") and discharge ("DC") for 6 imaginary patients who responded to questions about their perceived level of difficulty performing 21 functional tasks. Each row corresponds to a single patient's response and each column indicates one of 21 questions identifying a particular task in the OPTIMAL tool. Data for task questions 4 through 18 are not shown due to space limitations. OPTIMAL questions 22 and 23 reflect global status measured on a scale that differs from task difficulty and were not included in this demonstration. (Download the entire data set "*Ch10-Optimal Outcomes*" with either the NCSS or SPSS label on the bound-in disk.)

In order to compare scores across patients, the scores are adjusted to the number of completed questions using the following equations:

(A) Maximum Possible Score = Number of
Questions Completed * 5   **eq 10-1**
(B) % Difficulty =
Sum of Completed Question Ratings/Patient's
Maximum Possible Score

The constant 5 is used in **equation 10-1** because 5 is the maximum score for each response in the assessment tool.[c] For example, maximal possible disability at the initial evaluation for patient #2 is:

Maximum Possible Score = Number of Questions
Completed * 5 = (18 * 5) = **90**   **eq 10-2**
% Difficulty = Sum of Completed Question
Ratings/Patient's Maximum Possible Score
= (21/90) = 23%

In contrast, using the same tabulation procedures (**equations 10-1** and **10-2**), patient #1 at the initial evaluation had 77% difficulty (81/105) in performing the tasks. These calculations are repeated for each patient at the baseline and in the reevaluation phase of their care.

Effect Size: Assessment of Treatment Effect

The effect size (ES) was first introduced in Chapter 5 as an index to measure the relative responsiveness of a clinical assessment tool (ES$_{responsiveness}$; see equation 5-3). In that context, the average change scores from a single group of patients (initial minus reevaluation) are in a ratio with the standard deviation (SD) of the initial scores. The rationale for the calculation is that the score difference across sessions, when normalized to the variability of the scores at baseline, provides a standard measure of the detected treatment effect. This measure, in effect, shows the number of standard deviations that the treatment effect is located from a reference point of change = 0. Depending on the scale direction (do higher scores mean more or less impairment?) and the method of subtraction (initial vs. follow-up or reverse?), the meaning of a positive or negative ES will vary. In this demonstration, a +ES indicates improvement from initial to discharge assessments.

In responsiveness research, a unique ES$_{responsiveness}$ is calculated for each assessment tool. The ES for one tool can be compared with other assessment tools administered in the same time frame to the same patients. The clinical tool with the larger

ES$_{responsiveness}$ is presumed to have better responsiveness in a descriptive evaluation of measurement qualities.[d] In other words, a tool that can detect a bigger treatment effect on the same group of patients is more responsive to measuring the value of intervention than a different tool that detects a smaller effect.[e]

For evaluating a treatment effect, similar logic applies. The initial vs. discharge outcome scores for a particular patient group can be compared descriptively using an ES index. This analysis is referred to as a *within group* analysis because a single group of patients is evaluated over *two points in time*. For example, if the clinical data set has outcome measures for patients with shoulder dysfunction as well as patients with back pain, a within group analysis might address the outcome for only one of these groups at a time. The within group analysis can be repeated with each patient group if deemed appropriate by the research question. In this way, patients with shoulder dysfunction can be evaluated separately from those with back dysfunction (Table 10-2).

The ES in the context of a group of patients tested twice is called a *d index* (or difference index).[17] The d index is one type of ES that can be used both descriptively and in a statistical test to evaluate the outcome of care. Descriptively, large ESs in relation to smaller ESs indicate larger treatment effects. According to Cohen,[17] the d index can be loosely described as either small, medium, or large according to the following convention:

Small ES = 0.20
Medium ES = 0.50
Large ES = 0.80

The formula for the treatment effect size is:

$$ES = d\ index = \frac{\text{Mean of (Baseline – Follow-up)}}{\text{Standard Deviation of Initial Scores}}$$
eq 10-3

In the demonstration exercise (see Table 10-2), the imaginary patients with shoulder dysfunction had an ES related to their average OPTIMAL scores:

$$ES_{shoulder} = \frac{72\text{-}26}{1.73} = 26.6 \text{ standard deviations}$$

The ES = 26.6 is considered a very large treatment effect (**Fig. 10-4A**). Clinicians could use this

---

[c] When patient scores are entered into an Excel spreadsheet, the number of questions that have been rated by the subject can be found by the "COUNT" function.

[d] This assumes that higher scores on the assessment tool = more disability. Thus, subtraction of initial-discharge scores is positive with improvement at the follow-up.

[e] Often, only the point estimates of ES are used in descriptive analyses, ignoring confidence intervals.

preliminary information to suggest that their approach to patients with shoulder dysfunction might prove to be very effective in larger intervention studies.

In contrast, the ES for imaginary patients with back dysfunction derived from Table 10-2 is:

$$ES_{Back} = \frac{56-23}{28.73} = 1.15 \text{ standard deviations}$$

An ES of 1.15 is still considered a large treatment effect by the Cohen Descriptive Scale. However, the treatment effect for imaginary patients with back dysfunction is markedly smaller than for patients with shoulder impairment **(Fig. 10-4A)**.

Small Sample Size and Bias

When calculating effect size with small paired samples ($n \leq 20$), there is considerable bias in the outcome. Specifically the d index shows an upward bias with small sample sizes.[18] The correction for bias specified by Hedges and Olkin[19] is:

$$d\text{ unbiased} = d\text{ biased} \left[1 - \frac{3}{8(n-1)} \right] \quad \textbf{eq 10-4}$$

As the demonstration effect sizes each have $n = 3$, the unbiased ES for imaginary patients with shoulder and back dysfunction is:

ES Unbiased$_{shoulder}$ = **21.61**
ES Unbiased$_{back}$ = **0.93**

The ES and the unbiased ES are compared for each patient group in **Figure 10-4A**. The unbiased d index or ES in each case is lower than the ES without correction for small sample size. It is recommended that the **unbiased ES** be used for patient samples with $n \leq 20$.[18]

Statistical Analysis of Treatment Effect

When clinicians use descriptive procedures such as the Cohen scale for estimating the magnitude of the treatment effect, the occurrence of that effect due to chance is ignored.

Statistical analysis of change in the patient group function allows the clinician to address the likelihood that the treatment effect occurred by chance. For a single group of patients (e.g., those with shoulder or back dysfunction in the demonstration exercise) the question is: did the patients improve in self-perceived function from the initial to the discharge evaluation beyond chance improvements? The initial evaluation provides a control or reference point for comparing the same patient's function at the time of reevaluation or discharge **(Fig 10-4B)**.

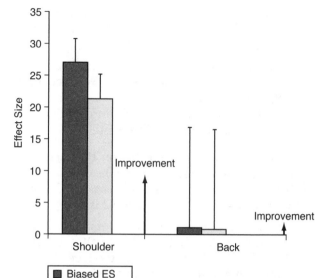

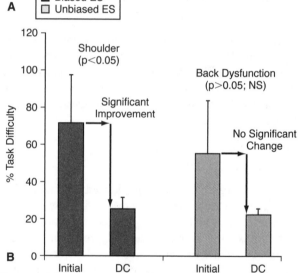

Figure 10-4 (A) Standardized ESs for each cohort (all positive ESs in this demonstration reflect improvement, but improvement for the shoulder cohort is much greater than for the back cohort). Unbiased ESs are ESs corrected for small sample *n*. Error bars are standard errors. (B) Statistical analysis—Subgroup changes on self-perceived task difficulty from initial evaluation to discharge for imaginary patients in the demonstration exercise. Lower OPTIMAL scores for task difficulty indicate less disability. Error bars are standard deviations. Abbreviations: DC = discharge, p = probability that the improvement occurred by chance, NS = not statistically significant, ES = effect size.

The creation of confidence intervals surrounding the ES provides essential information about the treatment effect by answering the following questions:[18]

1. Was the magnitude of the treatment effect significantly different than 0?
2. Was there a high level of precision when estimating the magnitude of the treatment effect

(the point estimate)? A confidence interval tests the hypothesis that initial and follow-up assessment scores differ significantly from 0. A 95% confidence interval for small samples of patients (e.g., $n \leq 20$) uses a critical t ratio that is similar to the critical z-score but adjusted for the number of subjects through a simple degrees of freedom (DF) calculation ($n-1$ for paired t-test, **Fig. 10-5**). The critical t ratio is used in a confidence interval for small samples **(eq 10-5B)** just as the critical z-score is used with larger samples (eq 10-5A) to define the area of the normal curve where the true results of the clinical test can vary due to sampling error (the error due to theoretical replication of the study using different patients from the target population).

The calculation of the 95% ES confidence interval for large and small sample sizes is based on the following formulas:[18]

Large Samples ($n > 20$)

95% CI

$$\text{Upper Boundary} = \text{ES} + (1.96 * \text{se}) \qquad \textbf{eq 10-5A}$$
$$\text{Lower Boundary} = \text{ES} - (1.96 * \text{se})$$

where "se" is the standard error of the change scores for the patient group and 1.96 is the critical z-score that corresponds with a two-tailed hypothesis test at $\alpha = 0.05$.

Small Samples ($n < 20$)[f]

95% CI

$$\text{Upper Boundary} = \text{ES Unbiased} +$$
$$(\text{critical t} * \text{se}) \qquad \textbf{eq 10-5B}$$
$$\text{Lower Boundary} = \text{ES Unbiased} - (\text{critical t} * \text{se})$$

where "se" is the standard error of the change scores for the patient group and t corresponds to the critical t-score for a two-tailed hypothesis test at a probability threshold or alpha level of 5% (written as $\alpha_2 = 0.05$) and at the appropriate df (Fig. 10-5).

For example, in the demonstration data set there are three patients with shoulder dysfunction ($n = 3$). The same three patients were tested twice (initial and discharge assessments). In this case of paired observations, $df = n - 1 = 3 - 1 = 2$. Thus, the clinician enters the table of critical t values at $df = 2$ (see Fig. 10-5). If

[f] t distributions, like z-score distributions, are standard scores "centered" around 0 (refer to Fig, A4-13). However, effect sizes are a ratio of difference scores and have a "noncentered" and skewed distribution referenced to the distance from 0. This distance is defined as $\Delta = d$ index/$\sqrt{N}$. When df is low (around 5, for example), visible skewing is not apparent until $\Delta = 2$. Therefore, the method used here is not a precise calculation of all effect size CIs. The approximation improves as df increases and as Δ decreases. For additional reading, refer to Cumming G, Finch S. A primer on the understanding, use, and calculation of confidence intervals that are based on central and non-central distributions. Educ Psych Meas 2001; 61:532–574.

df	Z score		t ratio	
	Critical z (90% CI)	Critical t (95% CI)	Critical t (90% CI)	Critical t (95% CI)
>20	1.645	1.96	Same as z	Same as z
2	--------	--------	2.920	4.303
5	--------	--------	2.015	2.571

A

df	α_2	.20	.10	.05
1		3.078	6.314	12.706
2		1.886	2.920	4.303
3		1.638	2.353	3.182
4		1.533	2.132	2.776
5		1.476	2.015	2.571

Enter the Table with appropriate df ($n-1$)

B

Figure 10-5 (A) Comparison of critical z- and t-scores for constructing confidence intervals. Abbreviations: df = degrees of freedom which are $n - 1$ for paired t-test, CI = confidence interval. Critical t ratios for other df can be found in Appendix B, Table B-2. (B) Arrows show the origin of two-tailed (α_2) critical t values that are used to calculate the 90% ($\alpha_2 = 0.10$) and 95% ($\alpha_2 = .05$) confidence intervals that test the significance of the effect size index or the treatment effect in original units of the assessment tool. (Table in B is adapted from StatSoft, Inc. (2010). Electronic Statistics Textbook. Tulsa, OK: StatSoft. WEB: http://www.statsoft.com/textbook/. Reprinted with permission from Statsoft, Inc. The online version of this table can be found at http://www.statsoft.com/textbook/distribution-tables/?button=3.)

a 95% CI is desired, then the column under alpha = 0.05 holds the critical t values that are used to form the CI boundaries. In this demonstration example, enter the critical t table at df = 2 and under the column $\alpha_2 = 0.05$ find the critical t value = 4.303. This will be the t value used in equation 10-5B.

The standard error (SE) was first introduced in the appendix to Chapter 4 (eq A4-4), and in Chapter 7 related to the kappa statistic. Additional details about the SE are discussed in the appendix to this chapter. In the current demonstration exercise, the SE is an estimate of the variability of difference scores (initial minus discharge OPTIMAL scores) for the universe of patients with shoulder or back dysfunction. If there is large variance of difference scores relative to the mean treatment effect, then the width of the confidence interval increases (reducing the precision of the point estimate or mean effect). In order to demonstrate a statistically significant change in the status of a group of patients from the initial to discharge evaluation, the CI should not hold a 0.

For this demonstration, the 95% CIs for the unbiased ESs in the shoulder and back group using equation 10-5B are:

ES Unbiased$_{shoulder}$ = **21.61**
95% CI (5.64 to 37.58)
ES Unbiased$_{back}$ = **0.93**
95% CI (–66.67 to 68.53)

The results indicate that there is a statistically significant treatment effect for patients with shoulder dysfunction, but not for patients with back problems (the 95% CI holds a 0).

Confidence Intervals in Clinic-Friendly Units

The use of the ES provides units that are compatible with a quantitative review or meta-analysis. These types of literature reviews use a standard metric (e.g., the d index) to combine the results of many studies. However, because the d index is unitless (it represents the number of standard deviations on a standardized probability distribution), the results may not easily translate into a meaningful clinical metric.

A 95% CI can be estimated that is clinic-friendly by keeping the original units of the assessment tool (in this case, the OPTIMAL tool). The components needed to calculate the 95% CI are found Table 10-2 (produced in a spreadsheet) but can also be generated in the output of statistical software **(Fig. 10-6)**.[g] The mean (SD) of the treatment effect based on the OPTIMAL assessment

for the shoulder subgroup of patients is a change of 46% in task difficulty (SD = 6.43%; see Table 10-2). The 95% CI is calculated by:

$$95\% \ CI \ for \ treatment \ effect = \text{Mean Difference Score} \pm (t) * \frac{SD}{\sqrt{N}}$$

eq 10-6

Lower Boundary of 95% CI = 46-(4.303* (6.43/SQRT(3)))= **30**	Point Estimate of Treatment Effect = **46**	Upper Boundary of 95% CI = 46+(4.303* (6.43/SQRT(3)))= **62**

The 95% confidence interval for the imaginary patients with shoulder dysfunction shows that the true change in function for the demonstration data set can vary from a mean change score of 30% to 63% on the OPTIMAL scale for task difficulty. The hypothesis of no difference would be supported only if a 0 were found in the interval. Because 0 is not in the interval, this means that the point estimate of a change of 46% on the OPTIMAL assessment represents a statistically significant improvement in self-perceived function. Note that the last term in **equation 10-6** is actually the SE (SD/√N).

For the imaginary patients in the demonstration who have back dysfunction (n = 3), the mean (SD) of the difference score on the OPTIMAL assessment for this subgroup of patients is 33% improvement in task difficulty (SD = 27.21%). The 95% CI for the group of patients with back dysfunction is (see equation 10-6):

Lower Boundary of 95% CI = 33 – (4.303 * (27.21/ SQRT(3))) = **-35**	Point Estimate of Treatment Effect = **33**	Upper Boundary of 95% CI = 33 + (4.303 * (27.21/SQRT(3))) **101**

Here, the 95% CI includes the value of 0, which means that it is possible the true result would show no improvement in self-perceived task difficulty (the initial task difficulty could equal the follow-up task difficulty) for patients in this subgroup. Therefore, the "large treatment effect" that was found when using the ES as a descriptive method of evaluating patient progress for imaginary patients with back dysfunction does not automatically translate into a statistically significant improvement in function (Fig. 10-4B). This means that the treatment effect for the imaginary patients with back dysfunction is not likely to be different from initial to follow-up assessment.

A calculator to check hand calculations of effect size point estimates and their 95% CIs is available on the bound-in disk (*"P_Effect Size Calculator"*). The

[g]Rounding errors create a slight difference between Excel outputs in Table 10-3 and statistical software output in Table 10-5.

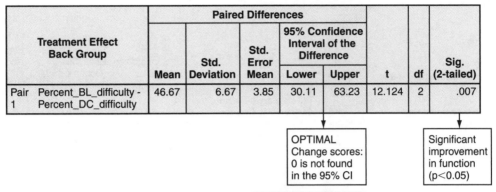

Figure 10-6 Within group analysis using a paired t-test and 95% confidence interval generated from statistical software (edited SPSS v18 output). Data filtered first for patients with shoulder dysfunction (A) and then back dysfunction (B). The dependent measure is the OPTIMAL % difficulty score at baseline ("Percent_BL_difficulty") minus discharge ("Percent_DC_difficulty"). (A) Results of paired t-test on patients with shoulder dysfunction show a 95% CI that *does not* include 0; thus a significant improvement in self-perceived task difficulty from initial to discharge evaluations (p value shows a low probability of occurring by chance). (B) Results of paired t-test on patients with back dysfunction show a 95% CI that does include 0; thus, no significant improvement in self-perceived task difficulty from initial to discharge evaluations (p value shows a high probability of occurring by chance). The data set on the bound-in disk is "*Ch10-Optimal Outcomes*" with the NCSS or SPSS label.

output of this calculator is applied to the back dysfunction subgroup of imaginary patients and is illustrated in **Figure 10-7**.

Precision of Estimating Patient Change

The precision of the 95% CIs for patients with shoulder vs. back dysfunction is measured by the width of each CI. Precision increases as width of the CI decreases **(Fig. 10-8)**. The range of possible values surrounding the point estimate is much larger than for the back dysfunction group compared to that of the shoulder group. Therefore, the precision of estimating the true treatment effect in the back group is low compared to the shoulder group.

Paired t-test: Same Patients Tested Twice

The *paired t-test* utilizes paired data (initial and follow-up scores) to calculate a difference score for each patient. The paired t ratio is the test statistic and the numerator is the mean treatment effect (similar to the effect size numerator). The feature that makes the t ratio distinct from the effect size is that the denominator of the t ratio uses the standard error of difference scores rather than the standard deviation:

$$t\,ratio = \frac{\text{Mean of (Baseline-Follow-up)}}{\text{Standard Error of (Baseline-Follow-up)}}$$
$$= \frac{\text{Mean of Difference Scores}}{\text{Standard Error of Difference Scores}}$$

eq 10-7

EFFECT SIZE CIs for Paired Measures on the Same Patients
(Outcomes may differ slightly from statistical software due to rounding of input data)

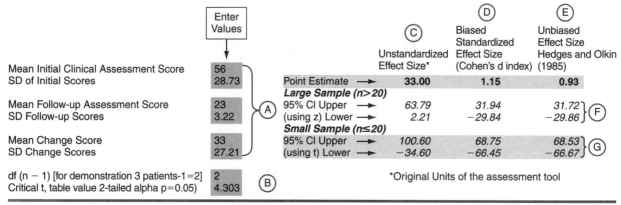

Figure 10-7 Calculator created in Excel for effect size point estimates and 95% CIs. (A) Enter means and standard deviations for each assessment. (B) refers to the critical t value for two-tailed test and df = *n* – 1; see Table B-2 or Figure 10-5B. Items C through G are calculated automatically. (C) Point estimate for the unstandardized treatment effect (mean initial assessment minus mean follow-up), (D) Cohen's d index, equation 10-3, (E) Unbiased effect size, equation 10-4, (F) 95% CI for large samples. (G) 95% CI for small samples.

Traditional Statistics: Alternatives to the 95% CI for Finding Statistical Significance

When evaluating a treatment effect, some authors caution against using traditional statistical analysis (accepting or rejecting the null hypothesis) because the outcome of this analysis provides only a dichotomous answer (statistically significant: yes or no) and the data presentation does not easily lend itself to meta-analytic procedures that incorporate data from multiple studies.[18]

Statistical significance of clinical change in traditional statistical procedures is determined by comparing the calculated t ratio with the critical t ratio. The calculated t ratio is always derived from the patients' scores. The critical t ratio is always found in a statistical table (e.g., Fig. 10-5B), which is transparent to the user of statistical software. In the table of critical t values, critical t is found by the number of statistical degrees of freedom (in this case, df = *n* – 1, or 3 – 1 = 2 for either patients in the demonstration with back or shoulder problems). The df are found in the row of the table and the alpha level in the column of the table. The column selected for probability threshold in this example is a two-tailed alpha level ("α_2") of p = 0.05. The row and column intersect at the critical t value = 4.303 for this demonstration. The alpha level is a probability threshold. It simply means that in order to be statistically significant, the result should rarely occur in a population

where it is known that there is no difference in performance between the initial and discharge evaluations (the "null distribution"). A 2-tailed alpha level for the test is selected because the practitioner does not know if the intervention will improve or degrade the patient's status (thus 2 "tails" or 2 possible outcomes). A two-tailed hypothesis test allows for either positive or negative results. An expanded table of critical t values is found in Appendix B (Table B-2).

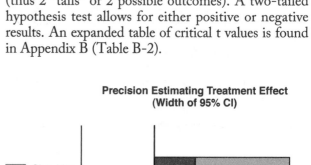

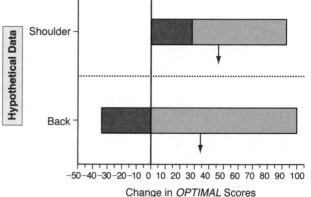

Figure 10-8 The width of the 95% confidence intervals for imaginary patients with shoulder or back dysfunction in the demonstration exercise. The precision for estimating the treatment effect is higher for the shoulder group because the 95% CI is smaller compared to the back group. Arrows indicate location of the point estimate (mean) treatment effect.

If the calculated t ratio exceeds the critical t ratio, then the difference in group performance from initial evaluation to discharge is statistically significant. In this demonstration with imaginary patients with shoulder dysfunction, the calculated t ratio = 12.12 and the critical t ratio for $N = 3$, df = 2, $\alpha_2 = 0.05$ is the table value of 4.303. The result is that calculated t (12.12) > critical t (4.303), indicating the average OPTIMAL change score for percent of difficulty shows a significant improvement in group function (the same result found when using the CI for hypothesis testing).

The positive therapeutic effect of "improvement" is noted by inspecting the sign on the calculated t statistic (or the ES, for that matter). The subtraction of initial-discharge scores from a tool that assigns more disability to higher scores means that a positive result shows improvement. For example, if the initial OPTIMAL score was 50% perceived task difficulty and the final score was 25%, then the difference score (50% − 25%) shows +25%. Thus, a drop in the task difficulty score at discharge creates a positive value when subtracted from baseline.

Power for Paired t-test

When OPTIMAL scores for only the patients with back dysfunction were evaluated, there was no statistically significant difference in the perception of task difficulty from initial evaluation to discharge (Fig. 10-4B). The relatively small treatment effect (the numerator of the t ratio) and the large variance of individual change scores (the denominator of the t ratio; SE from Fig. 10-6B) accounts for the finding that patient improvement was likely due to sampling error (a chance finding of change due to selecting only three patients, who might not be representative of the population where change occurs).

Whenever there is a finding of no difference, regardless of the statistical test, the question of statistical power must be addressed. Was there sufficient power in the analysis to find a difference if one truly existed? The number of patients as well as the variability of the scores have marked influence on the amount of statistical power. As the sample size increases and the variability of scores decreases, power increases.

A widely accepted standard level of power is 80%. This means that with theoretical replication of the study with different samples from the target population, a significant treatment effect will be found 80% of the time (if an effect truly exists). If an analysis has 80% power and there is no finding of a significant treatment effect, then clinical researchers conclude that the finding of no difference is likely to be true.

Regarding the critical number of patients needed to reach a sufficient level of power (80%), the ES with a slight modification is entered into a power table (Appendix B, Table B-7). An unbiased ES entered in the power table for the power of a paired t-test is (see Cohen[17]):

$$ES\ power\ paired\ t-test = unbiased\ d\ index * \sqrt{2}$$

eq 10-8

The unbiased ES is calculated using equation 10-4. For the imaginary patients with low back dysfunction, the ES used to determine the critical number of subjects needed for 80% power is:

$$ES\ power\ paired\ t-test = 0.93 * \sqrt{2} = 1.32$$

Power tables for t-tests are set up for independent two-group comparisons. Because the effect size for a paired t-test measures the same patients twice, the addition of the $\sqrt{2}$ element at the end of the ES equation is needed to make a correction for the way that error variance (the denominator of the t ratio) and degrees of freedom (reflecting the number of patients used for finding critical t values) are calculated.[17]

An excerpt from the power table for a two-tailed paired t-test at $\alpha = 0.05$ is shown in **Figure 10-9**. This table shows n down the left column and ES along the top row. The body of the table holds the power values. Linear interpolation is used to approximate the power of an ES that is not in the table. In our example, ES = 1.30 is not listed in the table, but

Power of Paired t-test α_2=0.05											
				Effect Size							
n	.10	.20	.30	.40	.50	.60	.70	.80	1.00	1.20	1.40
8	05	07	09	11	15	20	25	31	46	60	73
9	05	07	09	12	16	22	28	35	51	65	79
10	06	07	10	13	18	24	31	39	56	71	84
11	06	07	10	14	20	26	34	43	61	76	87
12	06	08	11	15	21	28	37	46	65	80	90
13	06	08	11	16	23	31	40	50	69	83	93
14	06	08	12	17	25	33	43	53	72	86	94

Figure 10-9 Power of the t-test for a two-tailed hypothesis test (α_2) at alpha = 0.05. An average is used to approximate the power of an ES not in the table. More precise methods are available in some statistical software programs. Long arrows point to the number of patients needed to achieve 80% power with ESs of 1.20 and 1.40 power in a two-tailed t-test at alpha = 0.05. The unbiased ES used to enter the table is adjusted by √2, as shown in **equation 10-8**. The full table can be found in Appendix B, (Table B-7) (Adapted from Statistical Power Analysis for the Behavioral Sciences by Cohen, Jacob. Copyright 1988 in the format Textbook via Copyright Clearance Center.[17]).

the *n* for an ES = 1.20 is 12 patients and the *n* for ES = 1.40 is 9 patients. The average n is 10.5 ~ 11 patients. Because only 3 patients participated in the demonstration analysis, and no statistical difference was found, the statistical test did not have sufficient power to find a difference if one truly existed.

Why Was n = 3 Sufficient for Detecting Significant Improvement in the Shoulder Group?

The reason that three patients with shoulder dysfunction were sufficient to find a difference in initial versus final assessments, but the same test on patients with back pain was not, is related to the large variance in the individual difference scores for those with back dysfunction (see the SEs in Fig. 10-6). As the SE increases relative to the pre/post OPTIMAL difference, the power of the statistical test decreases.

The type of power analysis generated in this example is a post-hoc power analysis, meaning that the assessment of patients already took place. The clinician then looks back in time to determine how many patients would have been needed to reach statistical significance given the known pattern of results. A post-hoc power analysis is needed only when there is a finding of no difference. In clinical research where studies are planned with specific recruitment targets, formal power analyses are done a priori using power tables that are specific to the statistical test that is proposed for the research project. Additional reading on the topic of power and alternative methods of estimating power using power tables can be found in Cohen.[17]

Assumptions Underlying the Use of Confidence Intervals

The primary assumption underlying the use of a confidence interval is that the treatment effect scores are distributed in the form of a normal bell-shaped curve. When this assumption is violated, inferring the results of the test to the population of patients in the target group may be unreliable and inaccurate.[18] Tests for the normality of the score distribution were discussed in Chapter 7 (Fig. 7-7) and guided the selection of correlation coefficients for clinical research. Here, tests for normality give confidence that the use of CIs is appropriate.[h]

If the distribution of the treatment effect scores (initial–discharge) is not normally distributed, however,

and the use of data transformation to "force" a normal distribution of scores fails (Chapter 7, Fig. 7-12), then CI might still be used in some cases.[20] The use of parametric test on treatment effects like the t-test even when the underlying assumptions are violated might be appropriate because these tests are considered robust, yielding similar results regardless of violating assumptions.[20] The complexity of assessing just how robust a parametric test is for each application requires in-depth analysis that is beyond the scope of this primer.

Alternatively, nonparametric tests such as the sign test could be used to determine the statistical significance of the number of responders versus nonresponders. This type of test is not dependent upon a normal probability distribution. However, the statistical power of this nonparametric test is lower than the parametric counterpart (t ratio). A demonstration of the sign test is in the appendix to this chapter. Some authors do not recommend the use of nonparametric tests because of the concern regarding low power. [20]

In routine clinical practice it is usually not feasible to randomly select patients for outcome assessment. The patients included in outcome assessments typically represent samples of convenience. Random selection of patients is not feasible in most clinical environments and the practitioner should be aware that the results most accurately apply to the patients in the sample and not the universe of patients with the target disorder.

Clinical Outcome Assessment Is *Not* Efficacy Assessment

Determining the change in patient function over time is not a test of efficacy because outcome assessment in the clinic does not control for confounding factors that might influence the result of treatment. Clinical outcomes might be influenced by factors other than the rehabilitation intervention.[21] For example, the natural history of some disorders reveals spontaneous recovery over time.[22] When natural history is not controlled, practitioners might incorrectly assume that rehabilitation was responsible for a positive (or negative) outcome. Regardless of this limitation, clinical outcome assessments have an important role in reducing the uncertainty of results from randomized controlled trials (RCTs) by offsetting the limitations of RCTs and systematic reviews.[23]

Limitations of RCTs and Systematic Reviews

Research designs that involve random assignment of patients to treatment and control groups are called

[h]There are many tests that are used to evaluate the normality of the distribution of scores, including tests for skewness, kurtosis, Shapiro, Wilk, and Kolmogorov-Smirnov. There is no widely held standard for the best normality test(s) and therefore, conflicting results about the conclusion of a normality analysis can occur.

randomized controlled trials (RCTs). The goal of many RCTs is to test new therapies and create a high level of certainty that the treatment of interest likely caused a positive effect in the treatment group that was not observed to the same extent in the control group. The rigorous controls found in high-quality RCTs give clinicians confidence that the results are true for the patient groups selected for study.[24]

Implementation of RCTs by practitioners is generally not feasible because the design of RCTs requires an experimental protocol where some interventions might not conform to accepted standards of practice (e.g., a control group of patients receiving "sham" therapy).[i] The amount of resources needed to initiate an RCT may also be prohibitive.[25] Clinicians, therefore, usually rely on published results from RCTs as one aspect of evidence for practice. The advantage to citing published results from RCTs is that factors such as the effects of selection bias (e.g., tendency to select less involved patients to receive the treatment of interest) and the natural history of the disease process (e.g., spontaneous recovery over time regardless of intervention efficacy) are uniformly controlled.

Systematic reviews are created from groups of RCTs to increase the certainty that the results are valid and reliable.[26] A systematic review is a pooling of many RCTs addressing the same topic.[27] Each RCT is rated for methodological quality, and the common results from RCTs deemed to be high quality are used as the recommendation for treatment. For example, a study that blinded therapists to patient group assignment might receive a higher "quality score" than a study that did not. Examples of systematic reviews related to rehabilitation can be found in PubMed (www.pubmed.gov, key search phrase "systematic review") and on various web sites, including the Cochrane library (http://www.cochrane.org) and a site developed by the *British Medical Journal* entitled "Clinical Evidence" (www.clinicalevidence.org).

There are several important limitations to consider when using RCTs and systematic reviews as the sole source to determine the best treatment for the individual patient in the clinic.

- There is no consensus on the best method to grade the quality of a RCT.[28]
- The results of the systematic review could change depending upon the method used to score methodological quality of each RCT.[28]
- RCTs may focus on homogeneous groups of patients, whereas in clinical practice, different symptom profiles and multiple co-interventions exist that could compromise the generalization of RCT results to the treatment of your patient.[23]
- Accuracy of diagnostic tests and prediction of the patient's prognosis cannot be determined from RCTs.[24]

SUMMARY

Supplementing the findings in published literature with analysis of data in local clinics can offset the limitations in generalizing RCT results to the individual patient. For the individual patient, documented clinical change following rehabilitation can provide evidence to support the use of procedures that were found helpful to the "average patient" in RCTs. Assessment of outcomes in local clinics might also increase awareness of additional factors that could influence generalization of RCT results to individual patients, such as acuity, functional level at the initial evaluation, specific types of co-interventions, or experience level of the clinician.

[i]When clinical facilities elect to participate in multicenter controlled trials, clinic patients might volunteer to be enrolled in a research study that is separate from the routine assessment and treatment. This type of trial is not within the scope of clinic-centered research because data collection and treatment are not under the direct control of the practitioner.

Appendix
Technical Details Regarding Measurement of Treatment Effects

Key Terms
- Standard Error (SE)
- t ratio vs. F ratio
- t ratio vs. Sign Test

Calculation of the t Ratio (The Small-Sample "z-score" for Paired Observations)

The SD is derived as follows:

From Chapter 4 Appendix:
$$SD = \sqrt{SS/n - 1} \qquad \textbf{eq A4-3}$$

where SS is the sum of the squared deviations of each difference score from the mean difference score. Using raw data from Figure 10-3, "Shoulder Dysfunction":

Similarity of the t Ratio to the F Ratio: Within Group Repeated Measures

Assume that patients showed improvement from the initial to the discharge evaluation (numerator of the paired t ratio).ʲ This improvement could be diminished by large variability of individual difference scores (denominator of the ratio). The concept is similar to that presented in the appendix to Chapter 6 for the repeated measures F ratio, where "group" is thought of

---

ʲThe term *between group* factor is a source of confusion when doing a "within group" analysis. When the *same patients* are evaluated over time, then "TIME" becomes the group (e.g., initial vs. discharge scores are the two levels of the TIME factor).

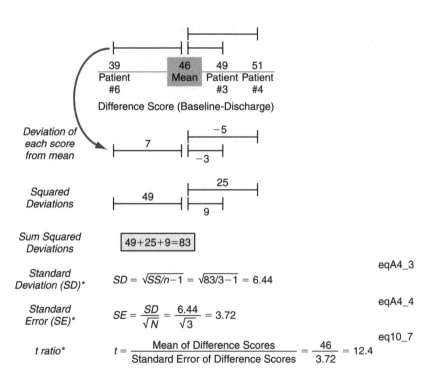

Calculation of SD and SE to form the t ratio. *The values differ slightly from those produced by statistical software due to rounding.

$$SD = \sqrt{SS/n-1} = \sqrt{83/3-1} = 6.44 \qquad \text{eqA4\_3}$$

$$SE = \frac{SD}{\sqrt{N}} = \frac{6.44}{\sqrt{3}} = 3.72 \qquad \text{eqA4\_4}$$

$$t = \frac{\text{Mean of Difference Scores}}{\text{Standard Error of Difference Scores}} = \frac{46}{3.72} = 12.4 \qquad \text{eq10\_7}$$

as time (baseline vs. follow-up status) for the same patients. In other words, "group" in this context is the *time* when the evaluation took place:

$$F\ ratio = \frac{Between\ "Group"\ Variance}{Within\ "Group"\ Variance}$$
$$= \frac{(Baseline - Follow\text{-}up)\ Variance}{Within\ Time\ Variance}$$

Eq A6-21 (modified)

The magnitude of the treatment effect is represented by the numerator, and the amount of measurement error (fluctuations of the outcome scores not related to treatment) is represented in the denominator. The denominator of the F ratio is also referred to as "error variance" or "unexplained variance." Thus, the paired t ratio is conceptually a special case of the repeated measures F ratio with a single factor that has only two levels of the independent variable. In this example, "Time" is the independent variable, with initial and discharge times as the levels of that factor. The same results would be expected when either the paired t-test or the within group repeated measures ANOVA is applied to the same data set.

t Ratio Versus Sign Test

The Sign Test is a procedure that is not dependent upon the assumption of a normal distribution of scores, but the procedure allows for a z-score approximation to estimate statistical significance of the proportion of (+) and (−) signs. In this case, positive therapeutic effects are denoted by plus signs and negative clinical effects are denoted by minus signs.

This test requires only the observation of direction of change in outcome for each patient. In Table 10-2, the direction (sign) of OPTIMAL score change in each imaginary patient with shoulder dysfunction is positive (+). In other scenarios, the subtraction of scores could yield negative (−) or no difference (0) values. The hypothesis of "no difference" (H_0) is that positive and negative signs will occur with the same frequency (50% for each sign). The alternative hypothesis (H_a) is that one sign occurs more frequently than the other beyond chance occurrences.

The count of *fewer* signs is designated x (so here $x = 0$ because all three patients had a positive outcome). The probability that this proportion (0 out of 3) occurs by chance is derived from a table of binomial probabilities. This can be done through an Excel spreadsheet using the function BINOMDIST.

In our example the entries are:

Numbers: the number of "successes" in the trial (**3** in our problem)

Trials: the number of trials in our experiment (**3** in our problem)

Probability: the probability of a success in a trial (**0.5** in our problem)

Cumulative: the probability to be calculated cumulative or not (**false** in the example = not cumulative)

The Excel entry in a blank cell is:

=BINOMDIST(3,3,0.5,FALSE)

This returns a two-tailed probability $p = 0.125$.

The result is that the probability that 3 positive outcomes occurred by chance with n = three patients is $p = 0.125$. In other words, when the critical p value is set at $p = 0.05$, the result we found is $p > 0.05$ and shows that the findings are likely to occur by chance. It may seem counterintuitive that the entire sample of patients had positive change, yet the Sign Test failed to reach statistical significance. For the imaginary patients with shoulder dysfunction (Table 10-2), the t ratio and 95% CI revealed a significant improvement in the treatment effect from the initial evaluation to discharge from the clinic. This highlights the fact that nonparametric tests like the Sign Test have low power in comparison to parametric tests like the t ratio because the count of signs did not yield a significant difference in either patient subgroup. The implication of low power is that a finding of "no treatment effect" may be incorrect.

PRACTICE

1. Confidence intervals apply to many aspects of evidence-based practice. In order to interpret confidence intervals properly, the context of this statistical method must be identified and the rules guiding the interpretation of each type of confidence interval must be applied. Using the knowledge gained in this text, complete the shaded boxes in the following table. The first row is labeled as a guide to the remainder of the table.

Application	Point Estimate	What the CI Tells You	Which Value Nullifies the Point Estimate (Creating a Nonsignificant Finding)?	What Is the Rationale for the Nullifying Value?
Diagnostic Validity	Positive Likelihood Ratio	The range of possible values surrounding the "true" LR		A patient is only 1 time more likely than prevalence to have a disorder
Meaningful Clinical Change		The level of confidence that the MDC is accurate	Any assessment score less than the MDC could be due to measurement error	The MDC defines a range where scores on a clinical assessment tool are due to error
Responsiveness of Clinical Assessment Tools	Responsiveness Indices		When comparing the width of the CI across responsiveness indices, overlap indicates no significant difference in responsiveness of the tools being compared.	Overlapping CIs for a responsiveness index between two assessment tools means that each index is likely to come from a population having the same level of responsiveness
Responsiveness of Clinical Assessment Tools	ROC Curve	Is the responsiveness capacity of the assessment tool any better than meaningless?		If the area under the ROC curve is different than meaningless (0.5), the CI will not hold the meaningless value
Consensus	Kappa	Determines if the "true" value of kappa falls in a range that indicates statistical significance		A CI holding $k = 0.40$ suggests that the true value of kappa may be too low to indicate consensus
Consensus	ICC	Variation of scores surrounding any patient's score (an index of measurement error)	No specific value but the wider the range, the more error is associated with the clinical tool	

Application	Point Estimate	What the CI Tells You	Which Value Nullifies the Point Estimate (Creating a Nonsignificant Finding)?	What Is the Rationale for the Nullifying Value?
Risk	Odds Ratio	The range of odds ratios that could occur with theoretical replication of the study using different patients, thus accounting for sampling error		A patient with a clinical sign or symptom could be only 1 time more likely to have the target condition (disease or disability) compared to those without the sign or symptom
Treatment Effect	Effect Size	The range of values surrounding clinical change scores		If the CI contains 0, it is possible that the true treatment effect could be 0

2. Applying a confidence interval for measuring treatment effect on the same patients tested twice (e.g., initial evaluation vs. follow-up) using ES assumes that the underlying data are normally distributed. Why?

3. Using the demonstration data set on the bound in disk (*Ch10-Optimal Outcomes*), were the initial and discharge outcomes (% task difficult) for each subgroup of patients and each assessment time (considered separately) normally distributed? Yes or No (show work)?
   Shoulder Group
   Initial evaluation?_____
   Discharge evaluation?___
   Back Group
   Initial evaluation?_____
   Discharge evaluation?___

4. If treatment effect outcomes are not normally distributed and a CI is desired to evaluate the treatment effect, what is the remedy?

5. In a study of 10 patients assessed at the initial and discharge evaluations, the biased effect size = 1.12. What would the unbiased effect size be?

6. What is the 95% CI surrounding the unbiased ES in question 5 if the standard deviation of the change scores was SD = 3?
   Upper Limit_____
   Lower Limit_____
   Is the treatment effect statistically different from 0 (and why)?

7. If the outcome measure was range of motion of the elbow in degrees, and the average change in ROM for 15 patients pre- vs. post-treatment was 24 degrees (SD = 6 degrees), then what is the 95% CI of the treatment effect in real units?
   Upper Limit_____
   Lower Limit_____
   Is the treatment effect statistically different from 0 (and why)?

REFERENCES

1. Randall KE, McEwen IR. Writing patient-centered functional goals. Phys Ther 2000; 80:1197–1203.
2. Skinner A, Turner-Stokes L. The use of standardized outcome measures in rehabilitation centres in the UK. Clin Rehab 2006; 20:609–615.
3. Jebsen RH, Taylor N, Trieschmann RB, et al. An objective and standardized test of hand function. Arch Phys Med Rehabil 1969; 50:311–319.
4. Ware JE, Sherbourne CD. A 36-item short form health survey (SF-36): I. Conceptual framework and item selection. Med Care 1992; 30:473–483.
5. Goetz CG, Fahn S, Martinez-Martin P, et al. Movement Disorder Society-sponsored revision of the Unified Parkinson's Disease Rating Scale (MDS-UPDRS): Process, format, and clinimetric testing plan. Movement Disorders 2007; 22:41–47.
6. Fugl-Meyer AR, Jaasko L, Leyman I, et al. The post-stroke hemiplegic patient. Scand J Rehabil Med 1975; 7:13–31.
7. Roland M, Fairbank J. The Roland–Morris Disability Questionnaire and the Oswestry Disability Questionnaire. Spine 2000; 25:3115–3124.
8. Guccione AA, Mielenz TJ, DeVellis R, et al. Development and testing of a self-report instrument to measure actions: Outpatient Physical Therapy Improvement in Movement Assessment Log (OPTIMAL). Phys Ther 2005; 85:515–530.
9. Lipsett PA, Swoboda SM, Campbell KA, et al. Sickness Impact Profile Score versus a Modified Short-Form survey for functional outcome assessment: acceptability, reliability, and validity in critically ill patients with prolonged intensive care unit stays. J Trauma 2000; 49:737–743.
10. Granger CV, Hamilton BB, Linacre JM, et al. Performance profiles of the Functional Independence Measure. Arch Phys Med Rehabil 1993; 72:84–89.
11. Granger CV. The emerging science of functional assessment: our tool for outcomes analysis. Arch Phys Med Rehabil 1998; 79:235–240.
12. Jette AM, Tao W, Norweg A, et al. Interpreting rehabilitation outcome measurements. J Rehabil Med 2007; 39:585–590.
13. Centers for Medicare & Medicaid Services. Medicare Benefit Policy Manual: Chapter 15—Covered medical and other health services. Rev. 106, 04-24-09, http://www.cms.hhs.gov/manuals/Downloads/bp102 c15.pdf.
14. Freeman JA, Hobart JC, Playford ED, et al. Evaluating neurorehabilitation: lessons from routine data collection. J Neurol Neurosurg Psych 2005; 76:723–728.
15. Horn SD, Gassaway J. Practice-based evidence study design for comparative effectiveness research. Med Care 2007; 45:S50–S57.
16. Marsh NV, Kersel DA. Screening tests for visual neglect following stroke. Neuropsych Rehab 1993; 3:245–257.
17. Cohen J. Statistical Power Analysis for the Behavioral Sciences. Hillsdale, NJ: Lawrence Erlbaum Associates, 1988.
18. Nakagawa S, Cuthill IC. Effect size, confidence interval and statistical significance: a practical guide for biologists. Biol Rev 2007; 82:591–605.
19. Hedges L, Olkin I. Statistical Methods for Meta-Analysis. New York: Academic Press, cited in Nakagawa S, Cuthill IC. Effect size, confidence interval and statistical significance: a practical guide for biologists. Biol Rev 2007; 82:591–605.
20. Johnson DH. Statistical sirens: The allure of nonparametrics. Ecology 1995; 76:1998–2000.
21. Herbert R, Jamtvedt G, Judy Mead J, et al. Outcome measures measure outcomes, not effects of intervention. Austral J Physiother 2005; 51:3–4.
22. Hurri H. The Swedish back school in chronic low back pain. Part II. Factors predicting the outcome. Scand J Rehabil Med 1989; 21.
23. Horn SD. Performance measures and clinical outcomes. JAMA 2006; 296:2731–2732.
24. Sackett DL, Rosenberg WMC, Gray JAM, et al. Evidence based medicine: what it is and what it isn't. BMJ 1996; 312:71–72.
25. Cicerone KD. Evidence-based practice and the limits of rational rehabilitation. Arch Phys Med Rehabil 2005; 86:1073–1074.
26. Cook DJ, Mulrow CD, Haynes RB. Systematic reviews: synthesis of best evidence for clinical decisions. Ann Intern Med 1997; 126:376–380.
27. Glasziou P, Irwig L, Bain C, et al. Systematic Reviews in Health Care. New York: Cambridge University Press, 2001.
28. Juni P, Witschi A, Bloch R, et al. The hazards of scoring the quality of clinical trials for meta analysis. JAMA 1999; 282:1054–1060.

Clinical Practice Guidelines

Clinical Questions
- What are clinical practice guidelines?
- Will clinical practice guidelines be useful to guide care for individual patients in my rehabilitation practice?

Introduction

Searching the literature to find rehabilitation assessments and treatments that are considered best practice can yield ambiguous results and leave practitioners in a quandary about which procedures have sound, evidenced-based support. Clinical practice guidelines are statements based on literature reviews conducted by experts in the field. These guidelines have been developed to assist clinicians to make choices about the care of patients in a specific population and circumstance.

Ideally, the clinical practice guidelines "contain recommendations that are based on evidence from a rigorous systematic review and synthesis of the published medical literature."[a] Expert panels should be formed to create clinical practice guidelines (see, for example, the Ottawa Panel practice guideline for adult rheumatoid arthritis[1]). External reviewers, including expert clinicians in the community, evaluate and provide peer review concerning the quality and clinical applicability of the recommendations in the guideline statement.

While clinical practice guidelines have the potential to improve the quality of clinical practice, Scalzitti[2] emphasizes that "it is the responsibility of the individual clinician ... to determine the applicability of the evidence from these guidelines to individual patients."[p.1622] Practice guidelines are time-delimited, can vary across cultures, and require updates.[3] This means that statements of best practice will change as new evidence and application considerations emerge in the literature.

Thus, practitioners should be aware of the dynamic nature of clinical practice guidelines and seek current valid statements as potential guides to patient care.

Where to Find Clinical Practice Guidelines

A primary site storing clinical practice guidelines is the National Guideline Clearing House: www.guideline.gov/. This site is searchable, and the entry of key topic words into the search box will yield all practice guidelines containing those terms.

Evaluating the Validity and Applicability of Practice Guidelines

Not all practice guidelines represent good practice decisions. One factor influencing the quality of any practice guideline is the quality of the literature review process that provides the underpinning for the statement of practice recommendations. However, there are other issues that influence the validity and applicability of practice guidelines. An appraisal instrument developed by the AGREE Collaboration[4] contains six domains that are independent and are intended to capture a separate dimension of guideline quality (Table 11-1).

At the end of the appraisal process an overall judgment is requested:

- Strongly recommend
- Recommend (with provisos or alterations)
- Would not recommend
- Unsure

Input From Stakeholders

Multiple appraisers (those who might be responsible for implementing the guideline, including therapists, physicians, and clinic administrators) should review the guideline. The agreement among these appraisers

[a]From the National Heart, Lung, and Blood Institute, National Institutes of Health web site http://www.nhlbi.nih.gov/guidelines/about.htm#what (accessed February 4, 2011).

Table 11-1	**Assessment Tool for Evaluating Clinical Practice Guidelines.** This instrument is adapted from the original AGREE II Instrument (http://www.agreetrust.org/). For more information about the ongoing research with the AGREE instrument, please visit the AGREE Research Trust Web site.[4]

APPRAISAL OF GUIDELINES FOR RESEARCH & EVALUATION (AGREE)

Domain	Items*	Item and Domain Score Total
A. Scope and purpose	1. The overall objective(s) of the guideline is (are) specifically described.	__/4
	2. The clinical question(s) covered by the guideline is (are) specifically described.	__/4
	3. The patients to whom the guideline is meant to apply are specifically described.	__/4
		Domain Total Score: __/12 possible = ____%
B. Stakeholder involvement	4. The guideline development group includes individuals from all the relevant professional groups.	__/4
	5. The patients' views and preferences have been sought.	__/4
	6. The target users of the guideline are clearly defined.	__/4
	7. The guideline has been piloted among target users.	__/4
		Domain Total Score: __/16 possible = _____%
C. Rigor of development	8. Systematic methods were used to search for evidence.	__/4
	9. The criteria for selecting the evidence are clearly described.	__/4
	10. The methods used for formulating the recommendations are clearly described.	__/4
	11. The health benefits, side effects and risks have been considered in formulating the recommendations.	__/4
	12. There is an explicit link between the recommendations and the supporting evidence.	__/4
	13. The guideline has been externally reviewed by experts prior to its publication.	__/4
	14. A procedure for updating the guideline is provided	__/4
		Domain Total Score: __/28 possible = _____%
D. Clarity and presentation	15. The recommendations are specific and unambiguous.	__/4
	16. The different options for management of the condition are clearly presented.	__/4
	17. Key recommendations are easily identifiable.	__/4
	18. The guideline is supported with tools for application.	__/4
		Domain Total Score: __/16 possible = _____%
E. Applicability	19. The potential organizational barriers in applying the recommendations have been discussed.	__/4
	20. The potential cost implications of applying the recommendations have been considered.	__/4
	21. The guideline presents key review criteria for monitoring and/or audit purposes.	__/4
		Domain Total Score: __/12 possible = _____%

Table 11-1	**Assessment Tool for Evaluating Clinical Practice Guidelines.** This instrument is adapted from the original AGREE II Instrument (http://www.agreetrust.org/). For more information about the ongoing research with the AGREE instrument, please visit the AGREE Research Trust Web site.[4]—**cont'd**

APPRAISAL OF GUIDELINES FOR RESEARCH & EVALUATION (AGREE)		
Domain	**Items***	**Item and Domain Score Total**
F. Editorial independence	22. The guideline is editorially independent from the funding body.	__/4
	23. Conflicts of interest of guideline development members have been recorded.	__/4
		Domain Total Score: __/8 possible = _____%

*Score each item, using the following scale: 4 for Strongly Agree, 3 for Agree, 2 for Disagree, 1 for Strongly Disagree.

can be tallied and compared against the maximum possible score for each domain. The level of agreement among raters is reflected by a standardized domain score:

$$Standardized\ Domain\ Score = \frac{Obtained\ Score - Minimum\ Possible\ Score}{Maximum\ Possible\ Score - Minimum\ Possible\ Score}$$

eq11-1

For example,[b] Domain A-Scope and Purpose has three items (Table 11-1). Using an example with three imaginary appraisers, their independent assessments of a practice guideline are:

Domain A-Scope and Purpose	Item #1	Item #2	Item #3	Total
Appraiser 1	4	3	2	**9**
Appraiser 2	2	1	3	**6**
Appraiser 3	2	1	2	**5**
Total	**8**	**5**	**7**	**20**

Maximum Possible Score = 4 (strongly agree)
× 3 (items) × 3 (appraisers) = 36
Minimum Possible Score = 1 (strongly disagree)
× 3 (items) × 3 (appraisers) = 9

Using **equation 11-1**, the standardized domain score for *domain A* is:

$$Standardized\ Domain\ Score = \frac{20 - 9}{36 - 9} = 0.41 * 100$$
$$= 41\%$$

[b]Adapted from *Appraisal Of Guidelines For Research & Evaluation (AGREE), The AGREE Collaboration,* September 2001, p. 5; www.agreecollaboration.org

The standardized domain score for practice guideline appraisal provides a relative index of the amount of agreement among raters for each domain. Because domains are evaluated separately, low levels of agreement in one domain (defined by the appraisers a priori; e.g., <60%) can help identify features of the practice guideline that could be improved, altered, or deleted.

Assessing Clinical Practice Guidelines

Target Population and the Clinical Intervention

In order to be useful, a practice guideline must specifically identify a target population as well as the goal of therapy or assessment. For example, a guideline intended to outline cognitive training for people with stroke as a general statement might not be as effective or meaningful as a guideline that outlines cognitive training protocols for people with an acute ischemic stroke involving partial anterior circulation of the brain as measured by the Bamford classification scheme.[5] In the latter scenario, both the target population and the intervention are not ambiguous.

Classifying patients in a way that potentially guides care can help define specific patient populations that form an unambiguous target population. Fritz et al.,[6] for example, conducted a randomized controlled trial comparing care recommended by a practice guideline with care deemed appropriate by classifying people with back pain into more distinct diagnostic categories. Patients receiving care according to their distinct profile of signs and symptoms had better outcomes than those who received a "one-size-fits-all" treatment recommended by the practice guideline.[6] Thus, clear definitions of the target population can lead to a focused guideline. It has been suggested that practice guidelines that are clear and unambiguous are more readily implemented in clinical settings than those with ambiguities.[7]

Level of Evidence Used to Support the Practice Guideline

Clinicians reviewing practice guidelines should note if systematic methods were used to search for evidence and if there is a clear and unambiguous link between the recommendations and the supporting evidence. The type and quality of literature supporting the practice guideline provide the clinician with a sense of the scientific rigor used to test the treatment procedure or assessment strategy. The levels of evidence supporting a practice guideline related to therapeutic interventions are shown in **Figure 11-1.** Literature classified as level I is scientifically stronger and provides more rigorous support for a practice recommendation compared to levels II through V.

Systematic reviews involve a comprehensive search of existing literature addressing the therapeutic approach in question. These reviews can take various forms, such as a narrative review concerning treatment efficacy or a quantitative review (also called a meta-analysis). Meta-analyses provide a quantitative measure of treatment effectiveness by combing data from trials that meet the requirements for inclusion in the review (e.g., target population and type of study design). Data synthesis is done using standardized indices such as the d index (see Chapter 10). When

Levels of Evidence	
I-A	Systematic reviews (including meta analysis) of RCTs
I-B	Single RCT with narrow confidence interval
II-A	Systematic reviews (including meta analysis) of cohort studies
II-B	Individual cohort study or single RCT rated low quality
II-C	Outcomes research (including retrospective chart reviews)
III-A	Systematic review of case-control studies
III-B	Individual case-control study
IV	Poor quality case control and cohort studies
V	Expert opinion

Stronger ⟶

Figure 11-1 Levels of evidence associated with each type of literature supporting practice recommendations related to therapeutic interventions. (Adapted with permission from the Center for Evidence Based Medicine, University of Oxford.) Abbreviations: RCT = randomized controlled trial. See text for definitions of study designs.

all relevant data are combined across studies, the meta-analysis provides a combined measure of the overall treatment effect.

One common criticism of meta-analyses is that the pool of studies included in the review are not really similar. Trials may differ on the age, gender, severity of the target condition, or the length of treatment, for example.[8] Higgins et al.[9] note that some degree of heterogeneity (differences in the results across reviewed studies) would be expected in meta-analyses simply because of variations among studies such as length of follow-up, study quality, and inclusion criteria for enrolled patients.

In order to address the issue of conflicting results among pooled studies, a test of heterogeneity may be useful.[10] The results of a test of heterogeneity will inform the reader if the different results in a pool of studies were likely due to differences in study methodology and clinical approach, or simply due to chance. Commonly used heterogeneity indices are the Cochran's Q (based on the chi-square distribution) and the "inconsistency index," or "I^2."[9,10]

When significant heterogeneity is found (based on Cochrane's Q index, $p < 0.20$), or when high values for the inconsistency index are reported (e.g., >50%), these findings generally indicate that there are marked inconsistencies among study results.[9,10] The question for practitioners evaluating the literature review component of a practice guideline is: Is it valid to combine studies with significant methodological or clinical differences? The appraiser of the clinical practice guideline should determine the amount of tolerance for heterogeneity in meta-analyses when deciding if the literature review component of the practice guideline has applicability to treating patients locally. In other words, if your patient is mildly involved, but the studies address a greater level of severity, or if your patient receives outpatient care, but the studies emphasize inpatient intervention, or if your patient is under 50 years of age and the preponderance of studies in the review address patients over 60 years of age, is the practice guideline useful? The calculation of a homogeneity index is beyond the scope of this text but readers can find computational details elsewhere.[11]

Systematic reviews are not limited to randomized controlled trials. For example, separate systematic reviews including meta-analyses can focus on nonrandomized designs including paired test-retest designs (such as those described in Chapter 10) or observational studies (see Fig. 11-1; levels II-A and III-A).

Nonrandomized Trials

A cohort study looks at a group of people (the "cohort") either forward (prospective) or backward (retrospective) in time. Some people in the group are exposed to an event while others are not. Outcomes are compared across "exposed" and "nonexposed" subgroups. For example, one study examined a group of patients with spinal cord injuries followed monthly over 1 year.[12] The authors found that the patients who experienced ("exposed to") injurious wheelchair-related falls were those who had pain, relatively good motor function, previous falls, and an inaccessible home entrance compared to those without these conditions ("nonexposed").[12]

A case-control study looks at "cases" (those who have the target condition or those exposed to a type of treatment) matched to "controls" (those who do not have the target condition or those exposed to a standard or traditional treatment). The assignment to groups in case-control studies is not randomized. However, case-control studies match cases to control subjects on key variables. For example, to evaluate the effectiveness of a new method of treating dysphagia, "cases" (those receiving a new treatment) were compared to "controls" (patients who received traditional therapy in the same clinic, but in the past).[13] Cases were matched to controls on the basis of age, gender, and primary diagnosis. Other forms of matching can include performance measures. A case-control study of neurobehavioral sequelae following traumatic brain injury in children compared the performance of "cases" (children ages 6 to 15 years who had a documented loss of consciousness) with "controls" (children individually matched to the cases based on a teacher's assessment of preinjury behavior and academic performance in reading and math, among other variables).[14]

Evaluating the Quality of Randomized Controlled Trials and Observational Studies

Randomized Controlled Studies

A systematic review may include a grade reflecting the quality of research. For example, a randomized controlled trial that specifies an appropriate method of randomization, uses double blinding, and addresses the number of patients who dropped out of the study would receive a higher grade than a study that misses one or more of these items (refer to Jadad et al.[15] for this assessment scale). These three items evaluate the control of bias.[16] Randomized controlled trials that do not address bias are at risk of reporting inaccurate findings contaminated with:

• Rater bias (changes in outcome because the person evaluating the patient is aware of the treatment rendered),

• Randomization bias (changes in outcome because the randomization method did not afford an equal chance of patient assignment to the treatment or control group),

• Study bias (the number of dropouts and the groups from which dropouts occurred potentially changes the results).

Care should be taken when grading the quality of any clinical trial because different methods of quality assessment can yield different results.[17] In addition, many scales may lack reliability and have not been validated.[16] Also, scales designed for a drug trial may not be as appropriate as scales designed to assess the quality of some therapeutic interventions used in the field of rehabilitation.[16]

The size of confidence intervals reported in RCTs is noted in level of evidence I-B (see Fig. 11-1). When a CI is narrow, this indicates that the variability of the results for a particular outcome measure is small (indicating less measurement error). Thus, RCTs reporting results that have narrow CIs provide a stronger level of evidence than those with wide CIs. Another factor influencing the width of the CI is the number of subjects participating in each study; as N increases, the CIs tend to get smaller.

Data from a hypothetical group of RCTs addressing the effect of biofeedback on habitual shoulder dislocation are shown in **Figure 11-2**.[18] The odds ratio (OR) in this example is a measure of the likelihood of achieving a positive outcome when exposed to biofeedback compared to those who received a control intervention (see Chapter 8 and equation 8-9). This outcome measure is appropriate for studies that use dichotomous variables. Here the recurrence of dislocation (yes or no) was the primary outcome.[18] Whereas the OR for "study C" closely approximates the OR for all studies combined in this hypothetical meta-analysis (OR = ~0.68; see Fig. 11-2), the width of the CI for "study C" is very large and includes the null value of 1. In contrast, the width of the 95% CI in "study B" is very precise (narrow) and provides a relatively greater level of confidence in the results (OR = ~0.6; those receiving biofeedback are less likely to experience a recurrence of shoulder dislocation compared to those who received the sham condition).

Nonrandomized Studies

The quality of studies that do not randomly assign patients to groups is determined by evaluating presence of bias, confounding variables, and chance findings.[19]

• Bias and confounding variables[c] in observational studies occur because the study design or

---

[c]Brennan and Croft (BMJ. 1994) provide separate definitions for bias and confounding variables, but for the purpose of this text, confounding variables are considered factors that create bias.

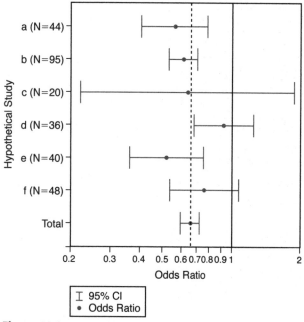

Figure 11-2 A plot of the odds ratios and corresponding 95% confidence intervals for 6 hypothetical studies with different numbers of patients. A CI containing an OR = 1 is considered not significant or clinically meaningful. The overall OR is indicated by the vertical dotted line. The solid line indicates the meaningless OR. (Reprinted from Sim J, Reid N. Statistical inference by confidence intervals: issues of interpretation and utilization. Phys Ther. 1999; 79: 186–195, with permission of the American Physical Therapy Association. This material is copyrighted, and any further reproduction or distribution requires written permission from APTA.)

existence of important, but unidentified, factors obscures the relationship between "exposure" and "dysfunction." For example, when assessing treatment effectiveness in a case-control trial, if the controls are not properly matched on all key variables except for the intervention, then factors omitted from matching (such as age or gender) could be the real cause of the study outcome. This scenario creates a false conclusion because age or gender were the variables explaining changes in dysfunction rather than the intervention per se.

• Chance findings in randomized controlled trials relate to the p values found during statistical analyses and confidence intervals. In observational studies, however, subjects are not randomly assigned to groups and thus confounding effects cannot be nullified by the randomization process. Therefore, the p values and confidence intervals in cohort studies may not accurately depict the degree of chance that exposure to the intervention is related to the occurrence of dysfunction. In other

words, p <0.05 does not necessarily indicate that there is a treatment or "exposure" effect.

Thus, a fundamental aspect of quality assessment in cohort studies is the possible presence of bias and confounding variables. If practitioners find that bias and confounding variables are present, then the impact of a "statistically significant effect" and the quality of the study are judged to be low.

Grading Specific Recommendations Within the Practice Guideline

Once the *levels* of evidence are established for specific recommendations within a clinical practice guideline (Table 11-1), each recommendation is graded to illustrate how well the practice statement is supported by the literature. A general template for grading recommendations in clinical practice guidelines is presented by the Oxford University Center of Evidence Based Medicine (**Table 11-2**). Their grading overview provides a clear conceptual model to judge the level of support for each practice recommendation.

Grading systems do vary in practice, however, and there are modifications to the theme presented in a general template (see Table 11-2) that are specific to practice topics. For example, a practice guideline for neuroprotective strategies and alternative therapies for Parkinson's disease (Guideline Summary NGC-4936)[20] graded recommendations on a 4-point scale of A-B-C-U, reflecting the range of

Table 11-2	**A General Format to Grade Specific Practice Recommendations Contained Within Practice Guidelines.** The level of studies refers to the definitions in Table 11-1.

Grades of Recommendation

A	consistent level 1 studies
B	consistent level 2 or 3 studies or extrapolations* from level 1 studies
C	level 4 studies or extrapolations* from level 2 or 3 studies
D	level 5 evidence or troublingly inconsistent or inconclusive studies of any level

*Extrapolations are where data are used in a situation that has potentially clinically important differences than the original study situation.
Reprinted with permission from the Center for Evidence Based Medicine, University of Oxford.

"A" = supported by level I studies to "U" = insufficient evidence to support the recommendation. In this guideline, it was stated that exercise therapy may be considered to improve function for patients with Parkinson's disease. This recommendation was graded "C." In the context of this practice guideline, "C" means that at least one level II study or two consistent level III studies were found to support the recommendation.[d] By contrast, the recommendation to use acupuncture to improve motor function in Parkinson's disease was graded "U" (data inadequate or conflicting). The grade of U does not necessarily mean that acupuncture is ineffective, but it does indicate that more study is needed before this treatment can be supported and recommended.

A different grading system was implemented by Brosseau et al.[21] as they developed recommendations to treat balance dysfunction following stroke (Guideline Summary NGC-5310). They used an 8-point scale with the grades A-B-C-D as a base, but then added a plus and a minus to the C and D grades. This range reflected "A" = one or more level I studies with >15% benefit to the treatment group through "D-" = evidence from one or more randomized controlled trials where the *controls benefited* more than the treatment group by at least 15%. This practice guideline graded balance training with visual feedback versus control as an "A" when treating standing balance (clinically important benefit demonstrated) but assigned a grade of "C" for rehabilitation of sitting balance following treatment (no benefit demonstrated).[c]

The grading protocols for each practice guideline are embedded in the summary statements that can be found at the National Guideline Clearing House (http://www.guideline.gov/). Each grading system is clearly defined in the context of the literature available to support the guideline. Clinicians should note, however, that similar grades are not comparable across clinical practice guidelines. The grade of "C," for example, as shown earlier for two different practice guidelines is not equivalent.

[d]Grades were inferred to fit the lexicon in Table 11-1. Refer to the actual practice guideline for precise definitions of grades.

Demonstration: Assessing Practice Guidelines

This demonstration is designed to encourage the evaluation of a real clinical practice guideline using the AGREE instrument)[4] (see Table 11-1). The reader should select a practice guideline of interest from and then review the practice guideline with the AGREE[4] template. Results should be compared with other appraisers. This exercise can be performed by students reviewing the guideline during clinical internships or among clinicians contemplating a partial or full implementation of the guideline. Some key questions to consider once the evaluation is complete:

- Do the recommendations within the guideline have adequate support in the literature?
- Are the recommendations feasible for implementation in your clinical setting?
- Do the benefits outweigh the risks or potential harm?
- If not feasible as presented, what changes should be made in the guideline to adapt the recommendations for your clinical practice?

SUMMARY

Clinical practice guidelines have the potential to guide and improve the care of patients in rehabilitation settings. However, not all guidelines are good guidelines and it is important that practitioners and other stakeholders carefully evaluate any practice guideline for relevance, feasibility of implementation, and the potential effectiveness for positive outcome.

With the focus on evaluating clinical practice guidelines and the emphasis on high-quality research to support practice recommendations, it could be assumed that level I research is increasing in the fields of rehabilitation. This assumption may not be true, [22] and more work is required to advance clinical research agendas.[23,24] Practicing clinicians have a role in generating clinical research that answers important clinical questions. Clinical practice *is* clinical research in many respects.

PRACTICE

Visit the National Guideline Clearing House web site (http://www.guideline.gov/), and review the following rehabilitation-related clinical practice guidelines using the AGREE assessment template[4] (see Fig. 11-1). Recruit multiple appraisers and calculate the Standardized Domain Score (see equation 11-1) for each domain in the AGREE tool.

Guideline Title

1. Occupational therapy practice guidelines for individuals with work-related injuries and illnesses (**NGC-7510**)
2. Practice parameter: assessing patients in a neurology practice for risk of falls (an evidence-based review; **NGC-6655**).
3. Evidence-based care guideline for pediatric constraint-induced movement therapy (CIMT; **NGC-7162**).

REFERENCES

1. Ottawa Panel Evidence-Based Clinical Practice Guidelines for Therapeutic Exercises in the Management of Rheumatoid Arthritis in Adults. Phys Ther 2004; 84:934–972.
2. Scalzitti DA. Evidence-based guidelines: application to clinical practice. Phys Ther 2001; 81:1622–1628.
3. DiCenso A, Guyatt G. Evidence-Based Nursing: A Guide to Clinical Practice. St Louis, MO: Elsevier Mosby, 2005.
4. AGREE Collaboration. Appraisal of Guidelines for Research and Evaluation (AGREE) Instrument. www.agreecollaboration.org.
5. Bamford J, Sandercock P, Dennis M, et al. Classification and natural history of clinically identifiable subtypes of cerebral infarction. Lancet 1991; 337:1521–1526.
6. Fritz JM, Delitto A, Erhard RE. Comparison of classification-based physical therapy with therapy based on clinical practice guidelines for patients with acute low back pain: a randomized clinical trial. Spine 2003; 28:1363–1372.
7. Grol R, Dalhuijsen J, Thomas S, et al. Attributes of clinical guidelines that influence use of guidelines in general practice: observational study. Brit Med J 1998; 317:858–861.
8. Di Fabio RP. Myth of evidence-based practice. J Orthop Sports Phys Ther 1999; 29:632–634.
9. Higgins JPT, Thompson SG, Deeks JJ, et al. Measuring inconsistency in meta-analyses. Brit Med J 2003; 327:557–560.
10. Jones JB, Blecker S, Shah NR. Meta-analysis 101: what you want to know in the era of comparative effectiveness. American Health and Drug Benefits 2008; 1:38-43.
11. Higgins JPT, Thompson SG. Quantifying heterogeneity in a meta-analysis. Statistics in Medicine. 2002; 21:1539–1558.
12. Nelson AL, Groer S, Palacios P, et al. Wheelchair-related falls in veterans with spinal cord injury residing in the community: a prospective cohort study. Arch Phys Med Rehabil 2010; 91:1166–1173.
13. Carnaby-Mann GD, Crary MA. McNeill Dysphagia Therapy Program: a case-control study. Arch Phys Med Rehabil 2010; 91:743–749.
14. Massagli TL, Jaffe KM, Fay GC, et al. Neurobehavioral sequelae of severe pediatric traumatic brain injury: a cohort study. Arch Phys Med Rehabil 1996; 77:223–231.
15. Jadad AR, Moore AP, Carroll D, et al. Assessing the quality of reports of randomized clinical trials: is blinding necessary? Controlled Clinical Trials 1996; 17:1–12.
16. Armijo Olivo S, Macedo LG, Gadottil C, et al. Scales to assess the quality of randomized controlled trials: a systematic review. Phys Ther 2008; 88: 156–175.
17. Juni P, Witschi A, Bloch R, et al. The hazards of scoring the quality of clinical trials for meta analysis. JAMA 1999; 282:1054–1060.
18. Sim J, Reid N. Statistical inference by confidence intervals: issues of interpretation and utilization. Phys Ther 1999; 79:186–195.
19. Brennan P, Croft P. Interpreting the results of observational research: chance is not such a fine thing. Brit Med J 1994; 309:727–730.
20. Suchowersky O, Gronseth G, Perlmutter J, et al. Quality Standards Subcommittee of the American Academy of Neurology. Practice parameter: neuroprotective strategies and alternative therapies for Parkinson disease (an evidence-based review): report of the Quality Standards Subcommittee of the American Academy of Neurology. Neurology 2006; 66:976–982.
21. Brosseau L, Wells GA, Finestone HM, et al. Clinical practice guidelines for balance training. Top Stroke Rehabil 2006; 13:41-5.
22. Dirette D, Rozich A, Viau S. Is there enough evidence for evidence-based practice in occupational therapy? Am J Occup Ther 2009; 63:782–786.
23. Clinical Research Agenda for Physical Therapy. Phys Ther 2000; 80:499–513.
24. Goldstein MS, Scalzitti DA, Craik RL. The Revised Research Agenda for Physical Therapy. Phys Ther 2011; 91:165–174.

Clinical Application of Statistical Analyses With Interactive Practice

Clinical Question
• How do statistics guide clinical practice?

Demonstration Practice Exercises

The goal of the problem-solving exercises in this chapter is to stimulate discussion and a broad understanding about the clinical application of statistical methodologies covered in this primer. The structure of each practice exercise is:

1. **Summary of a Real Study**—Studies picked from the rehabilitation literature are summarized in abstract form and selected real results are presented. Readers are encouraged to search the literature and read each article cited in this appendix for a complete perspective of the outcome measures and research design.

2. **Hypothetical Studies**—A hypothetical study is presented with imaginary data and imaginary patients. The selected variables and research methods used in the real study (i.e., a pre- and post-test on patients evaluated with measures of strength or function that are common in rehabilitation practice) are also used in the hypothetical study, but the data values are made up and the patients are imaginary. The results obtained through the demonstration practice analyses of these hypothetical studies, therefore, are not real and may or may not agree with the original work. The practice exercises are designed to challenge the reader to independently perform analyses that are either similar to the types of analyses in the original article or analyses covered in this text, but not addressed in a real study.

3. **Solutions**—The answers to all of the demonstration exercises can be found at the end of Appendix C. The solutions use NCSS and SPSS or PSPP statistical software[a] (as indicated). The interpretation of the outcomes for the hypothetical demonstration exercises is guided by the appropriate chapters that address the topics covered in the demonstrations.

Practice Exercise 1: Manual Muscle Testing

Summary of Real Study 1

A study published in *Clinical Rehabilitation* addressed the diagnostic validity of manual muscle testing.[1] One purpose of that study was to determine if side-to-side differences in knee extension force detected by a dynamometer (the criterion standard) could also be detected by a clinical test (manual muscle testing). Any difference in manual muscle test (MMT) scores between lower extremities (e.g., a grade of 3 versus 3+) was considered a difference in side-to-side strength. Thus, the outcome for MMT was dichotomized as yes = side-to-side difference vs. no = muscle test scores are equal side-to-side. The author reports his results in **Table A-1.**

The dynamometer detected differences in knee extension force from side-to-side. A contingency table was developed to show how the classification by the dynamometer agreed or disagreed with manual muscle testing assessed by a clinician. The labels of the contingency table correspond to the standard contingency table labels A through D for diagnostic validity (Chapter 2, Fig. 2-1).

---

[a]PSPP has limited functionality and will run most but not all statistical analyses presented in this appendix.

| Table A-1 | | Results Reported by Bohannon[1] on the Accuracy of Manual Muscle Testing for Detecting Between-Side Differences in Muscle Force Identified by Dynamometry. The **bold row** shows the data of interest for discussion in this appendix. | | | | | | | |

Dynamometer Difference (%)	Cell Counts[a]				Sensitivity (%)	Specificity (%)	Predictive Value +(%)	Predictive Value −(%)	Diagnostic Accuracy (%)
	a	b	c	d					
15	**44**	**4**	**26**	**33**	62.9	89.2	91.7	55.9	72.0
20	43	5	20	39	68.3	88.6	89.6	66.1	76.6
25	39	9	15	44	72.2	83.0	81.2	74.6	77.6
30	34	14	13	46	72.3	76.7	70.8	78.0	74.8

[a] $n = 107$.

Reprinted from Bohannon RW. Manual muscle testing: does it meet the standards of an adequate screening test? Clin Rehabilitation 2005; 19:662–667 with permission.

Hypothetical Study 1

The data for the hypothetical study with imaginary patients is shown in **Figure A-1** and relate to the condition where the dynamometer identifies a 15% side-to-side difference in knee extension force.

NCSS	SPSS (or PSPP)
Manual Muscle Testing.S0	*Manual Muscle Testing.sav*

Exercises for Hypothetical Study #1

Open the demonstration data set that matches your statistical software:

1-1. Diagnostic Validity

    a. From the hypothetical data set, generate a 2 2 contingency table (criterion standard MMT) using a cross-tabulation procedure that shows the frequency of patient counts in each cell (see Chapter 6).

    b. How does this contingency table in the hypothetical study compare to the real study?

    c. What is the sensitivity, specificity, and +Likelihood ratio generated from the hypothetical study contingency table?

    d. Is the +likelihood ratio statistically significant?

    e. There are different ways to define diagnostic accuracy. Assuming a prevalence (pretest probability) of 65%, what is the approximate diagnostic accuracy (post-test probability) of MMT in determining side-to-side differences in knee extensor force?

Hypothetical Data

Variable name	Definition		Patient_num	criterion_standard	MMT	MMT_R_Knee_Ext	MMT_L_Knee_Ext	ABS_MMT_R_minus_L
Criterion standard	Dynamometer detecting side-to-side differences or not		1	zNO_side_sde_diff	detected	6	8	2
			2	zNO_side_sde_diff	detected	7	5	1
			3	side_sde_diff	detected	6	8	2
			4	side_sde_diff	detected	5	8	3
			5	side_sde_diff	detected	6	8	3
MMT	Manual muscle test detecting side-to-side differences or not		6	side_sde_diff	detected	5	6	1
			7	side_sde_diff	detected	4	7	2
			8	side_sde_diff	detected	7	8	1
			9	side_sde_diff	detected	6	7	1
			10	side_sde_diff	detected	6	5	1
			11	side_sde_diff	detected	4	8	4
MMT R knee ext	Manual muscle test grade for R knee extension		12	side_sde_diff	detected	6	9	3
			13	side_sde_diff	detected	6	9	3
			14	side_sde_diff	detected	6	7	1
			15	side_sde_diff	detected	7	8	1
			16	side_sde_diff	detected	7	9	2
			17	side_sde_diff	detected	5	7	2
MMT L knee ext	Manual muscle test grade for L knee extension		18	side_sde_diff	detected	5	8	3
			19	side_sde_diff	detected	5	7	2
			20	side_sde_diff	detected	5	8	3
			21	side_sde_diff	detected	6	8	2
			22	side_sde_diff	detected	7	12	5
ABS_MMT_R_minus_L	Absolute difference in MMT grades R minus L		23	side_sde_diff	detected	7	8	1
			24	side_sde_diff	detected	7	8	1
			25	side_sde_diff	detected	5	9	4
			26	side_sde_diff	detected	6	8	2

Figure A-1 Data definitions and values for a hypothetical study on manual muscle testing based on selected methods and outcome variables described by Bohannon.[1] Only 26 of 107 rows are displayed (the full data set is available on the bound-in disk in the file entitled "Manual Muscle Testing" with either the NCSS or SPSS extension).

f. Using the diagnostic accuracy method described by the author,[1] what is the result for the hypothetical data?

g. How do the interpretations of outcome vary by the method of calculating diagnostic accuracy?

1-2. Assume an additional research question for this hypothetical study: "Is there an *association* between the criterion standard demonstrating side-to-side differences in knee extension force and the detection of side-to-side differences by the clinical test?" (Both variables are categorical; refer to Chapter 7.)

a. What is (are) the name(s) of the most appropriate statistics to measure this association? (Provide the values for each statistic, the df where appropriate, and the p value for the hypothesis test, H_0 correlation = 0.)

b. Is the association statistically significant?

c. What is the percent shared variance between the criterion standard and clinical test results?

d. What is the direction and descriptive strength of the relationship?

e. Explain the results of a residual analysis of the contingency table "criterion standard" versus "MMT."

Practice Exercise #2: Developmental Assessment

Summary of Real Study #2

The Pediatric Evaluation of Disability Inventory (PEDI) is an assessment instrument that is designed to measure functional status in children and youth between the ages of 6 months and 7.5 years in the three domains: Self-care, Mobility, and Social Function.[2] This assessment tool can also be used with older children who have developmental delays.[3] There are 73 items in the self-care domain, and each item is scored as "unable/limited in capability to perform in most situations" or "capable of performing the item in most situations."[3] The composite score for the self-care scale varies from 0 (worse) to 100 (best function).[4]

To determine the minimal clinically important difference (MCID) for the PEDI, a retrospective chart review is done for 53 children who received inpatient rehabilitation services. Iyer et al.[4] compared Likert scale ratings from physical, occupational, and speech therapists with the PEDI self-care change scores

(initial versus discharge).[b] The clinicians were blinded from the PEDI scores and used clinical summaries from the patient's chart to make their judgment of functional change. The Likert scale used by the clinicians to register their opinion of clinical change is illustrated in **Figure A-2.**

Likert ratings were converted to four classifications:

- 0 and all of the negative Likert ratings = "no change,"
- +1 to +3 = MCID,
- ratings of +4 to +5 represented "moderate change,"
- ratings of +6 to +7 represented "large change."

The authors evaluated how MCID (derived from the Likert scale) corresponded with the actual PEDI change scores for patients in each change classification (no change through large change). A selection of their results relating to the domain of self-care functional skills is shown in Table A-2. As the patients classified by the clinicians' Likert rating as MCID had a mean PEDI change score of 10 points (see "minimal change" in Table A-2), it was suggested that the

[b]Additional procedures and analyses were done by Iyer et al. (2003). The description of only the PEDI functional skills in the Self-Care Scale domain and the Likert scale were highlighted in the text to simplify the development of the corresponding hypothetical replication study.

15-Point Likert Scale
Please indicate how much this child changed from admission to discharge in ___ (capability/level of independence) in the area of ___ (self-care, mobility, or social function) by choosing one of the options from the sheet in front of you.

 7 A very great deal better
 6 A great deal better
 5 A good deal better
 4 Moderately better
 3 Somewhat better
 2 A little better
 1 About the same, hardly any better at all
 0 No change
-1 About the same, hardly any worse at all
-2 A little worse
-3 Somewhat worse
-4 Moderately worse
-5 A good deal worse
-6 A great deal worse
-7 A very great deal worse

Figure A-2 Likert scale used by clinicians to judge clinical improvement of 53 children admitted to a rehabilitation hospital. (Reprinted from Iyer LV, Haley SM, Watkins MP, Dumas HM. Establishing minimal clinically important differences for scores on the Pediatric Evaluation of Disability Inventory for inpatient rehabilitation. Phys Ther 2003; 83:888–898, with permission of the American Physical Therapy Association. This material is copyrighted, and any further reproduction or distribution requires written permission of the APTA.)

Table A-2	Average *Change* in the Pediatric Evaluation of Disability Inventory (PEDI) Scores for Likert Scale Categories Relating to Self-Care															
PEDI Scale	No Change (0)				Minimal Change (1–3)				Moderate Change (4–5)				Large Change (6-7)			
	N	X	SD	Range	N	X	SD	Range	N	X	SD	Range	N	X	SD	Range
Self-care FS (n = 53)	7	3.2	7.5	−3.9–8.6	15	10.1	9.3	0–34.2	21	24.3	17.5	4.2–62.5	10	55.0	22.1	15.7–85.1

Reprinted from Iyer LV, Haley SM, Watkins MP, Dumas HM. Establishing minimal clinically important differences for scores on the Pediatric Evaluation of Disability Inventory for inpatient rehabilitation. Phys Ther 2003; 83:888–898, with permission of the American Physical Therapy Association. This material is copyrighted, and any further reproduction or distribution requires written permission of the APTA.

MCID for the PEDI was a change of 10 points on a scale from 0 to 100 for this particular domain.

Hypothetical Study #2

A hypothetical data set is illustrated in **Figure A-3**. To emphasize the point that the data set is fabricated, the outcome measures are from a hypothetical instrument similar to the PEDI and are referred to here as the PEDO.

Exercises for Hypothetical Study #2

Open the demonstration data set that matches your statistical software:

NCSS	SPSS
PEDO.S0	PEDO.sav

2-1. Minimal Clinically Important Difference or Meaningful Clinical Change

  a. Determine the number of imaginary patients classified as having MCID using descriptive statistics modules on the variable "Convert Likert Rating."

  b. What is the average change score for those classified as having MCID on the PEDO (use descriptive statistics with a filter)?

  c. How do the hypothetical study results for the PEDO compare with the results reported by Iyer et al.[4] for the PEDI?

  d. Alternatively, determine MCID for the PEDO by running a ROC curve (criterion standard vs. PEDO change scores; make sure statistical software filters are off). What

Hypothetical Data

Variable name	Definition
PEDO_change_score	Pre-post rehabilitation change
Likert rating	Imaginary clinician rating of change when blind to PEDO scores
Convert_Likert rating	Likert ratings converted to classify imaginary patients as "no, minimal, moderate or large change"
Criterion_standard	Dichotomized Likert rating: no change vs better

PEDO_Change_Score	Likert_rating	Convert_Likert_rating	Criterion_Standard
1	0	no_change	no_change
1	−6	no_change	no_change
1	0	no_change	no_change
0	−4	no_change	no_change
1	0	no_change	no_change
6	−2	no_change	no_change
1	−1	no_change	no_change
4	1	MCID	better
3	1	MCID	better
11	3	MCID	better
7	1	MCID	better
24	2	MCID	better
16	2	MCID	better
23	2	MCID	better
9	2	MCID	better
19	3	MCID	better
28	1	MCID	better
10	3	MCID	better
19	2	MCID	better
17	1	MCID	better
29	2	MCID	better
25	3	MCID	better

Figure A-3 Data definitions and values for a hypothetical replication study of meaningful clinical change using fabricated values for a hypothetical assessment tool called the PEDO (based on selected methods and outcome variables of a study by Iyer et al.[4]). Only 22 of 53 rows are displayed (the full data set is available on the bound-in disk; file name "PEDO" with either the NCSS or SPSS extension).

is the MCID using the ROC methodology (Chapter 4)?

e. Is it possible to calculate MDC, Chapter 4 using the hypothetical PEDO data set? Explain.

f. What is the MCID *proportion*?

Practice Exercise 3: Hand Function

Summary of Real Study 3

The modified Kapandji Index (MKI) assesses opposition of the thumb and flexion and extension of the long fingers.[5] This measure provides an index of overall hand mobility and, therefore, supplements the hand mobility assessment provided by goniometry. The test has three components:[5]

- Opposition of the thumb—scored from 0 (impossible to do) to 10 (completely accomplished)
- Flexion of each long finger—scored from 0 (impossible to do) to 5 (completely accomplished; range 0–20 for 4 fingers)
- Finger extension—scored from 0 (impossible to do) to 5 (completely accomplished; range, 0–20 for 4 fingers)

The composite score for the MKI is 50 points (*higher scores indicate greater function*).

The Cochin rheumatoid hand disability scale was used to assess disability of the hand.[5] The scale has 18 questions concerning activities of daily living; each question is scored from 0 (performed without difficulty) to 5 (impossible to do). Disability is assessed by adding the scores of all questions (range 0–90) to obtain a total score. *The highest score indicates maximum disability.*

Lefevre-Colau et al.[5] studied the responsiveness of the MKI and the Cochin disability scale using the effect size ($ES_{responsiveness}$) and the standardized response mean (SRM; see Chapter 5). Patients with rheumatoid arthritis were evaluated before and then 6 months after surgery to improve hand function. A selection of their results is shown in Table A-3.

Responsiveness was calculated by baseline minus postsurgery scores. Negative responsiveness indices for the MKI indicate improvement after surgery compared to baseline, whereas positive responsiveness indices for the Cochin scale indicate improvement (Table A-3).

Hypothetical Study 3

The hypothetical data set is illustrated in **Figure A-4**. Descriptor variables indicated if the measures improved or got worse (the variables "iMKI_improved" and "iCochin_improved" with responses in each row of either

Table A-3	Responsiveness of Selected Outcome Measures			
Variable	Mean of the Differences ± SD	Paired *t*-Test *P* Value	SRM	Effect Size
MKI	−1.10 ± 5.54	.167	−.19	−.10
Cochin scale	7.92 ± 12.45	.0001	.66	.58

Reprinted from Arch Phys Med Rehabil 2003, 84, Lefevre-Colau MM, Poiraudeau S, Oberlin C, Demaille S, Fermanian F, Rannou F, Revel M. Reliability, validity, and responsiveness of the modified Kapandji index for assessment of functional mobility of the rheumatoid hand, Pp. 1032–8, Copyright (2003), with permission from Elsevier.

yes or no).[c] Each descriptor is coded so improvement = 1 and no improvement = 2 (see the variables iMKI_improved_**coded**" and "iCochin_improved_**coded**").

Exercises for Hypothetical Replication Study #3

Open the demonstration data set that matches your statistical software:

NCSS	SPSS
Hand Function.S0	Hand Function.sav

3-1. Group-Level Responsiveness Indices
a. Follow the methods discussed in Chapter 5 to determine $ES_{responsiveness}$ and the SRM for the imaginary MKI and Cochrin variables using the demonstration data set (you should calculate an ES and SRM for each of these variables).
b. How do the hypothetical study results compare with the results reported by Lefevre-Colau et al.?[5]
c. Why are the iMKI responsiveness indices negative?

3-2. Individual-Level Responsiveness Indices
a. Using the imaginary patient satisfaction variable as the criterion standard, run ROC analyses on the change scores for the iMKI and iCochin variables (the variable columns labeled "inverted_iMKI_change" and "iCochin_change").[d] Show the ROC plots[e] for each change score.

[c]NCSS statistical software sorts by alpha numeric characters. A "z" is placed in front of the entry "no" so that any resulting contingency table will show "yes" in the first column or row and "zNo" in the second column or row.
[d]The sign of the iMKI has been reversed so that a positive number indicates improvement in both measures of hand function (see the variable "invert _iMKI_change").
[e]For SPSS, the variable "Satisfaction_*code*" was added to the hypothetical data set so that the required numeric values could be used for the criterion standard ("State Variable" in the SPSS ROC dialog box).

Hypothetical Data

Patient_num	pre_iMKI	post_iMKI	pre_iCochin	post_iCochin	iMKI_change	iCochin_change	iMKI_improved	iMKI_improved_code	iCochin_improved	iCochin_improved_code	Satisfaction
1	26	49	20	25	-23	-5	Yes	1	zNo	0	zNo
2	3	21	32	46	-18	-14	Yes	1	zNo	0	zNo
3	9	28	6	2	-19	4	Yes	1	Yes	1	Yes
4	7	18	19	32	-11	-13	Yes	1	zNo	0	zNo
5	28	40	43	5	-12	38	Yes	1	Yes	1	Yes
6	4	44	34	5	-40	29	Yes	1	Yes	1	Yes
7	34	22	21	47	12	-26	zNo	0	zNo	0	zNo
8	48	29	36	37	19	-1	zNo	0	zNo	0	zNo
9	38	39	39	58	-1	-19	Yes	1	zNo	0	Yes
10	17	19	32	28	-2	4	Yes	1	Yes	1	Yes
11	36	49	11	11	-13	0	Yes	1	zNo	0	zNo
12	17	39	56	10	-22	46	Yes	1	Yes	1	Yes
13	45	20	22	10	-5	12	zNo	0	Yes	1	zNo
14	35	40	42	5	-5	37	Yes	1	Yes	1	Yes
15	32	49	31	0	-17	31	Yes	1	Yes	1	Yes
16	49	41	57	37	8	20	zNo	0	Yes	1	zNO
17	13	47	31	29	-34	2	Yes	1	Yes	1	Yes
18	40	50	59	49	-10	10	Yes	1	Yes	1	Yes
19	27	50	40	56	-23	-16	Yes	1	zNo	0	zNo
20	47	15	25	14	32	11	zNo	0	Yes	1	zNo
21	35	41	56	11	-6	45	Yes	1	Yes	1	Yes
22	48	22	35	12	26	23	zNo	0	Yes	1	zNo

Variable name	Definition
pre_iMKI post_iMKI	Imaginary Kapandji index pre and post surgery
pre_iCochin post_iCochin	Imaginary Cochin index pre and post surgery
iMKI_change iCochin_change	Imaginary change scores for each index
iMKI_improved iMKI_improved_code iCochin_improved iCochin_improved_code	Indication if change score showed improvement Code for improvement 1=yes, 0=no
Satisfaction	Hypothetical satisfaction survey results
Invert_iMKI_changePED O_change_score	Changes sign so that positive number=improvement

Figure A-4 Hypothetical data description and values for an imaginary study designed to measure the responsiveness of two hand function scales based on selected methods and outcome variables described by Lefevre-Colau et al.[5] Only 22 of 50 rows are displayed (the full data set is available on the bound-in disk in the file "Hand Function" with either the NCSS or SPSS extension).

b. For the *optimal point* on each curve determine (1) the sensitivity for meaningful clinical change, (2) the false positive rate, and (3) the specificity for meaningful clinical change.

c. What is the estimated MCID for the inverted iMKI and iCochin change scores from the ROC plots?

d. Do each of these change scores identify the greatest number of true positives + true negatives in their respective ROC analyses?

e. For inverted iMKI and iCochin separately, what is the change score that has the highest +LR and lowest −LR?

f. Define the LRs in terms of meaningful clinical change research (Chapter 4). Then compare the statistical and clinical significance of the LRs identified in the previous question.

g. Is responsiveness (area under the ROC curve) of hand function tools statistically different when comparing the inverted iMKI vs. the iCochin change scores[f] and comparing each hand function tool with meaningless area ($AUC_{meaningless} = 0.50$)?

[f]Hint: In order to compare two ROC curves simultaneously, the outcome variables must change in the same direction. As negative change scores show improvement for the MKI and positive change scores show improvement for the Cochin disability index, use the column in the hypothetical data set that "inverts" the MKI scores so that positive MKI changes from pre- to postsurgery would reflect improvement (see the variable column "Invert_MKI_change").

Practice Exercise 4: Shoulder Sick Leave

Summary of Real Study 4

Kuijpers et al.[6] developed a clinical prediction rule for determining the risk of sick leave use related to shoulder dysfunction in workers during a 6-month period following the first health-care consultation. The goal was to accurately predict the risk of sick leave related to shoulder pain so that early intervention strategies might be designed to reduce this risk. Thus, sick leave due to shoulder pain was the primary outcome measure and was dichotomized (coded "Yes" if ≥1 sick day; coded "No" if sick days = 0).

The clinical prediction rule for sick leave risk due to shoulder pain is summarized in the score chart shown in **Figure A-5**. For example, a patient with 3 days of sick leave during 2 months preceding the initial evaluation, a self-reported shoulder pain intensity of 5 points (on a numeric scale of 0 to 10), who perceives the cause of pain due to typical overuse and who has no anxiety or distress, receives 7 points. This total score = 7 translates to a risk of taking sick leave for shoulder pain of 40% to 50% compared with those who had a reference score of 0.

The authors arrived at this prediction rule by first entering many psychological, physical, and work environment variables into a multiple logistic regression analysis. The logistic regression procedure selected the best set of predictor variables (**Table A-4**).

Using the optimal predictors in the logistic prediction equation to predict sick leave use (the variables listed in Table A-4), the authors generated a ROC curve that analyzed the accuracy of prediction. The ROC curve plots true positive rate versus false-positive rate, or, in other words, a plot of sensitivity (those who were accurately described by the prediction equation as sick leave users) compared with the false-positive rate (those *not* using sick leave who were classified as sick leave users by the prediction equation). They reported an AUC of 0.70 (95% CI 0.64–0.76) and concluded that this result represents satisfactory discrimination between patients who did or did not use sick leave.[6]

Hypothetical Study #4

The hypothetical data set is illustrated in **Figure A-6**:

- Dichotomous predictor variables:
  - The number of sick days recorded for a 6-month period ("Sick_days_6mo_after_BL"), then

Table A-4	The Optimal Set of Predictors for Sick Leave Use Due to Shoulder Pain Derived from Multiple Logistic Regression

Variable	OR	95% CI
Sick Leave at Baseline in Preceding 2 Months		
0 weeks*		
≤ 1 week	1.7	0.8–3.6
> 1 week	2.2	1.0–4.7
Shoulder pain (0–10)		
0–3 points*		
4–6 points	1.7	0.9–3.2
7–10 points	1.9	0.9–3.9
Strain, overuse: usual activities (yes/no)	1.9	1.1–3.5
Coexisting psychological complaints (yes/no)	4.0	1.5–10.8

* Reference category

From Kuijpers T, AWM van der Windt D, van der Heijden GJMG, Twisk JWR, Vergouwe Y, Bouter LM. A prediction rule for shoulder pain related sick leave: a prospective cohort study. BMC Musculoskelet Disord 2006; 7:doi: 10.1186/1471-2474-7-97.[6] © 2006 Kuijpers et al; licensee BioMed Central Ltd.

Sick leave in the preceding 2 months	
none	0 ---
0-1 week	2 ---
>1 week	3 ---
Intensity of shoulder pain (0-10)	
0-3 points	0 ---
4-6 points	2 ---
7-10 points	3 ---
Perceived cause: strain or overuse during regular activities	3 ---
Reported psychological problems (anxiety, distress, depression)	6 ---
	+
Total score	---

Total score	Risk
≤1	10% - 20%
2 – 3	20% - 30%
4 – 5	30% - 40%
6 – 7	40% - 50%
8	50% - 60%
9 – 10	60% - 70%
11 – 12	70% - 80%
13 – 15	80% - 90%

Figure A-5 Score chart for determining risk of sick leave during 6 months following consultation in workers who initially present with shoulder dysfunction. (From Kuijpers T, AWM van der Windt D, van der Heijden GJMG, Twisk JWR, Vergouwe Y, Bouter LM. A prediction rule for shoulder pain related sick leave: a prospective cohort study. BMC Musculoskelet Disord 2006; 7:doi: 10.1186/1471-2474-7-97.[6] © 2006 Kuijpers et al; licensee BioMed Central Ltd.)

Hypothetical Data

Patient_num	Sick_days_6mo_after_BL	Dichotomous_sick_days	Coded_Dichotomous_sick_days	Psych_complaints	Perceived_Cause	Previous_neck_sympt	BL_Sick_days_num	Shoulder_Pain_score	Age_yrs
1	13	Yes	1	zNo	Typical_overuse	Yes	9	10	32
2	19	Yes	1	zNo	Unusual_overuse	zNo	29	10	54
3	12	Yes	1	zNo	Typical_overuse	Yes	21	10	31
4	10	Yes	1	zNo	Unusual_overuse	Yes	28	7	61
5	14	Yes	1	zNo	Typical_overuse	Yes	8	9	39
6	12	Yes	1	zNo	Unusual_overuse	zNo	30	7	27
7	11	Yes	1	zNo	Unusual_overuse	zNo	11	8	27
8	14	Yes	1	zNo	Typical_overuse	Yes	28	5	44
9	14	Yes	1	zNo	Unusual_overuse	Yes	23	10	50
10	0	zNo	0	zNo	Typical_overuse	zNo			
11	0	zNo	0	zNo	Unusual_overuse	zNo			
12	0	zNo	0	zNo	Unusual_overuse	Yes			
13	0	zNo	0	zNo	Typical_overuse	zNo			
14	0	zNo	0	zNo	Unusual_overuse	Yes			
15	0	zNo	0	zNo	Typical_overuse	zNo			
16	0	zNo	0	zNo	Typical_overuse	Yes			
17	0	zNo	0	zNo	Typical_overuse	Yes			
18	0	zNo	0	zNo	Unusual_overuse	Yes			
19	19	Yes	1	zNo	Typical_overuse	zNo			
20	11	Yes	1	zNo	Unusual_overuse	zNo			
21	12	Yes	1	zNo	Typical_overuse	Yes			
22	13	Yes	1	zNo	Typical_overuse	Yes			
23	10	Yes	1	zNo	Typical_overuse	Yes			
24	16	Yes	1	zNo	Typical_overuse	zNo			
25	13	Yes	1	zNo	Unusual_overuse	zNo			
26	17	Yes	1	zNo	Unusual_overuse	zNo			

	Psych_coded	Cause_coded	Neck_coded
1	0	1	1
2	0	0	0
3	0	1	1
4	0	0	1
5	0	1	1
6	0	0	0
7	0	0	0
8	0	1	1
9	0	0	1
10	0	1	0
11	0	0	1
12	0	0	1
13	0	1	0
14	0	0	1
15	0	1	0
16	0	1	1
17	0	1	1
18	0	0	1
19	0	1	0
20	0	0	0
21	0	1	1
22	0	1	1
23	0	1	1
24	0	1	0
25	0	0	0
26	0	0	0

Variable name	Definition
Sick_days_6mo_after_BL	Sick days 6 months after initial evaluation
Dichotomous_sick_days Coded_Dichotomous_sick_days	Sick days after initial evaluation dichotomize (yes or no) and coded 1 or 0 respectively
Psych_complaints Perceived_Cause Previous_neck_sympt BL_sick_days_num	Dichotomous—yes or no Cause of shoulder complaints Dichotomous—yes or no Number of sick days prior to initial evaluation
Shoulder_pain_score	Sum of pain scores during shoulder mobility tests Higher scores=more pain
Age_yrs	Age in years
Psych_coded Cause_coded	Psych complaints coded 1=yes, 0=no Cause of shoulder complaint coded 1=strain due to typical (1) or unusual (0) activities
Neck_coded	Neck complaints in the past 1=yes, 0=no
Variables not shown in figure Present_BL_sick_days_GTE1	Dichotomous—if sick days are greater than or equal to ("GTE") 1, then code=1, if not, then code=0
Present_Shoulder_Pain_GTE6	Dichotomous—coded 1 if patient presents with pain score greater than or equal to 6, if not, then code=0
Sum_predictors_present At_least_3_present At_least_2_present At_least_1_present	Number of predictor variables present when patient has initial evaluation Patient has at least 3 predictor variables at initial evaluation Patient has at least 2 predictor variables at initial evaluation Patient has at least 1 predictor variable at initial evaluation

Figure A-6 Data for a hypothetical study of sick leave use due to shoulder dysfunction based on selected methods and outcome variables described by Kuijpers et al.[6] Only 26 of 298 rows are displayed (the full data set is available on the bound-in disk in the file "Shoulder Sick Leave" with either the NCSS or SPSS extension).

dichotomized to classify patients as either a user or nonuser of sick leave (see the variable "Dichotomous_sick_days"; the variable "Coded_Dichotomous_sick_days" translates the classification into 0 = no sick leave or 1 = yes, sick leave).

- Reports of anxiety or other psychological complaints ("Psych_complaints" yes or no coded as 1 or 0, respectively, in the variable "Psych_coded"), the perceived cause of injury. ("Perceived_Cause" typical or atypical overuse coded as 1 or 0, respectively, in "Cause_Coded"),

and a history of previous neck symptoms ("Previous_neck_sympt" yes or no coded as 1 or 0, respectively, in the variable "Neck_coded").
- Continuous predictor variables
- The number of sick days taken prior to the initial evaluation ("BL_Sick_days_num"); the shoulder pain score on a scale of 0 (no pain) to 10 (maximum pain; see the variable column labeled "Shoulder_Pain_score").
- Age ("Age_yrs")

Exercises for Hypothetical Study #4

Open the demonstration data set that matches your statistical software:

NCSS	SPSS
Shoulder Sick Leave.S0	*Shoulder Sick Leave.sav*

4-1. Identify the optimal set of predictors for sick leave use.
  a. Use the methods described in Chapter 8 for multiple logistic models to determine the optimal set of sick leave predictors. The dependent variable is "Coded_Dichotomous _sick_days." Potential predictor variables to enter are:
    - BL_SICK_DAYS_NUM
    - SHOULDER_PAIN_SCORE
    - AGE_YRS
    - PSYCH_CODED
    - CAUSE_CODED
    - NECK_CODED
  b. Which variables from this set of potential predictors should be included in the hypothetical study prediction model and why?
  c. What is the optimal prediction model (equation) using only Wald score significant predictors?
  d. What is the goodness-of-fit for this model?
  e. If a new imaginary patient enters the clinic with the following profile (three findings at the initial evaluation), what is the probability that he will use sick leave related to shoulder pain in the future?
    - 10 days of sick leave prior to baseline evaluation
    - Shoulder pain score of 8
    - Has anxiety and depression
4-2. The use of a logistic regression prediction equation to determine the probability of sick leave due to shoulder pain is cumbersome in a clinical setting. Create a clinical prediction rule based on the number of clinical traits with predictive value that are present in the model.

In order to do this, the continuous variables in the model—baseline sick days ("BL_Sick_days_num"), shoulder pain score ("Shoulder_Pain_score")—must be dichotomized to find the cut-point for each variable.
  a. Run a ROC analysis on each continuous variable in the optimal model (using "Coded_Dichotomous_sick_days" as the criterion standard) and create a table showing the optimal cut-point for each continuous variable in the decision rule.
4-3. Find the variable columns in the hypothetical data set that show the following for each patient (refer to Chapter 9, Fig. 9-3 for other examples): (1) at least two predictors present; (2) at least one predictor present
  a. Show the plot of a ROC analysis for the number of clinical traits present ("at least 1 trait present" and "at least 2 traits present") using the criterion standard of "Coded_Dichotomous_sick_days."
  b. Create a table showing sensitivity, specificity, and the +LR (plus 95% CIs) for each level of the new decision rule (refer to Chapter 9, Table 9-7).
  c. Assuming a prevalence of 35%, compare the estimated post-test probability of sick leave use when an imaginary patient presents with at least two clinical sign variables at the initial evaluation versus one clinical sign (use Fagan's nomogram and refer to Chapter 9, Fig. 9-5 for an example).
  d. How would these hypothetical results guide the care of the patient?

Practice Exercise #5: Pull Test

Summary of Real Study #5

Visser et al.[7] sought to identify a reliable clinical test measuring postural instability in patients with Parkinson's disease. Their goal was to find a credible test that was easy to use in a clinical environment. The general format of all tests was to evaluate the stability of a patient who was standing and receiving a quick pull backward by a therapist behind the patient. The results showed that a pull test scored using the Nutt method had excellent inter-rater reliability (weighted kappa = 0.93 using a squared weighting scheme to weight the disagreements among raters).[8] The Nutt method for scoring the pull test is shown in **Figure A-7**.

9A "squared" method of rating is the same as the "quadratic method." The value of the disagreement between rater1 and rater2 is squared.

Ratings (and the accompanying test condition):
1. Nutt (shoulder pull, unexpected)
   0=Normal, may take 2 steps to recover
   1=Takes 3 or more steps; recovers unaided
   2=Would fall if not caught
   3=Spontaneous tendency to fall or unable to stand unaided
   (test not executable)

Figure A-7 The Nutt method of scoring the pull test in patients with Parkinson's disease. (From Visser M, Marinus J, Bloem BR, Kisjes H, van den Berg BM, van Hilten JJ. Clinical tests for the evaluation of postural instability in patients with Parkinson's disease. Arch Phys Med Rehabil 2003; 84:1669–1674[7]).

Hypothetical Study 5

The focus of this hypothetical study is on the reliability of the Nutt scoring method (ordinal-level data). Two imaginary raters, not randomly selected, evaluated the results of a pull test from video of each imaginary patient. It is known that weighting disagreements in reliability studies might bias results. The goal here is to demonstrate the outcome of consensus measures using a "squared" method to weight the kappa versus an $ICC_{interrater\ fixed}$. The hypothetical data sets are illustrated in **Figure A-8**.

The variables are a criterion standard for assessing postural stability (e.g., two falls within 6 months of the study), rater number, and the pull test scored using the Nutt method.

Exercises for Hypothetical Study #5

Open the demonstration data sets that match your statistical software:

NCSS	SPSS
Pull Test-ICC.S0	Pull Test-ICC.sav
Pull Test-weighted Kappa.S0	Pull Test-weighted Kappa.sav

5-1. Follow the procedure outlined in Chapter 6 and calculate the $ICC_{interrater\ fixed}$ using data set *Pull Test-ICC*.
  a. What is the descriptive value of the $ICC_{inter\ rater\ fixed}$?
  b. If a patient receives an average pull test rating of "2" (*"would fall if not caught"*), then what is the range of error associated with this measurement?

5-2. Run statistical software to obtain the contingency tables for calculating weighted kappa using the data set *Pull Test-weighted Kappa* (refer to Chapter 6, Fig. 6-5). Note that the weighting method described there as a quadratic weighting scheme is the same as the "squared" weighting scheme used by Visser et al.[7]

  a. What is the value for the weighted kappa?
  b. Compare the magnitude of weighted kappa with $ICC_{inter\ rater\ fixed}$. Was there bias in the weighting scheme?

Practice Exercise 6: Treatment Effect

Summary Real Study 6

Di Fabio et al.[8] conducted an in-clinic study to determine disability and functional status of patients with low-back pain receiving worker's compensation. One of the goals of the study was to describe the effect of compliance with therapeutic exercise on patient outcome (measured by changes in the Oswestry scale, fingertip-to-floor distance, and maximum isometric lift). Compliance was defined as the number of treatments divided by the scheduled number of treatments, expressed as a percent. High compliance was defined as ≥80%, whereas low compliance was defined as <80%. To answer the key question "Did patients improve after receiving treatment?" the treatment effects were quantified by a paired t-test (refer to Chapter 10).

Outcomes were measured at the initial evaluation and then again after 1 month and at the time of discharge from the clinic. For this demonstration only, the initial versus 1-month assessments will be considered. The difference between the outcomes from initial evaluation to follow-up was the treatment effect. A summary of results is shown in **Table A-5**.[8]

When the goal is to identify the treatment effect from data presented in a literature review targeting studies designed to compare initial versus posttreatment follow-up, the average change in performance normalized to the standard deviation of the initial assessment score provides the magnitude of change, or the effect size (refer to Chapter 10, eq 10-3). For example, from Table A-5, the mean Oswestry Disability Score at the initial evaluation was 38% disability compared to a mean of 28% following treatment. Because $n > 20$ and the table shows the SD of the initial Oswestry scores (14%), the magnitude of the treatment effect is:

High-Compliance Group Self-Perceived Disability:
$$ES = d\ index = 38 - 28/14 = 0.71\ (eq\ 10-3)$$

According to Cohen's scale for describing the magnitude of the d index, ES = 0.71 approaches a large treatment effect.[9] Lower scores on the Oswestry scale indicate less self-perceived disability,[h] so there was a

hThe complete Oswestry tool can be found in Chapter 5.

Hypothetical Data

Patient_num	Criterion_Standard	Rater	Nutt_score
1	Unstable	1	3
2	Unstable	1	3
3	Unstable	1	1
4	Unstable	1	3
5	Unstable	1	2
6	Unstable	1	1
7	Unstable	1	2
8	Unstable	1	3
9	Unstable	1	2
10	Unstable	1	2
11	Unstable	1	1
12	Unstable	1	3
13	Unstable	1	3
14	Unstable	1	1
15	Unstable	1	1
16	Unstable	1	2
17	Unstable	1	1
18	Unstable	1	2
19	Unstable	1	1
20	Unstable	1	3
21	Unstable	1	2
22	Unstable	1	1
23	Stable	1	0
24	Stable	1	2
25	Stable	1	0
26	Stable	1	1

A

Hypothetical Data

Patient_num	Criterion_Standard	Rater1_Nutt_score	Rater2_Nutt_score
1	Unstable	3	2
2	Unstable	3	2
3	Unstable	1	0
4	Unstable	3	2
5	Unstable	2	1
6	Unstable	1	0
7	Unstable	2	1
8	Unstable	3	2
9	Unstable	2	1
10	Unstable	2	1
11	Unstable	1	0
12	Unstable	3	2
13	Unstable	3	2
14	Unstable	1	0
15	Unstable	1	0
16	Unstable	2	1
17	Unstable	1	1
18	Unstable	2	1
19	Unstable	1	0
20	Unstable	3	2
21	Unstable	2	1
22	Unstable	1	1
23	Stable	0	0
24	Stable	2	1
25	Stable	0	0
26	Stable	1	1

B

Figure A-8 Data for a hypothetical study based on selected methods and outcome variables described by Visser et al.[7] (A) Setup for ANOVA and ICC-rater designation in a single column. (B) Same data setup for weighted kappa but with rater designation in two columns (one for each rater). Only 26 of 42 rows are displayed (the full data set is available on the bound-in disk; file names "Pull Test-ICC" and "Pull Test-weighted Kappa" with the NCSS or SPSS extension).

large positive effect of treatment (less perceived disability following treatment) in the group that complied with the therapeutic intervention.

If this study were included in a meta-analysis, data would be extracted from Table A-5 and the ES would be calculated for each outcome measure and each cohort grouped by compliance to therapy (meta-analyses are discussed in Chapter 11). The ES provides a standard metric that can be used to describe the magnitude of the treatment effect for every similar study included in the quantitative review.

Table A-5	Means (SDs) of Outcome Measures for Patients in High and Low Compliance With a Therapeutic Intervention for the Treatment of Low Back Pain			
	Outcome Measure Initial Evaluation vs. 1-Month Reassessment		**Unbiased Effect Size**	
	Initial Assessment	1-Month Reassessment	N[a]	Paired *t* Value
High compliance				
Oswestry scores (%)	38 (14)	28 (19)	28	3.08[b]
Fingertip-to-floor distance (cm)	30 (18)	17 (18)	33	4.06[b]
Maximum isometric lift (lb)	82 (80)	132 (83)	26	−5.75[b]
Maximum isometric lift (N)	364 (355)	586 (369)		
Low compliance				
Oswestry scores (%)	43 (16)	40 (21)	14	NS[c]
Fingertip-to-floor distance (cm)	44 (21)	30 (19)	13	4.91[b]
Maximum isometric lift (lb)	70 (64)	110 (88)	10	−3.27[b]
Maximum isometric lift (N)	311 (284)	488 (391)		

[a]Number of patients with paired scores who had values for both the initial and 1-month

[b]P < .025

[c]NS = not significant; P >.025

Adapted from Di Fabio RP, Mackey G, Holte J. Disability and functional status in patients with low back pain receiving worker's compensation: a descriptive study with implications for the efficacy of physical therapy. Phys Ther 1995; 75:180–193, with permission of the American Physical Therapy Association. This material is copyrighted, and any further reproduction or distribution requires written permission from APTA.

Hypothetical Study #6

A hypothetical quantitative review is being conducted by a team of clinicians to determine if rehabilitation for people receiving worker's compensation is effective. The data in Table A-5 represent one of the studies that meet the requirements for inclusion in this imaginary systematic literature review.

Exercises for Hypothetical Study #6

6-1a. Refer to Chapter 10 and then create a table of effect sizes (treatment effects or d indexes) for each paired comparison in Table A-5. Use equations 10-3 or 10-4, where appropriate, to fill in the template shown in **Table A-6** (recall that for $N > 20$, the unbiased effect size is derived from equation 10-3).

6-1b. Why are the effect sizes for maximum isometric lift negative?

6-2a. The statistical significance of the change in function for each outcome measure in the real study[8] was measured using a paired t-test generated by statistical software (Table A-5). This practice question will use the change score and a confidence interval in clinic-friendly units to determine statistical significance at $\alpha = 0.05$ (refer to **equation 10-6** and **Table A-7**). If there is *no difference beyond sampling error* between the patient's status at the initial assessment versus the 1-month post-treatment

follow-up, then the 95% CI of the change in the patient's status will hold the value of 0.

Mean change scores are derived from **Table A-5** by simple subtraction: mean of initial evaluation minus mean 1-month follow-up. Assume that the standard error of the change scores (needed for the confidence intervals) is that presented in **Table A-7**.

Specifically for the Oswestry scores, did patients make statistically significant improvements from the initial evaluation to the 1-month follow-up in their self-perceived disability? (1) Did the *highly compliant*

Table A-6	Template to Complete an Effect Size Extraction from Di Fabio et al.[8] Summary Data on High and Low Compliance Outcomes When Comparing the Initial With the Post-treatment 1-Month Follow-up (see Table A-5)
High Compliance	
Oswestry scale (% disability)	
Fingertip-floor distance (cm)	
Maximum isometric lift (lbs)	
Low Compliance	
Oswestry scale (% disability)	
Fingertip-floor distance (cm)	
Maximum isometric lift (lbs)	

Table A-7	**Point Estimates of Treatment Effect (Mean Change Scores) and Hypothetical Standard Errors of Change Scores When Comparing Initial Evaluation to the Post-treatment 1-Month Follow-up.** Based on selected methods and outcome variables described by Di Fabio et al.[8]		
		Mean Change Score (Point Estimate)	**Hypothetical SE of Change Scores**
HIGH Compliance			
Oswestry scale (% disability)		• 10	• 3.43
Fingertip-floor distance (cm)		• 13	• 3.42
Maximum isometric lift (lbs)		• −50	• 10.46
LOW Compliance			
Oswestry scale (% disability)		• 3	• 2.77
Fingertip-floor distance (cm)		• 14	• 1.6
Maximum isometric lift (lbs)		• −40	• 9.23

- Hypothetical studies were based on selected methods and outcome measures presented in the real studies.
- This format provides an opportunity for clinicians to practice becoming active participants in data analysis and interpretation of statistical analyses.

REFERENCES

1. Bohannon RW. Manual muscle testing: does it meet the standards of an adequate screening test? Clin Rehabil 2005; 19:662–667.
2. Haley SM, Dumas HM, Ludlow LH. Variation by diagnostic and practice pattern groups in the mobility outcomes of inpatient rehabilitation programs for children and youth. Phys Ther 2001; 81:1425–1436.
3. Tokcan G, Haley SM, Gill-Body KM, et al. Item-specific functional recovery in children and youth with acquired brain injury. Pediatr Phys Ther 2003; 15:16–22.
4. Iyer LV, Haley SM, Watkins MP, et al. Establishing minimal clinically important differences for scores on the Pediatric Evaluation of Disability Inventory for inpatient rehabilitation. Phys Ther 2003; 83:888–898.
5. Lefevre-Colau MM, Poiraudeau S, Oberlin C, et al. Reliability, validity, and responsiveness of the modified Kapandji index for assessment of functional mobility of the rheumatoid hand. Arch Phys Med Rehabil 2003; 84:1032–1038.
6. Kuijpers T, AWM van der Windt D, van der Heijden GJMG, et al. A prediction rule for shoulder pain related sick leave: a prospective cohort study. BMC Musculoskelet Disord 2006;7.
7. Visser M, Marinus J, Bloem BR, et al. Clinical tests for the evaluation of postural instability in patients with Parkinson's disease. Arch Phys Med Rehabil 2003; 84:1669–1674.
8. Di Fabio RP, Mackey G, Holte J. Disability and functional status in patients with low back pain receiving worker's compensation: a descriptive study with implications for the efficacy of physical therapy. Phys Ther 1995; 75:180–193.
9. Cohen J. Statistical Power Analysis for the Behavioral Sciences. Hillsdale, NJ: Lawrence Erlbaum Associates, 1988.

patients improve significantly with respect to self-perceived disability following treatment? (2) Did the group of patients with *low compliance* show significant improvement in their disability scores with treatment?

6-2b. Plot the point estimates of the treatment effect (mean change scores) and the 95% confidence intervals for each outcome measure. (1) Which 95% CI among all the outcome measures contains the null value of 0 (no treatment effect)? (2) Do the tests of significance using 95% CI correspond to the paired t-test results in the real study?

6-3. What is the level of evidence provided by the pretest–post-test cohort study by Di Fabio et al.[8]?

SUMMARY

- Selected studies in the rehabilitation literature were picked to illustrate concepts in rehabilitation research covered in this primer.

Appendix B
Statistical Tables

| Table B-1 | **Area Between 0 and z.** First column contains the root z and first row contains the decimal place. For example, the area covered by critical z = 1.96 is found by the intersection of the row labeled 1.9 ("z root value") and the column labeled "0.06." Note that the two-tail area for commonly used critical z = 1.96 and z = 1.645 are table values. |

Area between 0 and z

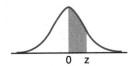

0   z

Z root value ↓ Decimal→	0.00	0.01	0.02	0.03	0.04	0.05	0.06	0.07	0.08	0.09
0.0	0.0000	0.0040	0.0080	0.0120	0.0160	0.0199	0.0239	0.0279	0.0319	0.0359
0.1	0.0398	0.0438	0.0478	0.0517	0.0557	0.0596	0.0636	0.0675	0.0714	0.0753
0.2	0.0793	0.0832	0.0871	0.0910	0.0948	0.0987	0.1026	0.1064	0.1103	0.1141
0.3	0.1179	0.1217	0.1255	0.1293	0.1331	0.1368	0.1406	0.1443	0.1480	0.1517
0.4	0.1554	0.1591	0.1628	0.1664	0.1700	0.1736	0.1772	0.1808	0.1844	0.1879
0.5	0.1915	0.1950	0.1985	0.2019	0.2054	0.2088	0.2123	0.2157	0.2190	0.2224
0.6	0.2257	0.2291	0.2324	0.2357	0.2389	0.2422	0.2454	0.2486	0.2517	0.2549
0.7	0.2580	0.2611	0.2642	0.2673	0.2704	0.2734	0.2764	0.2794	0.2823	0.2852
0.8	0.2881	0.2910	0.2939	0.2967	0.2995	0.3023	0.3051	0.3078	0.3106	0.3133
0.9	0.3159	0.3186	0.3212	0.3238	0.3264	0.3289	0.3315	0.3340	0.3365	0.3389
1.0	0.3413	0.3438	0.3461	0.3485	0.3508	0.3531	0.3554	0.3577	0.3599	0.3621
1.1	0.3643	0.3665	0.3686	0.3708	0.3729	0.3749	0.3770	0.3790	0.3810	0.3830
1.2	0.3849	0.3869	0.3888	0.3907	0.3925	0.3944	0.3962	0.3980	0.3997	0.4015
1.3	0.4032	0.4049	0.4066	0.4082	0.4099	0.4115	0.4131	0.4147	0.4162	0.4177
1.4	0.4192	0.4207	0.4222	0.4236	0.4251	0.4265	0.4279	0.4292	0.4306	0.4319
1.5	0.4332	0.4345	0.4357	0.4370	0.4382	0.4394	0.4406	0.4418	0.4429	0.4441
1.6	0.4452	0.4463	0.4474	0.4484	0.4495	0.4505	0.4515	0.4525	0.4535	0.4545
(1.645)					0.4500					
1.7	0.4554	0.4564	0.4573	0.4582	0.4591	0.4599	0.4608	0.4616	0.4625	0.4633

Continued

Table B-1

Area Between 0 and z. First column contains the root z and first row contains the decimal place. For example, the area covered by critical z = 1.96 is found by the intersection of the row labeled 1.9 ("z root value") and the column labeled "0.06." Note that the two-tail area for commonly used critical z = 1.96 and z = 1.645 are table values.**—cont'd**

Z root value ↓ Decimal→	0.00	0.01	0.02	0.03	0.04	0.05	0.06	0.07	0.08	0.09
1.8	0.4641	0.4649	0.4656	0.4664	0.4671	0.4678	0.4686	0.4693	0.4699	0.4706
1.9	0.4713	0.4719	0.4726	0.4732	0.4738	0.4744	0.4750	0.4756	0.4761	0.4767
2.0	0.4772	0.4778	0.4783	0.4788	0.4793	0.4798	0.4803	0.4808	0.4812	0.4817
2.1	0.4821	0.4826	0.4830	0.4834	0.4838	0.4842	0.4846	0.4850	0.4854	0.4857
2.2	0.4861	0.4864	0.4868	0.4871	0.4875	0.4878	0.4881	0.4884	0.4887	0.4890
2.3	0.4893	0.4896	0.4898	0.4901	0.4904	0.4906	0.4909	0.4911	0.4913	0.4916
2.4	0.4918	0.4920	0.4922	0.4925	0.4927	0.4929	0.4931	0.4932	0.4934	0.4936
2.5	0.4938	0.4940	0.4941	0.4943	0.4945	0.4946	0.4948	0.4949	0.4951	0.4952
2.6	0.4953	0.4955	0.4956	0.4957	0.4959	0.4960	0.4961	0.4962	0.4963	0.4964
2.7	0.4965	0.4966	0.4967	0.4968	0.4969	0.4970	0.4971	0.4972	0.4973	0.4974
2.8	0.4974	0.4975	0.4976	0.4977	0.4977	0.4978	0.4979	0.4979	0.4980	0.4981
2.9	0.4981	0.4982	0.4982	0.4983	0.4984	0.4984	0.4985	0.4985	0.4986	0.4986
3.0	0.4987	0.4987	0.4987	0.4988	0.4988	0.4989	0.4989	0.4989	0.4990	0.4990

*Adapted from (Electronic Version): StatSoft, Inc. Electronic Statistics Textbook. Tulsa, OK: StatSoft, 2010. WEB: http://www.statsoft.com/textbook/. (Printed Version): Hill T Lewicki, P. STATISTICS Methods and Applications. Tulsa, OK: StatSoft, 2007. Reprinted with permission from Statsoft, Inc. The online version of this table can be found at http://www.statsoft.com/textbook/distribution-tables/?button=3.

Table B-2

Critical t Values. Calculated t must be greater than or equal to the table value to achieve statistical significance (rejecting H_0). When a paired t-test is used, df = n – 1.

t table with right tail probabilities

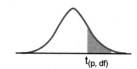

$t_{(p,\ df)}$

p→α₁ 0.40	0.25	0.10	0.05	0.025	0.01	0.005	0.0005
p→α₂ 0.80	0.50	0.20	0.10	0.05	0.02	0.01	0.001

Df↓								
1	0.324920	1.000000	3.077684	6.313752	12.70620	31.82052	63.65674	636.6192
2	0.288675	0.816497	1.885618	2.919986	4.30265	6.96456	9.92484	31.5991
3	0.276671	0.764892	1.637744	2.353363	3.18245	4.54070	5.84091	12.9240
4	0.270722	0.740697	1.533206	2.131847	2.77645	3.74695	4.60409	8.6103
5	0.267181	0.726687	1.475884	2.015048	2.57058	3.36493	4.03214	6.8688
6	0.264835	0.717558	1.439756	1.943180	2.44691	3.14267	3.70743	5.9588
7	0.263167	0.711142	1.414924	1.894579	2.36462	2.99795	3.49948	5.4079
8	0.261921	0.706387	1.396815	1.859548	2.30600	2.89646	3.35539	5.0413
9	0.260955	0.702722	1.383029	1.833113	2.26216	2.82144	3.24984	4.7809

| Table B-2 | **Critical t Values.** Calculated t must be greater than or equal to the table value to achieve statistical significance (rejecting H_0). When a paired t-test is used, df = $n - 1$.—**cont'd** | | | | | | | |

$p \rightarrow \alpha_1$ 0.40 $p \rightarrow \alpha_2$ 0.80 Df↓	0.25 0.50	0.10 0.20	0.05 0.10	0.025 0.05	0.01 0.02	0.005 0.01	0.0005 0.001
10	0.260185	0.699812	1.372184	1.812461	2.22814	2.76377	3.16927	4.5869
11	0.259556	0.697445	1.363430	1.795885	2.20099	2.71808	3.10581	4.4370
12	0.259033	0.695483	1.356217	1.782288	2.17881	2.68100	3.05454	4.3178
13	0.258591	0.693829	1.350171	1.770933	2.16037	2.65031	3.01228	4.2208
14	0.258213	0.692417	1.345030	1.761310	2.14479	2.62449	2.97684	4.1405
15	0.257885	0.691197	1.340606	1.753050	2.13145	2.60248	2.94671	4.0728
16	0.257599	0.690132	1.336757	1.745884	2.11991	2.58349	2.92078	4.0150
17	0.257347	0.689195	1.333379	1.739607	2.10982	2.56693	2.89823	3.9651
18	0.257123	0.688364	1.330391	1.734064	2.10092	2.55238	2.87844	3.9216
19	0.256923	0.687621	1.327728	1.729133	2.09302	2.53948	2.86093	3.8834
20	0.256743	0.686954	1.325341	1.724718	2.08596	2.52798	2.84534	3.8495
21	0.256580	0.686352	1.323188	1.720743	2.07961	2.51765	2.83136	3.8193
22	0.256432	0.685805	1.321237	1.717144	2.07387	2.50832	2.81876	3.7921
23	0.256297	0.685306	1.319460	1.713872	2.06866	2.49987	2.80734	3.7676
24	0.256173	0.684850	1.317836	1.710882	2.06390	2.49216	2.79694	3.7454
25	0.256060	0.684430	1.316345	1.708141	2.05954	2.48511	2.78744	3.7251
26	0.255955	0.684043	1.314972	1.705618	2.05553	2.47863	2.77871	3.7066
27	0.255858	0.683685	1.313703	1.703288	2.05183	2.47266	2.77068	3.6896
28	0.255768	0.683353	1.312527	1.701131	2.04841	2.46714	2.76326	3.6739
29	0.255684	0.683044	1.311434	1.699127	2.04523	2.46202	2.75639	3.6594
30	0.255605	0.682756	1.310415	1.697261	2.04227	2.45726	2.75000	3.6460
inf	0.253347	0.674490	1.281552	1.644854	1.95996	2.32635	2.57583	3.2905

Adapted from (Electronic Version): StatSoft, Inc.. Electronic Statistics Textbook. Tulsa, OK: StatSoft, 2010. WEB: http://www.statsoft.com/textbook/. (Printed Version): Hill, T, Lewicki, P. STATISTICS Methods and Applications. Tulsa, OK: StatSoft, 2007. Reprinted with permission from Statsoft, Inc. The online version of this table can be found at http://www.statsoft.com/textbook/distribution-tables/?button=3.

Table B-3

Critical Values for Chi Square. Df are calculated using the methods described in Chapter 7. The calculated chi square must be ≥ critical value to achieve statistical significance. Commonly used critical chi squares (for p = 0.05) are highlighted in bold.

Right tail areas for the
Chi-square Distribution

x^2

DF↓ area→	.995	.990	.975	.950	.900	.750	.500	.250	.100	.050	.025	.010	.005
1	0.00004	0.00016	0.00098	0.00393	0.01579	0.10153	0.45494	1.32330	2.70554	**3.84146**	5.02389	6.63490	7.87944
2	0.01003	0.02010	0.05064	0.10259	0.21072	0.57536	1.38629	2.77259	4.60517	**5.99146**	7.37776	9.21034	10.59663
3	0.07172	0.11483	0.21580	0.35185	0.58437	1.21253	2.36597	4.10834	6.25139	**7.81473**	9.34840	11.34487	12.83816
4	0.20699	0.29711	0.48442	0.71072	1.06362	1.92256	3.35669	5.38527	7.77944	**9.48773**	11.14329	13.27670	14.86026
5	0.41174	0.55430	0.83121	1.14548	1.61031	2.67460	4.35146	6.62568	9.23636	**11.07050**	12.83250	15.08627	16.74960
6	0.67573	0.87209	1.23734	1.63538	2.20413	3.45460	5.34812	7.84080	10.64464	**12.59159**	14.44938	16.81189	18.54758
7	0.98926	1.23904	1.68987	2.16735	2.83311	4.25485	6.34581	9.03715	12.01704	**14.06714**	16.01276	18.47531	20.27774
8	1.34441	1.64650	2.17973	2.73264	3.48954	5.07064	7.34412	10.21885	13.36157	**15.50731**	17.53455	20.09024	21.95495
9	1.73493	2.08790	2.70039	3.32511	4.16816	5.89883	8.34283	11.38875	14.68366	**16.91898**	19.02277	21.66599	23.58935
10	2.15586	2.55821	3.24697	3.94030	4.86518	6.73720	9.34182	12.54886	15.98718	**18.30704**	20.48318	23.20925	25.18818
11	2.60322	3.05348	3.81575	4.57481	5.57778	7.58414	10.34100	13.70069	17.27501	**19.67514**	21.92005	24.72497	26.75685
12	3.07382	3.57057	4.40379	5.22603	6.30380	8.43842	11.34032	14.84540	18.54935	**21.02607**	23.33666	26.21697	28.29952
13	3.56503	4.10692	5.00875	5.89186	7.04150	9.29907	12.33976	15.98391	19.81193	**22.36203**	24.73560	27.68825	29.81947
14	4.07467	4.66043	5.62873	6.57063	7.78953	10.16531	13.33927	17.11693	21.06414	**23.68479**	26.11895	29.14124	31.31935
15	4.60092	5.22935	6.26214	7.26094	8.54676	11.03654	14.33886	18.24509	22.30713	**24.99579**	27.48839	30.57791	32.80132
16	5.14221	5.81221	6.90766	7.96165	9.31224	11.91222	15.33850	19.36886	23.54183	**26.29623**	28.84535	31.99993	34.26719
17	5.69722	6.40776	7.56419	8.67176	10.08519	12.79193	16.33818	20.48868	24.76904	**27.58711**	30.19101	33.40866	35.71847
18	6.26480	7.01491	8.23075	9.39046	10.86494	13.67529	17.33790	21.60489	25.98942	**28.86930**	31.52638	34.80531	37.15645
19	6.84397	7.63273	8.90652	10.11701	11.65091	14.56200	18.33765	22.71781	27.20357	**30.14353**	32.85233	36.19087	38.58226
20	7.43384	8.26040	9.59078	10.85081	12.44261	15.45177	19.33743	23.82769	28.41198	**31.41043**	34.16961	37.56623	39.99685
21	8.03365	8.89720	10.28290	11.59131	13.23960	16.34438	20.33723	24.93478	29.61509	**32.67057**	35.47888	38.93217	41.40106
22	8.64272	9.54249	10.98232	12.33801	14.04149	17.23962	21.33704	26.03927	30.81328	**33.92444**	36.78071	40.28936	42.79565
23	9.26042	10.19572	11.68855	13.09051	14.84796	18.13730	22.33688	27.14134	32.00690	**35.17246**	38.07563	41.63840	44.18128
24	9.88623	10.85636	12.40115	13.84843	15.65868	19.03725	23.33673	28.24115	33.19624	**36.41503**	39.36408	42.97982	45.55851

Df↓ area→	.995	.990	.975	.950	.900	.750	.500	.250	.100	.050	.025	.010	.005
25	10.51965	11.52398	13.11972	14.61141	16.47341	19.93934	24.33659	29.33885	34.38159	**37.65248**	40.64647	44.31410	46.92789
26	11.16024	12.19815	13.84390	15.37916	17.29188	20.84343	25.33646	30.43457	35.56317	**38.88514**	41.92317	45.64168	48.28988
27	11.80759	12.87850	14.57338	16.15140	18.11390	21.74940	26.33634	31.52841	36.74122	**40.11327**	43.19451	46.96294	49.64492
28	12.46134	13.56471	15.30786	16.92788	18.93924	22.65716	27.33623	32.62049	37.91592	**41.33714**	44.46079	48.27824	50.99338
29	13.12115	14.25645	16.04707	17.70837	19.76774	23.56659	28.33613	33.71091	39.08747	**42.55697**	45.72229	49.58788	52.33562
30	13.78672	14.95346	16.79077	18.49266	20.59923	24.47761	29.33603	34.79974	40.25602	**43.77297**	46.97924	50.89218	53.67196

From (Electronic Version): StatSoft, Inc.. Electronic Statistics Textbook. Tulsa, OK: StatSoft, 2010. WEB: http://www.statsoft.com/textbook/. (Printed Version): Hill, T, Lewicki, P. STATISTICS Methods and Applications. Tulsa, OK: StatSoft, 2007. Reprinted with permission from Statsoft, Inc. The online version of this table can be found at http://www.statsoft.com/textbook/distribution-tables/?button=3.

| **Table B-4** | **Critical Values for F, $\alpha = 0.05$.** df1 is the between groups df as the numerator of the F ratio and df2 is the error df for the denominator of the F ratio. Calculated F ratio must be $\geq$ critical value to achieve statistical significance. |

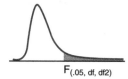

$F_{(.05, df, df2)}$

df1→(numerator)

df2 (denominator)↓	1	2	3	4	5	6	7	8	9
1	161.4476	199.5000	215.7073	224.5832	230.1619	233.9860	236.7684	238.8827	240.5433
2	18.5128	19.0000	19.1643	19.2468	19.2964	19.3295	19.3532	19.3710	19.3848
3	10.1280	9.5521	9.2766	9.1172	9.0135	8.9406	8.8867	8.8452	8.8123
4	7.7086	6.9443	6.5914	6.3882	6.2561	6.1631	6.0942	6.0410	5.9988
5	6.6079	5.7861	5.4095	5.1922	5.0503	4.9503	4.8759	4.8183	4.7725
6	5.9874	5.1433	4.7571	4.5337	4.3874	4.2839	4.2067	4.1468	4.0990
7	5.5914	4.7374	4.3468	4.1203	3.9715	3.8660	3.7870	3.7257	3.6767
8	5.3177	4.4590	4.0662	3.8379	3.6875	3.5806	3.5005	3.4381	3.3881
9	5.1174	4.2565	3.8625	3.6331	3.4817	3.3738	3.2927	3.2296	3.1789
10	4.9646	4.1028	3.7083	3.4780	3.3258	3.2172	3.1355	3.0717	3.0204
11	4.8443	3.9823	3.5874	3.3567	3.2039	3.0946	3.0123	2.9480	2.8962
12	4.7472	3.8853	3.4903	3.2592	3.1059	2.9961	2.9134	2.8486	2.7964
13	4.6672	3.8056	3.4105	3.1791	3.0254	2.9153	2.8321	2.7669	2.7144
14	4.6001	3.7389	3.3439	3.1122	2.9582	2.8477	2.7642	2.6987	2.6458
15	4.5431	3.6823	3.2874	3.0556	2.9013	2.7905	2.7066	2.6408	2.5876
16	4.4940	3.6337	3.2389	3.0069	2.8524	2.7413	2.6572	2.5911	2.5377
17	4.4513	3.5915	3.1968	2.9647	2.8100	2.6987	2.6143	2.5480	2.4943
18	4.4139	3.5546	3.1599	2.9277	2.7729	2.6613	2.5767	2.5102	2.4563
19	4.3807	3.5219	3.1274	2.8951	2.7401	2.6283	2.5435	2.4768	2.4227
20	4.3512	3.4928	3.0984	2.8661	2.7109	2.5990	2.5140	2.4471	2.3928
21	4.3248	3.4668	3.0725	2.8401	2.6848	2.5727	2.4876	2.4205	2.3660
22	4.3009	3.4434	3.0491	2.8167	2.6613	2.5491	2.4638	2.3965	2.3419
23	4.2793	3.4221	3.0280	2.7955	2.6400	2.5277	2.4422	2.3748	2.3201
24	4.2597	3.4028	3.0088	2.7763	2.6207	2.5082	2.4226	2.3551	2.3002
25	4.2417	3.3852	2.9912	2.7587	2.6030	2.4904	2.4047	2.3371	2.2821
26	4.2252	3.3690	2.9752	2.7426	2.5868	2.4741	2.3883	2.3205	2.2655
27	4.2100	3.3541	2.9604	2.7278	2.5719	2.4591	2.3732	2.3053	2.2501
28	4.1960	3.3404	2.9467	2.7141	2.5581	2.4453	2.3593	2.2913	2.2360
29	4.1830	3.3277	2.9340	2.7014	2.5454	2.4324	2.3463	2.2783	2.2229
30	4.1709	3.3158	2.9223	2.6896	2.5336	2.4205	2.3343	2.2662	2.2107
40	4.0847	3.2317	2.8387	2.6060	2.4495	2.3359	2.2490	2.1802	2.1240
60	4.0012	3.1504	2.7581	2.5252	2.3683	2.2541	2.1665	2.0970	2.0401
120	3.9201	3.0718	2.6802	2.4472	2.2899	2.1750	2.0868	2.0164	1.9588
inf	3.8415	2.9957	2.6049	2.3719	2.2141	2.0986	2.0096	1.9384	1.8799

Adapted from (Electronic Version): StatSoft, Inc. Electronic Statistics Textbook. Tulsa, OK: StatSoft, 2010. WEB: http://www.statsoft.com/textbook/.(Printed Version): Hill, T, Lewicki, P. STATISTICS Methods and Applications. Tulsa, OK: StatSoft, 2007. Reprinted with permission from Statsoft, Inc. The online version of this table can be found at http://www.statsoft.com/textbook/distribution-tables/?button=3.

10	12	15	20	24	30	40	60	120	INF
241.8817	243.9060	245.9499	248.0131	249.0518	250.0951	251.1432	252.1957	253.2529	254.3144
19.3959	19.4125	19.4291	19.4458	19.4541	19.4624	19.4707	19.4791	19.4874	19.4957
8.7855	8.7446	8.7029	8.6602	8.6385	8.6166	8.5944	8.5720	8.5494	8.5264
5.9644	5.9117	5.8578	5.8025	5.7744	5.7459	5.7170	5.6877	5.6581	5.6281
4.7351	4.6777	4.6188	4.5581	4.5272	4.4957	4.4638	4.4314	4.3985	4.3650
4.0600	3.9999	3.9381	3.8742	3.8415	3.8082	3.7743	3.7398	3.7047	3.6689
3.6365	3.5747	3.5107	3.4445	3.4105	3.3758	3.3404	3.3043	3.2674	3.2298
3.3472	3.2839	3.2184	3.1503	3.1152	3.0794	3.0428	3.0053	2.9669	2.9276
3.1373	3.0729	3.0061	2.9365	2.9005	2.8637	2.8259	2.7872	2.7475	2.7067
2.9782	2.9130	2.8450	2.7740	2.7372	2.6996	2.6609	2.6211	2.5801	2.5379
2.8536	2.7876	2.7186	2.6464	2.6090	2.5705	2.5309	2.4901	2.4480	2.4045
2.7534	2.6866	2.6169	2.5436	2.5055	2.4663	2.4259	2.3842	2.3410	2.2962
2.6710	2.6037	2.5331	2.4589	2.4202	2.3803	2.3392	2.2966	2.2524	2.2064
2.6022	2.5342	2.4630	2.3879	2.3487	2.3082	2.2664	2.2229	2.1778	2.1307
2.5437	2.4753	2.4034	2.3275	2.2878	2.2468	2.2043	2.1601	2.1141	2.0658
2.4935	2.4247	2.3522	2.2756	2.2354	2.1938	2.1507	2.1058	2.0589	2.0096
2.4499	2.3807	2.3077	2.2304	2.1898	2.1477	2.1040	2.0584	2.0107	1.9604
2.4117	2.3421	2.2686	2.1906	2.1497	2.1071	2.0629	2.0166	1.9681	1.9168
2.3779	2.3080	2.2341	2.1555	2.1141	2.0712	2.0264	1.9795	1.9302	1.8780
2.3479	2.2776	2.2033	2.1242	2.0825	2.0391	1.9938	1.9464	1.8963	1.8432
2.3210	2.2504	2.1757	2.0960	2.0540	2.0102	1.9645	1.9165	1.8657	1.8117
2.2967	2.2258	2.1508	2.0707	2.0283	1.9842	1.9380	1.8894	1.8380	1.7831
2.2747	2.2036	2.1282	2.0476	2.0050	1.9605	1.9139	1.8648	1.8128	1.7570
2.2547	2.1834	2.1077	2.0267	1.9838	1.9390	1.8920	1.8424	1.7896	1.7330
2.2365	2.1649	2.0889	2.0075	1.9643	1.9192	1.8718	1.8217	1.7684	1.7110
2.2197	2.1479	2.0716	1.9898	1.9464	1.9010	1.8533	1.8027	1.7488	1.6906
2.2043	2.1323	2.0558	1.9736	1.9299	1.8842	1.8361	1.7851	1.7306	1.6717
2.1900	2.1179	2.0411	1.9586	1.9147	1.8687	1.8203	1.7689	1.7138	1.6541
2.1768	2.1045	2.0275	1.9446	1.9005	1.8543	1.8055	1.7537	1.6981	1.6376
2.1646	2.0921	2.0148	1.9317	1.8874	1.8409	1.7918	1.7396	1.6835	1.6223
2.0772	2.0035	1.9245	1.8389	1.7929	1.7444	1.6928	1.6373	1.5766	1.5089
1.9926	1.9174	1.8364	1.7480	1.7001	1.6491	1.5943	1.5343	1.4673	1.3893
1.9105	1.8337	1.7505	1.6587	1.6084	1.5543	1.4952	1.4290	1.3519	1.2539
1.8307	1.7522	1.6664	1.5705	1.5173	1.4591	1			

Table B-5	Critical Values for Spearman Rank Correlation Coefficient (r_s) for Two-Tailed (α_2) and One-Tailed (α_1) Tests. n is the number of paired observations. Calculated r_s must be greater than or equal to table value in order to reject null hypothesis.							
α_2	0.50	0.20	0.10	0.05	0.02	0.01	0.005	0.002	0.001
α_1	0.25	0.10	0.05	0.025	0.01	0.005	0.0025	0.001	0.005
n									
4	0.600	1.000	1.000						
5	0.500	0.800	0.900	1.000	1.000				
6	0.371	0.657	0.829	0.886	0.943	1.000	1.000		
7	0.321	0.571	0.714	0.786	0.893	0.929	0.964	1.000	1.000
8	0.310	0.524	0.643	0.738	0.833	0.881	0.905	0.952	0.976
9	0.267	0.483	0.600	0.700	0.783	0.833	0.867	0.917	0.933
10	0.248	0.455	0.564	0.648	0.745	0.794	0.830	0.879	0.903
11	0.236	0.427	0.536	0.618	0.709	0.755	0.800	0.845	0.873
12	0.224	0.406	0.503	0.587	0.671	0.727	0.776	0.825	0.860
13	0.209	0.385	0.484	0.560	0.648	0.703	0.747	0.802	0.835
14	0.200	0.367	0.464	0.538	0.622	0.675	0.723	0.776	0.811
15	0.189	0.354	0.443	0.521	0.604	0.654	0.700	0.754	0.786
16	0.182	0.341	0.429	0.503	0.582	0.635	0.679	0.732	0.765
17	0.176	0.328	0.414	0.485	0.566	0.615	0.662	0.713	0.748
18	0.170	0.317	0.401	0.472	0.550	0.600	0.643	0.695	0.728
19	0.165	0.309	0.391	0.460	0.535	0.584	0.628	0.677	0.712
20	0.161	0.299	0.380	0.447	0.520	0.570	0.612	0.662	0.696
21	0.156	0.292	0.370	0.435	0.508	0.556	0.599	0.648	0.681
22	0.152	0.284	0.361	0.425	0.496	0.544	0.586	0.634	0.667
23	0.148	0.278	0.353	0.415	0.486	0.532	0.573	0.622	0.654
24	0.144	0.271	0.344	0.406	0.476	0.521	0.562	0.610	0.642
25	0.142	0.265	0.337	0.398	0.466	0.511	0.551	0.598	0.630
26	0.138	0.259	0.331	0.390	0.457	0.501	0.541	0.587	0.619
27	0.136	0.255	0.324	0.382	0.448	0.491	0.531	0.577	0.608
28	0.133	0.250	0.317	0.375	0.440	0.483	0.522	0.567	0.598
29	0.130	0.245	0.312	0.368	0.433	0.475	0.513	0.558	0.589
30	0.128	0.240	0.306	0.362	0.425	0.467	0.504	0.549	0.580
31	0.126	0.236	0.301	0.356	0.418	0.459	0.496	0.541	0.571
32	0.124	0.232	0.296	0.350	0.412	0.452	0.489	0.533	0.563
33	0.121	0.229	0.291	0.345	0.405	0.446	0.482	0.525	0.554
34	0.120	0.225	0.287	0.340	0.399	0.439	0.475	0.517	0.547
35	0.118	0.222	0.283	0.335	0.394	0.433	0.468	0.510	0.539
36	0.116	0.219	0.279	0.330	0.388	0.427	0.462	0.504	0.533
37	0.114	0.216	0.275	0.325	0.383	0.421	0.456	0.497	0.526
38	0.113	0.212	0.271	0.321	0.378	0.415	0.450	0.491	0.519
39	0.111	0.210	0.267	0.317	0.373	0.410	0.444	0.485	0.513
40	0.110	0.207	0.264	0.313	0.368	0.405	0.439	0.479	0.507
41	0.108	0.204	0.261	0.309	0.364	0.400	0.433	0.473	0.501
42	0.107	0.202	0.257	0.305	0.359	0.395	0.428	0.468	0.495
43	0.105	0.199	0.254	0.301	0.355	0.391	0.423	0.463	0.490
44	0.104	0.197	0.251	0.298	0.351	0.386	0.419	0.458	0.484
45	0.103	0.194	0.248	0.294	0.347	0.382	0.414	0.453	0.479
46	0.102	0.192	0.246	0.291	0.343	0.378	0.410	0.448	0.474
47	0.101	0.190	0.243	0.288	0.340	0.374	0.405	0.443	0.469
48	0.100	0.188	0.240	0.285	0.336	0.370	0.401	0.439	0.465
49	0.098	0.186	0.238	0.282	0.333	0.366	0.397	0.434	0.460
50	0.097	0.184	0.235	0.279	0.329	0.363	0.393	0.430	0.456

| Table B-5 | Critical Values for Spearman Rank Correlation Coefficient (r_s) for Two-Tailed (α_2) and One-Tailed (α_1) Tests. n is the number of paired observations. Calculated r_s must be greater than or equal to table value in order to reject null hypothesis.—cont'd | | | | | | | |

α_2	0.50	0.20	0.10	0.05	0.02	0.01	0.005	0.002	0.001
α_1	0.25	0.10	0.05	0.025	0.01	0.005	0.0025	0.001	0.005
n									
52	0.095	0.180	0.231	0.274	0.323	0.356	0.386	0.422	0.447
54	0.094	0.177	0.226	0.268	0.317	0.349	0.379	0.414	0.439
56	0.092	0.174	0.222	0.264	0.311	0.343	0.372	0.407	0.432
58	0.090	0.171	0.218	0.259	0.306	0.337	0.366	0.400	0.424
60	0.089	0.168	0.214	0.255	0.300	0.331	0.360	0.394	0.418
62	0.087	0.165	0.211	0.250	0.296	0.326	0.354	0.388	0.411
64	0.086	0.162	0.207	0.246	0.291	0.321	0.348	0.382	0.405
66	0.084	0.160	0.204	0.243	0.287	0.316	0.343	0.376	0.399
68	0.083	0.157	0.201	0.239	0.282	0.311	0.338	0.370	0.393
70	0.082	0.155	0.198	0.235	0.278	0.307	0.333	0.365	0.388
72	0.081	0.153	0.195	0.232	0.274	0.303	0.329	0.360	0.382
74	0.080	0.151	0.193	0.229	0.271	0.299	0.324	0.355	0.377
76	0.078	0.149	0.190	0.226	0.267	0.295	0.320	0.351	0.372
78	0.077	0.147	0.188	0.223	0.264	0.291	0.316	0.346	0.368
80	0.076	0.145	0.185	0.220	0.260	0.287	0.312	0.342	0.363
82	0.075	0.143	0.183	0.217	0.257	0.284	0.308	0.338	0.359
84	0.074	0.141	0.181	0.215	0.254	0.280	0.305	0.334	0.355
86	0.074	0.139	0.179	0.212	0.251	0.277	0.301	0.330	0.351
88	0.073	0.138	0.176	0.210	0.248	0.274	0.298	0.327	0.347
90	0.072	0.136	0.174	0.207	0.245	0.271	0.294	0.323	0.343
92	0.071	0.135	0.173	0.205	0.243	0.268	0.291	0.319	0.339
94	0.070	0.133	0.171	0.203	0.240	0.265	0.288	0.316	0.336
96	0.070	0.132	0.169	0.201	0.238	0.262	0.285	0.313	0.332
98	0.069	0.130	0.167	0.199	0.235	0.260	0.282	0.310	0.329
100	0.068	0.129	0.165	0.197	0.233	0.257	0.279	0.307	0.326

From Zar JH. Significance Testing of the Spearman Rank Correlation Coefficient. Journal of the American Statistical Association 1972; 67:578-580. Reprinted with permission from the Journal of the American Statistical Association, Copyright 1972 by the American Statistical Association, all rights reserved.

| Table B-6 | Critical Values for Pearson Product Moment Correlation Coefficient (r) for Two-Tailed (α_2) and One-Tailed (α_1) Tests. $df = n - 2$. Calculated **r** must be greater than or equal to table value in order to reject the null hypothesis. | | | | |

α_1	.05	.025	.01	.005	.0005
α_2	.10	.05	.02	.01	.001
df					
1	.988	.997	.9995	.9999	.9999
2	.900	.950	.980	.990	.999
3	.805	.878	.934	.959	.991
4	.729	.811	.882	.917	.974
5	.669	.755	.833	.875	.951
6	.622	.707	.789	.834	.925
7	.582	.666	.750	.798	.898
8	.549	.632	.716	.765	.872
9	.521	.602	.685	.725	.847
10	.497	.576	.658	.708	.823
11	.476	.553	.634	.684	.801

Continued

| Table B-6 | **Critical Values for Pearson Product Moment Correlation Coefficient (r) for Two-Tailed (α_2) and One-Tailed (α_1) Tests.** df = n − 2. Calculated **r** must be greater than or equal to table value in order to reject the null hypothesis.—**cont'd** | | | | |

α_1	.05	.025	.01	.005	.0005
α_2	.10	.05	.02	.01	.001
df					
12	.458	.532	.612	.661	.780
13	.441	.514	.592	.641	.760
14	.426	.497	.574	.623	.742
15	.412	.482	.558	.606	.725
16	.400	.468	.543	.590	.708
17	.389	.456	.529	.575	.693
18	.378	.444	.516	.561	.679
19	.369	.433	.503	.549	.665
20	.323	.381	.445	.487	.597
25	.360	.423	.492	.537	.652
30	.296	.349	.409	.449	.554
35	.275	.325	.381	.418	.519
40	.257	.304	.358	.393	.490
45	.243	.288	.338	.372	.465
50	.231	.273	.322	.354	.443
60	.211	.250	.295	.325	.406
70	.195	.232	.274	.302	.380
80	.183	.217	.257	.283	.357
90	.173	.205	.242	.267	.338
100	.164	.195	.230	.254	.321

From Fisher RA, Yates F. Statistical Tables for Biological, Agricultural, and Medical Research. Edinburg Tweed Court, London: Longman Group UK, Ltd, 1974. This table was reproduced from Page 64: Table VII 'The Correlation Coefficient' with permission.

| Table B-7 | **Power for t-Test Using a Two-Tailed Hypothesis Test at alpha 0.05** | | | | | | | | | | |

Power of t-test a_2 = 0.05
Effect Size

n	.10	.20	.30	.40	.50	.60	.70	.80	1.00	1.20	1.40
8	05	07	09	11	15	20	25	31	46	60	73
9	05	07	09	12	16	22	28	35	51	65	79
10	06	07	10	13	18	24	31	39	56	71	84
11	06	07	10	14	20	26	34	43	61	76	87
12	06	08	11	15	21	28	37	46	65	80	90
13	06	08	11	16	23	31	40	50	69	83	93
14	06	08	12	17	25	33	43	53	72	86	94
15	06	08	12	18	26	35	45	56	75	88	96
16	06	08	13	19	28	37	48	59	78	90	97
17	06	09	13	20	29	39	51	62	80	92	98
18	06	09	14	21	31	41	53	64	83	94	98
19	06	09	15	22	32	43	55	67	85	95	99
20	06	09	15	23	33	45	58	69	87	96	99
21	06	10	16	24	35	47	60	71	88	97	99
22	06	10	16	25	36	49	62	73	90	97	99
23	06	10	17	26	38	51	64	75	91	98	*
24	06	10	17	27	39	53	66	77	92	98	

| Table B-7 | Power for t-Test Using a Two-Tailed Hypothesis Test at alpha 0.05—cont'd |

Power of t-test $a_2 = 0.05$
Effect Size

n	.10	.20	.30	.40	.50	.60	.70	.80	1.00	1.20	1.40
25	06	11	18	28	41	55	68	79	93	99	
26	06	11	19	29	42	56	69	80	94	99	
27	06	11	19	30	43	58	71	82	95	99	
28	07	11	20	31	45	59	73	83	96	99	
29	07	12	20	32	46	61	74	85	96	99	
30	07	12	21	33	47	63	76	86	97	*	
31	07	12	21	34	49	64	77	87	97		
32	07	12	22	35	50	65	78	88	98		
33	07	13	22	36	51	67	80	89	98		
34	07	13	23	37	53	68	81	90	98		
35	07	13	23	38	54	70	82	91	98		
36	07	13	24	39	55	71	83	92	99		
37	07	14	25	39	56	72	84	92	99		
38	07	14	25	40	57	73	85	93	99		
39	07	14	26	41	58	74	86	94	99		
40	07	14	26	42	60	75	87	94	99		
42	07	15	27	44	62	77	89	95	99		
44	07	15	28	46	64	79	90	96	*		
46	08	16	30	48	66	81	91	97			
48	08	16	31	49	68	83	92	97			

Adapted from Statistical Power Analysis for the Behavioral Sciences by Cohen, Jacob. Copyright 1988 in the format Textbook via Copyright Clearance Center.

Appendix C
Answers to Practice Exercises

Chapter 2

1a. Top: Rating Therapist #1; Side: Rating Therapist #2

1b. Top: Standard for improvement; Side: Change score for improvement

1c. Top: Standard for improvement; Side: Change score for improvement (compare two or more contingency tables)

1d. Top: categorical variable #1; Side: categorical variable #2

1e. Top: standard for prognosis; Side: patient symptom or characteristic

1f. Top: standard for pathology; Side: clinical test of pathology

2a. Meaningful clinical change

2b. Consensus (IntER rater)

2c. Prediction of prognosis

2d. Responsiveness

2e. Diagnostic accuracy

Chapter 3

1.

Sensitivity (95% CI)	Specificity (95% CI)	+LR (95% CI)	−LR (95% CI)
EXAMPLE X 0.27(0.18–0.23(0.13–0.38)	0.31(0.17–0.37)	2.90 0.56)	2.90 (1.95–4.32)
EXAMPLE Y 0.63(0.56–0.73(0.59–0.84)	1.98(1.54–0.69)	1.98(1.54–2.54)	0.42 (0.26–0.70)
EXAMPLE Z 0.82(0.76–0.73(0.67–0.79)	3.97(2.95–0.86)	3.97(2.95–5.33)	0.33 (0.26–0.42)

Note that hand calculations may vary slightly from Excel-based calculations due to the level of precision used and rounding error.

2a. sensitivity EXAMPLE Z,

2b. specificity EXAMPLE Z
(these are the point estimates with the smallest 95% CI)

2c. First calculate prevalence for each table, then apply nomogram
EXAMPLE X–32%, +LR = 0.31, post-test probability approx = 10%

EXAMPLE Y–18%, +LR=0.98, posttest probability approx = 16%
EXAMPLE Z–49%, +LR= 3.97, posttest probability approx = 78%

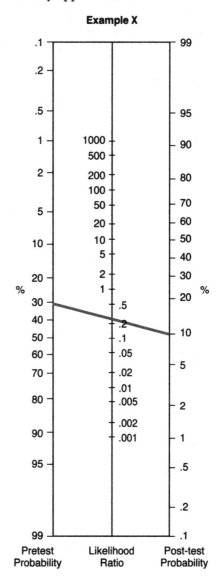

Example X

Pretest Probability — Likelihood Ratio — Post-test Probability

Example Y

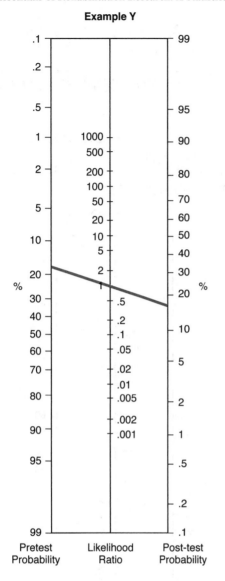

Example Z

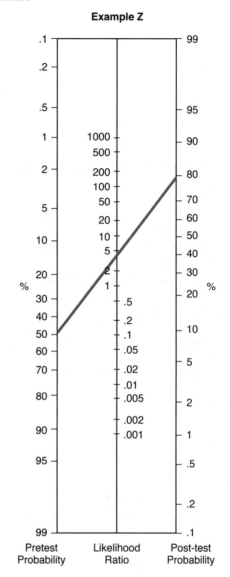

3. Pretest probability = prevalence = 18%

4. TUG = 9 s, Table 3-3–NCSS shows Sensitivity = 0.93, 1 – Specificity = 0.33. That point in the ROC plot is:

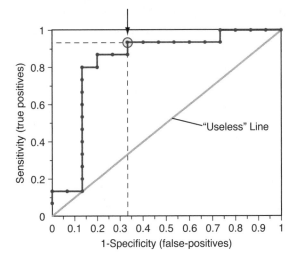

5a. PPV increases

5b. NPV decreases

Chapter 4

1a. $MDC_{90} = 18.13 \sim 18$

1b. Yes, $MDC_{95} = 21.61 \sim 22$

1c. $MDC_{90} = 18$ means that change scores less than 18 can be due to error inherent in the use of the assessment tool, so true change must equal or exceed 18 points from initial to follow-up assessment.

1d. SEM

1e. SEM = 7.79 ~ 8

1f. MCID = 8 means that the patient must change at least 8 points from the initial to follow-up evaluation in order to have clinically significant change.

2. +LR = 14 in general indicates that patients who have a positive result on the clinical test will have a "large" influence on the certainty that the target condition is present.

2a. In the context of diagnostic validity, the clinical test will greatly improve diagnostic certainty that the patient has a specific impairment or dysfunction.

2b. In the context of meaningful change, the clinical test will greatly improve the certainty that the subject has changed status in a clinically meaningful way.

3. A scatter plot of Sensitivity (true positive) vs. 1 – Specificity (false-positive) plotted in Excel. The optimal point is MCID = 5 change points.

This MCC threshold has a sensitivity of 0.97 and 3a. false-positive rate of 0.13 and correctly identifies true results (cell counts A + D) in 80 of 88 cases.

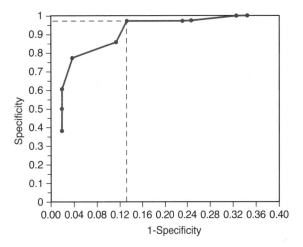

4. b

5. For initial RM scores ≤ 12,
$n = 27$
$SD_{initial} = 3.02$
$r_{Spearman} = -0.157$
critical z = 1.645
$MDC_{90} = 7.56 \sim 8$ RM change points
For initial RM scores ≥ 12,
$n = 61$
$SD_{initial} = 3.13$
$r_{Spearman} = 0.18$
critical z = 1.645
$MDC_{90} = 6.59 \sim 7$ RM change points

Chapter 5

1. 0.2 or 20%

2. 0.16–0.25 (bound-in disk, CI calculator)

3. b, c, e

4. Individual responsiveness indices show that tool #2 > tool#1; group responsiveness tool #1 > tool #2.

5. MCID proportion

6. Two things: the difference in responsiveness between the tools and the difference in responsiveness of each tool from a "useless" tool.

7a. Floor Effect = #Patients with worse possible score/Total number of patients = 22/50 = 44%

7b. Ceiling Effect = #Patients with best possible score/Total number of patients = 3/50 = 6%

8. Too difficult. The clinician does not know the true level of dysfunction in 44% of the patients who had severe difficulty performing the tasks.

Chapter 6

1a. $P_o = 0.57$
1b. kappa = 0.33
1c. "poor"
 2. Weights

		Clinician 1		
		Minimal	**Moderate**	**Severe**
Clinician 2	Minimal	0	1	4
	Moderate	1	0	1
	Severe	4	1	0

3a. fo*weight = wfo

10 * 0 = 0	3 * 1 = 3	2 * 4 = 8
5 * 1 = 5	5 * 0 = 0	1 * 1 = 1
3 * 4 = 12	1 * 1 = 1	5 * 0 = 0

SUM wfo = 5 + 12 + 3 + 1 + 8 + 1 = **30**

fc*weight = wfc

7.71 * 0 = 0	3.86 * 1 = 3.86	3.43 * 4 = 13.72
5.66 * 1 = 5.66	2.83 * 0 = 0	2.51 * 1 = 2.51
4.63 * 4 = 18.52	2.31 * 1 = 2.31	2.06 * 0 = 0

SUM wfc = 5.66 + 18.52 + 3.86 + 2.31 + 13.72 + 2.51 = **46.58**
kappa(w) = 1 – sum wfo/sum wfc = 1 – (30/46.58) = **0.36 (ans)**

3b. "poor"
4a.

Clinician 2	Clinician 1		
	Minimal–Moderate	Severe	Totals
Minimal–Moderate	23	3	26
Severe	4	5	9
Totals	27	8	35

4b. kappa = 0.46; Po = 0.80
4c. The prevalence index is >0.40 (unacceptable skew in cells A versus D). Raters have much higher agreement on minimal–moderate cases ($P_{pos} = 0.87$) compared with severe cases ($P_{neg} = 0.59$).

4d. No. Both the 90% and 95% CIs contain the threshold value of kappa = 0.40.
5a.

RM Analysis of Variance Table. Tone Score is the outcome measure.					
Source Term	**DF**	**Sum of Squares**	**Mean Square**	**F-Ratio**	**Prob Level**
A: Patient	26	25	0.9615384		
B: Clinicians	1	7.407E-02	7.407E-02	0.15	0.702636
AB	26	12.92593	0.497151		
S	0				
Total (Adjusted)	53	38			
Total	54				

PMS = 0.96 ⎫
RMS = 0.07 ⎬
EMS = 0.50 ⎭
#raters (Clinician df + 1) = 2
#patients (Patient df + 1) = 27

Enter mean square data into Consensus Calculator for Inter rater fixed ICC.

Icc inter rater fixed = **0.32 (ans)**

5b. "Poor"
5c. Selected Patient score = 2
SEM = sqrt(0.497) = 0.71
#replications = 2 (e.g., 2 raters)
eq 6-18→95% CI is:
2 ± 1.96 * 0.71/sqrt(2) = 0.98
2 + 0.98 = 2.98 ~ 3 ⎫
2 – 0.98 = 1.02 ~ 1 ⎬
True value can vary from 1 to 3; the full scale (ans).

Chapter 7

1. $\chi^2 = 8.64$, df = 3, critical $\chi^2_{alpha\ 0.05} = 7.81$, $p < 0.05$

Index	**Result**	**Interpretation**
Size and Sign	$r_{cv} = 0.38$	→ weak direct relationship
Coefficient of determination	$(r_{cv})^2 = 0.14$	→ 14% shared variance
Hypothesis test (H_0: $r_{cv} = 0$?)	$p < 0.05$	→ $r_{cv} \neq 0$

Residuals:

Largest Positive Residual Cane/Control Group: the count of people who used canes in the *control group* was significantly higher than would have occurred by chance.

Largest Negative Residual Cane/Treatment Group: the count of people who used canes in the *treatment group* was significantly lower than would have occurred by chance.

Combined Report (NCSS) Residual Group		
Assistive_Device	Control	Treatment
cane	1.63	−1.45
crutches	−1.30	1.16
none	−0.68	0.60
walker	−0.06	0.05
Total	0.00	0.00

The conclusion is that there were significantly more people in the control group with canes than in the treatment group. The association between group assignment and mobility device was statistically significant, but showed a weak relationship with only 14% shared variance.

2. Collapsing the table renders χ^2 not significant ($\chi^2 = 0.99$, df = 1, critical $\chi^2_{alpha\ 0.05} = 3.84$, p > 0.05). Residuals cannot be interpreted post-hoc because χ^2 does not show a significant association.

Index	Result	Interpretation
Size and Sign	$r_{cv} = 0.13$	→ little to no direct relationship
Coefficient of determination	$(r_{cv})^2 = 0.02$	→ 2% shared variance
Hypothesis test (H_0: $r_{cv} = 0$?)	p > 0.05	→ accept $r_{cv} = 0$

3. Test of Normality (NCSS)

Tests of Normality (SPSS)

Tests of Normality

	Kolmogorov-Smirnov[a]			Shapiro-Wilk		
	Statistic	df	Sig.	Statistic	df	Sig.
Berg	.157	13	.200*	.913	13	.201
Timed_UP_GO	.278	13	.007	.783	13	.004

[a.] Lilliefors Significance Correction
* This is a lower bound of the true significance

Significant violation of normality (sig or p<0.05)

Because one of the variables (TUG) is not normally distributed, a Spearman rank correlation coefficient is used.

Index	Result	Interpretation
Size and Sign	$r_s = -0.74$	→ moderate inverse relationship
Coefficient of determination	$(r_{cv})^2 = 0.55$	→ 55% shared variance
Hypothesis test (H_0: $r_s = 0$?)	p < 0.05	→ $r_s \neq 0$

NCSS Spearman Correlations Section (Row-Wise Deletion)		
	Berg	Timed_UP_GO
Berg	1.000000	**−0.741356**
	0.000000	0.003730
	13.000000	13.000000

Conclusion: There is a significant *inverse* association between these two clinical measures. As the Berg score increases (better performance) the Timed Up & Go decreases (becomes faster).

4. Yes, instead of $r_s = -0.74$, the Pearson r = −0.68.

Normality Tests Section									
	— Skewness Test —			——— Kurtosis Test ———-			- Omnibus Test -		
Variable	Value	Z	Prob	Value	Z	Prob	K2	Prob	Variable Normal?
Berg	−0.53	−1.01	0.3120	2.07	−0.60	0.5506	1.38	0.5020	Yes
Timed_UP_GO	1.79	2.99	0.0028	5.71	2.57	0.0103	15.54	0.0004	No

5. Yes

NCSS Normality Tests Section									
	—— Skewness Test ——-			——- Kurtosis Test ——-			Omnibus Test		
Variable	Value	Z	Prob	Value	Z	Prob	K2	Prob	Variable Normal?
Log_TUG	0.56	1.06	0.2872	3.26	1.01	0.3120	2.15	0.3405	Yes

6. Best correlation between two continuous variables normally distributed is Pearson r. Outcome:

(NCSS) Pearson Correlations Section (Row-Wise Deletion)		
	Log_Berg	Log_TUG
Log_Berg	1.000000	-0.722682
	0.000000	0.005260
	13.000000	13.000000

Note how close this result is to the Spearman rank coefficient calculated in Question 2.

Chapter 8

1. Step A

Regression Coefficient * Coded Value + Constant = logit

History of falling (coded 1) _____ $(1.55 * 1) + (-3.46) = -1.91$

Living alone (coded 1) _____$(0.56 * 1) + (-3.46) = -2.9$

Medications ≥ (coded 1) _____$(0.51 * 1) + (-3.46) = -2.95$

Sex female (coded 1) _____$(0.48 * 1) + (-3.46) = -2.98$

Step B: convert logit to predicted odds (eq 8-10)
Step C: convert predicted odds to predicted probability (eq 8-11)

Predicted Probability of Recurrent Falling				
	logit	Odds	Predicted Prob	Predicted Prob (%)
Hx falling	−1.91	0.14808	0.128981	12.90
Living alone	−2.9	0.055023	0.052154	5.22
Meds	−2.95	0.05234	0.049737	4.97
Sex female	−2.98	0.050793	0.048338	4.83

2.

Predicted Probability of Recurrent Falling			
logit	Odds	Prob	Prob (%)
−2.95	0.05234	0.049737	4.97

Probability of recurrent falls is 4.97% for a patient who does not have a history of falling (code = 0), but who is male (code = 0) and is living with someone (code = 0) and taking more than four medications (code = 1).

3. All of them. The contributions of each variable to the slope of the prediction line were all statistically significant ($p < 0.05$; reject H_0: slope contribution = 0)

4a.

	Imaginary Patient Profile (enter patient scores)	assumed code or units*
sex	0	0 female; 1 male
LOS	10	days
admission FIM	60	
admission FIM sq	3600	
interrupted stay	0	0 = No, 1 = Yes
= (3.585) + (0 * 7.4) + (10 * 0.279) + (60 * 0.855) + (3600 * −0.007) + (0 * −12.683)		
Predicted FIM change score		33

4b. Yes. The imaginary patient with this profile is predicted to have meaningful clinical change–improvement–following rehabilitation. Initial FIM = 60 and predicted FIM at discharge = 93 (a change of 33 points).

4c. Predicted FIM change score with interrupted stay = (3.585) + (0 * 7.4) + (10 * 0.279) + (60 * 0.855) + (3600 * –0.007) + (1 * –12.683) = **20**

Imaginary Patient Profile	(enter patient scores)
sex	0
LOS	10
admission FIM	60
admission FIM sq	3600
interrupted stay	1

5a.

Predicted Probability of Independence 2 Weeks Following Hip Surgery			
logit	Odds	Prob	Prob (%)
–3.1366	0.04343021	0.041623	4.16

Patient *not* able to walk >2 m but could move to sitting from supine is *not likely* to be functionally independent 2 weeks following surgery; probability to be in the target group <50%.

5b.

Predicted Probability of Independence 2 weeks following Hip Surgery			
logit	Odds	Prob	Prob (%)
0.5523	1.737244088	0.634669	63.47

A patient able to walk >2 m and who can move to sitting from supine is *likely* to be classified as functionally independent 2 weeks following surgery; probability to be in the target group >50%.

Chapter 9

1a. Predicting Responders = –11.9535043095852 + 5.49405923851886 * (Borg_Exertion_Scale_LT12 = 1) + 4.5479275113839 * (Joint_Space_Narrowing = 1) + 5.88660825711869 * (Pain = 1) + 4.43072060509002 * (Assist_Device = 1)

1b. Borg_Exertion_Scale_LT12—no
Joint_Space_Narrowing—yes
Assist_Device—yes
Pain— yes

logit	Odds	Probability
2.912	18.39	0.948424 = 95%

1c. approx 96%

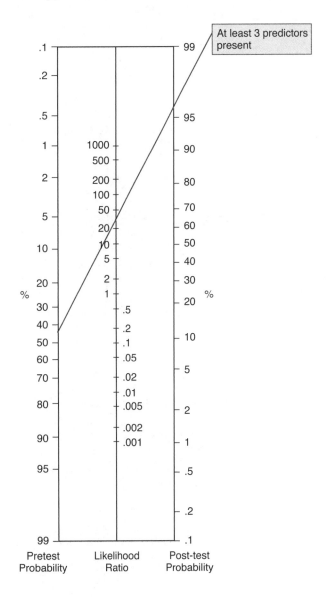

1d. No.

2. Univariate logistic regression generates unadjusted odds ratios. Multivariate logistic regression adjusts each odds ratio according to all remaining variables in the model.

3. ROC curve analyses.

4a.

At_least_2_Present	Count	Count	Count	Count			False+	Specificity
Cutoff Value	+|P A	+|A B	−|P C	−|A D	Sensitivity A/(A+C)	C/(A + C)	B/(B + D)	D/(B + D)
~~0.00~~	~~32~~	~~39~~	~~0~~	~~0~~	~~1.00000~~	~~0.00000~~	~~1.00000~~	~~0.00000~~
1.00	32	31	0	8	1.00000	0.00000	0.79487	0.20513

4b.

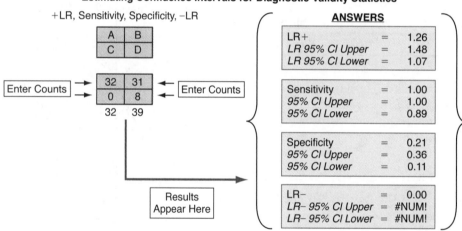

Estimating Confidence Intervals for Diagnostic Validity Statistics*

4c. Posttest Probability = Positive Predictive Value = A/(A + B) = 32/(32 + 31) = 51% (alternatively, use the nomogram).

5. Wald score = z score = 0.85, then 0 to z+ is p = 0.3023 (using **Table B-1**; area from 0 to z under the normal curve):
0 to z− is p = 0.3023.

p two-tail covers the bell curve area 2 * 0.3023 = 0.6046.

p that z = 0.85 occurs by chance in a two-tailed distribution is (1 − 0.6046) = 0.3954 (see also the Wald z probability value for the variable "Age" in Table 9-5).

5a. No. p = 0.3954 so p > 0.05.

Chapter 10

1.

Application	Point Estimate	What the CI Tells You	Which Value Nullifies the Point Estimate (Creating a Nonsignificant Finding)?	What Is the Rationale for the Nullifying Value?
Diagnostic Validity	Positive Likelihood Ratio	The range of possible values surrounding the "true" LR	1.0	A patient is only 1 time more likely than prevalence to have a disorder.
Meaningful Clinical Change	Minimal Detectable Change (MDC): MDC_{90} or MDC_{95}	The level of confidence that the MDC is accurate	Any assessment score less than the MDC could be due to measurement error.	The MDC defines a range where scores on a clinical assessment tool are due to error.
Responsiveness of Clinical Assessment Tools	Responsiveness Indices	The precision that each responsiveness index holds the "true" value of the index	When comparing the width of the CI across responsiveness indices, overlap indicates no significant difference in responsiveness of the tools being compared.	Overlapping CIs for a responsiveness index between two assessment tools means that each index is likely to come from a population having the same level of responsiveness.
Responsiveness of Clinical Assessment Tools	ROC Curve	Is the responsiveness capacity of the assessment tool any better than meaningless?	0.5	If the area under the ROC curve is different than meaningless (0.5), the CI will not hold the meaningless value.
Consensus	Kappa	Determines if the "true" value of kappa falls in a range that indicates statistical significance	Usually 0.40 but can be any reference value set by the practitioner	A CI holding k = 0.40 suggests that the true value of kappa may be too low to indicate consensus.
Consensus	ICC	Variation of scores surrounding any patient's score (an index of measurement error)	No specific value but the wider the range, the more error is associated with the clinical tool	A wide range of possible scores when repeating measures on a given patient do not give confidence in the assessment tool.

Continued

Application	Point Estimate	What the CI Tells You	Which Value Nullifies the Point Estimate (Creating a Nonsignificant Finding)?	What Is the Rationale for the Nullifying Value?
Risk	Odds Ratio	The range of odds ratios that could occur with theoretical replication of the study using different patients, thus accounting for sampling error	1.0	A patient with a clinical sign or symptom could be only 1 time more likely to have the target condition (disease or disability) compared to those without the sign or symptom.
Treatment Effect	Effect Size	The range of values surrounding clinical change scores	0	If the CI contains 0, it is possible that the true treatment effect could be 0.

2. A normal probability distribution has a fixed amount of probability linked to each standard deviation. This allows for a test of significance based on critical z values (large sample size) or critical t values (small sample sizes). The ES is based on a standardized normal distribution with a mean of 0 and an SD = 1. Thus, if the point estimate for an ES has a CI that does not include 0, then the treatment effect is statistically significant. The variation of possible point estimates for the ES, in other words, occurs far enough from the standard mean of 0 effect so that the observed treatment effect is not likely due to chance.

3. For both groups: Normal distribution by skewness, kurtosis
For Shoulder Not Normal by *Shapiro Wilk*
For Back Normal by *Shapiro Wilk*
NCSS: Filter Affected_Area = "Shoulder"

Normality Tests Section

Variable	—- Skewness Test —-			——— Kurtosis Test ———			- Omnibus Test -		Variable Normal?
	Value	Z	Prob	Value	Z	Prob	K2	Prob	
Percent_BL_difficult	0.00	0.00	1.0000	0.00	0.00	1.0000	1.00	0.6065	Yes
Percent_DC_difficult	0.00	0.00	1.0000	0.00	0.00	1.0000	1.00	0.6065	Yes

Filter Affected_Area = "Back"

Normality Tests Section

Variable	—- Skewness Test —-			——— Kurtosis Test ———			- Omnibus Test -		Variable Normal?
	Value	Z	Prob	Value	Z	Prob	K2	Prob	
Percent_BL_difficult	0.00	0.00	1.0000	0.00	0.00	1.0000	1.00	0.6065	Yes
Percent_DC_difficult	0.00	0.00	1.0000	0.00	0.00	1.0000	1.00	0.6065	Yes

SPSS *For Shapiro Wilk and Kolmogorov–Smirnov*
The null hypothesis for these tests is that the data are normally distributed. If the test result is significant (lower than or equal to 0.05), then the data are *not* normally distributed.

Tests of Normality

(Shoulder)	Kolmogorov-Smirnov[a]			Shapiro-Wilk		
	Statistic	df	Sig.	Statistic	df	Sig.
Percent_BL_difficulty	.385	3	.	.750	3	.000←——Not normally distributed
Percent_DC_difficulty	.227	3	.	.983	3	.747

[a]Lilliefors Significance Correction

Tests of Normality

(Back)	Kolmogorov-Smirnov[a]			Shapiro-Wilk		
	Statistic	df	Sig.	Statistic	df	Sig.
Percent_BL_difficulty	.316	3	.	.889	3	.353
Percent_DC_difficulty	.328	3	.	.871	3	.298

[a]Lilliefors Significance Correction

4. Attempt a transformation of data by using the square root or log of each data point, for example.

5. eq 10-4:

$$d\ unbiased = d\ biased \left[1 - \frac{3}{8(n-1)}\right]$$
$$1.12 * (1 - (3/8*9)) = 1.07$$

6. eq 10-5B
Small Samples ($n \le 20$)
95% CI
Upper Boundary = $ES_{unbiased}$ + (critical t * se)
Lower boundary = $ES_{unbiased}$ − (critical t * se)
Unbiased ES (from Question 5) = 1.07
$n = 10$ (given)
$df = n - 1 = 9$
Critical t at df = 9, $\alpha_2 = 0.05$ (Table B-2) = 2.26
SD = 3 (given)
SE = SD/$\sqrt{n}$ = 3/$\sqrt{10}$ = 0.95
Upper Boundary = 1.07 + (2.26 * 0.95) = 3.22
Lower Boundary = 1.07 − (2.26 * 0.95) = −1.08

6a. The treatment effect is not statistically different from 0 because the 95% CI holds a 0.

7. eq 10-6:

$$95\%\ CI\ for\ treatment\ effect = Mean\ Difference\ Score \pm (t) * \frac{SD}{\sqrt{N}}$$

Given:
Mean difference in ROM = 24 deg
SD of average change = 6 deg
$n = 15$
Calculated:
$df = n - 1 = 15 - 1 = 14$
Critical t at df = 14, $\alpha_2 = 0.05$ (Table B-2) = 2.15
SE = SD/$\sqrt{n}$ = 6/$\sqrt{15}$ = 3.87
Upper Boundary = 24 + (2.15 * 1.55) = 27.33 deg
Lower Boundary = 24 − (2.15 * 1.55) = 20.67 deg

7a. Yes, there is a significant change in elbow ROM following treatment because *0 is not* in the CI.

Chapter 11

The AGREE tool was designed to guide the appraisal of clinical practice guidelines and to help stakeholders form an opinion about the quality, applicability, and feasibility of implementation in local clinical settings. As such, there are no right or wrong answers. This exercise encourages a gathering of multiple appraisers to discuss, share opinions, and evaluate practice guidelines.

Appendix A

Hypothetical Study #1: Manual Muscle Testing
1-1a.

Cross-Tabulation Procedure

NCSS Counts	criterion_standard		
MMT	side_side_diff	zNO_side_side_diff	Total
detected	42	6	48
Not_detected	26	33	59
Total	68	39	107

Alternatively, PSPP (free at this writing):

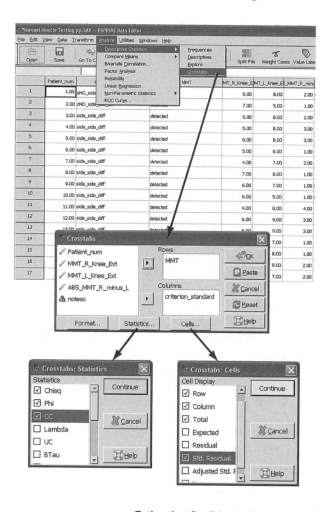

MMT * criterion_standard [count]			
	criterion_standard		
MMT	side_side_diff	zNO_side_sde_diff	Total
detected	42.0	6.0	48
Not_detected	26.0	33.0	59
Total	68.0	39.0	107.0

1-1b. Fewer true positives (cell A) and more false-positives (cell B)

1-1c. Using P_Calculator from Chapter 3, sensitivity = 0.66, specificity = 0.85, +LR = 4.27

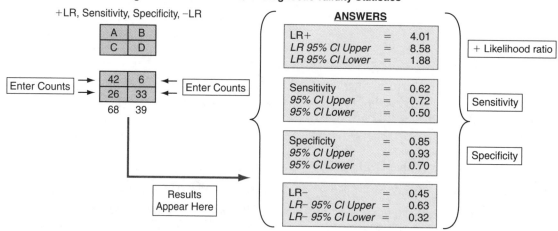

Estimating Confidence Intervals for Diagnostic Validity Statistics

+LR, Sensitivity, Specificity, −LR

ANSWERS

LR+	=	4.01
LR 95% CI Upper	=	8.58
LR 95% CI Lower	=	1.88

+ Likelihood ratio

Sensitivity	=	0.62
95% CI Upper	=	0.72
95% CI Lower	=	0.50

Sensitivity

Specificity	=	0.85
95% CI Upper	=	0.93
95% CI Lower	=	0.70

Specificity

LR−	=	0.45
LR− 95% CI Upper	=	0.63
LR− 95% CI Lower	=	0.32

1-1d. Yes, the value "1" does *not* appear in the +LR confidence interval (1.88–8.58).

1-1e. Using the Fagan nomogram, the post-test probability is approximately 90%. Alternatively, using the positive predictive value (**eq 3-7**; PVV = 88% = post-test probability)

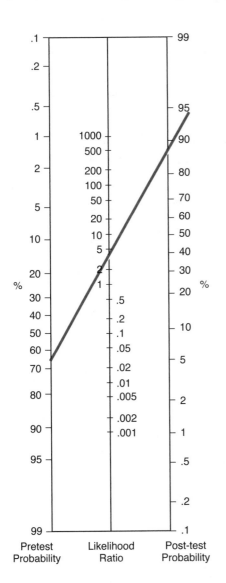

Pretest Probability — Likelihood Ratio — Post-test Probability

1-1f. Diagnostic accuracy method used by Bohannon[1] applied to theoretical data = $(a + d)/(a + b + c + d) = (42 + 33)/107 = 70\%$. *Note*: This formula shows the percent agreement of criterion standard with the clinical test (refer to **eq 6-1**).

1-1g. Diagnostic accuracy appears to be high using post-test probability and markedly lower using percent agreement. These hypothetical outcomes highlight the difference between post-test probability and percent agreement.

1-2a. Chi square converted to Cramer's V; chi square = 21.6, df = 1, p < 0.05, Cramer's V or $r_{cv} = 0.45$.

NCSS Statistical Software Output: Chi-Square Statistics		
Chi-Square	21.553968	
Degrees of Freedom	1	
Probability Level	0.000003	Reject H_0
Cramer's V	0.448820	

Alternatively, PSPP:

Chi-square tests.

Statistic	Value	df	Asymp. Sig. (2-sided)
Pearson Chi-Square	21.55	1	.00

Symmetric measures.

Category	Statistic	Value	Asymp. Std.	Approx.	Sig.
Nominal					
	Cramer's V	.45			

1-2b. Yes, p< 0.05.

1-2c. Percent shared variance is the coefficient of determination; $r^2_{cv} = (0.45)^2 = 0.20$, or 20% shared variance.

1-2d. Weak direct association

1-2e. Positive residuals in cell A (2.05) and cell D (2.48) indicate that there are more observations in these cells than expected by chance (thus more agreement with the criterion standard than expected by chance). Negative residuals in cell B (–2.75) and cell C (–1.88) indicate that there are fewer observations for the frequency of false-positives and false-negatives than expected by chance. The clinical test (MMT) identifies true results more than expected by chance.

Statistical Software Output: Residual Analysis		
	criterion_standard	
MMT	side_side_diff	zNO_side_sde_diff
detected	2.08	–2.75
Not_detected	–1.88	2.48

Alternatively, PSPP:

MMT * criterion_standard [std. resid.]			
	criterion_standard		
MMT	side_side_diff	zNO_side_sde_diff	Total
detected	2.1	−2.7	.0
Not_detected	−1.9	2.5	.0

Hypothetical Study #2: Developmental Assessment

2-1a. 15 imaginary patients classified as having meaningful clinical change. In NCSS, SPSS, and PSPP, follow Analyze→ Descriptive Statistics→ Frequencies (or Frequency Tables).

NCSS Frequency Table Report

Frequency Distribution of Convert_Likert_rating	
Convert_Likert_rating	Count
MCID	15
large_change	10
moderate_change	21
no_change	7

(output truncated)

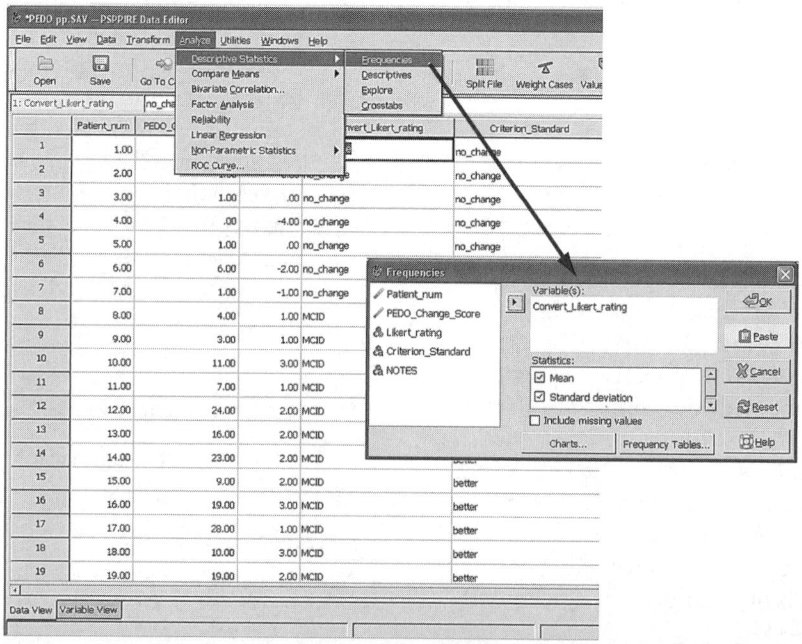

Convert_Likert_rating (edited)			
Value Label	Value Frequency	Percent	Cum. Percent
MCID	15	28.30	28.30
large_change	10	18.87	47.17
moderate_change	21	39.62	86.79
no_change	7	13.21	100.00

2-1b. NCSS: Filter→ Convert_Likert_rating = "MCID"

Summary Section of PEDO_Change_Score			
Count	Mean	Standard Deviation	Standard Error
15	16.26667	8.572936	2.213523

Alternatively, PSPP:

Alternatively, PSPP:

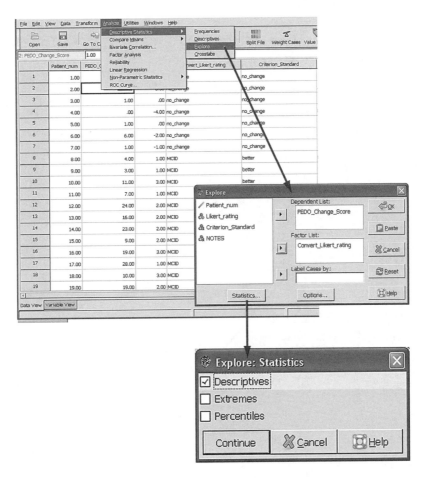

Convert_Likert_rating			Statistic	Std. Error
PEDO_Change_ Score	MCID	Mean	16.27	2.21

2-1c. Iyer et al.[4] reported MCID on the order of 10 PEDI points. The hypothetical results for the PEDO data yield an MCID of 16 PEDO points.

2-1d. Selected portions of statistical output are shown. The MCID according to this output is a PEDO change score of 3 points (the PEDO change score with the highest value of true results; cells A + D highlighted in the ROC data matrix).

NCSS: ROC Data for Condition = Criterion Standard Using the Empirical ROC Curve

PEDO_Change_Score								
Cutoff Value	Count+|P A	Count+|A B	Count −|P C	Count −|A D	Sensitivity A/(A + C)	C/(A + C)	False+ B/(B+D)	Specificity D/(B + D)
0.00	46	7	0	0	1.00000	0.00000	1.00000	0.00000
1.00	46	6	0	1	1.00000	0.00000	0.85714	0.14286
3.00	46	1	0	6	1.00000	0.00000	0.14286	0.85714
4.00	45	1	1	6	0.97826	0.02174	0.14286	0.85714
6.00	44	1	2	6	0.95652	0.04348	0.14286	0.85714

Continued

PEDO_Change_Score—cont'd

Cutoff Value	Count+|P A	Count+|A B	Count –|P C	Count –|A D	Sensitivity A/(A + C)	C/(A + C)	False+ B/(B+D)	Specificity D/(B + D)
7.00	**43**	**0**	**3**	**7**	0.93478	0.06522	0.00000	1.00000
9.00	**42**	**0**	**4**	**7**	0.91304	0.08696	0.00000	1.00000
10.00	**41**	**0**	**5**	**7**	0.89130	0.10870	0.00000	1.00000

"(output truncated)

Alternatively, PSPP:

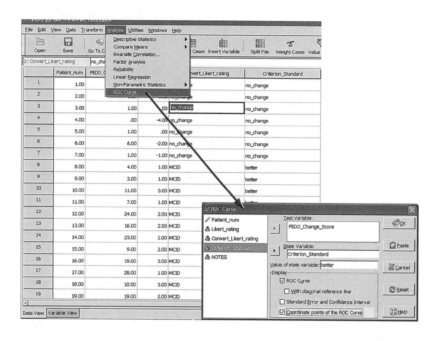

Coordinates of the Curve (PEDO_Change_Score)

Positive If Greater Than or Equal to	Sensitivity	1 – Specificity
–1.00	1.00	1.00
.50	1.00	.86
2.50	1.00	.14
3.50	.98	.14
7.00	.91	.00
9.00	.89	.00

Output truncated—Optimal cut-point rounded to nearest whole # = 3.

2-1e. No. The data set must display pre- and post-PEDO scores in order to calculate MDC. As it stands, the PEDO data set shows the PEDO change scores.

2-1f. MCID Proportion = Cell A + Cell D/N = (46 + 6/53) * 100 = 98% **eq 5-2**

Hypothetical Study #3: Hand Function

3-1a. Descriptive statistics modules in statistical software provide means and standard deviations for each variable to enable calculation of $ES_{responsiveness}$ and SRM.

Descriptive Statistics					
	N	Minimum	Maximum	Mean	Std. Deviation
pre_iMKI	50	.00	50.00	30.3400	15.25914
post_iMKI	50	10.00	50.00	33.6000	12.44416
pre_iCochin	50	3.00	59.00	29.5000	15.65867
post_iCochin	50	.00	58.00	24.2000	19.22265
iMKI_change	50	-40.00	36.00	-3.2600	19.15970
iCochin_change	50	-35.00	46.00	5.3000	20.56473
Valid *N* (listwise)	50				

Effect Sizes (ES):

iMKI $ES_{responsiveness} = -3.26/15.26 = -0.21$ **eq 5-3**
iCochin $ES_{responsiveness} = 5.3/15.66 = 0.34$

Standardized Response Mean (SRM):

iMKI $SRM = -3.26/19.16 = -0.17$ **eq 5–4**
iCochin $SRM = 5.3/20.57 = 0.26$

3-1b. The ES and SRM in the hypothetical study follow the same pattern reported by the results reported by Lefevre-Colau et al.[5] Descriptively, the iCochin Disability Scale appears to have greater group responsiveness to change than the iMKI.

3-1c. Because larger iMKI values reflect improvement, pre- minus post-test values yield negative responsiveness indices when patient status improves.

3-2a. (*Note*: ROC plot is made with iMKI with sign inverted so that both scales plotted have positive values = improvement.) Notations have been added to the ROC plots.

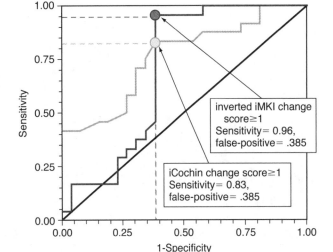

ROC Curve of Satisfaction

inverted iMKI change score≥1
Sensitivity= 0.96,
false-positive= .385

iCochin change score≥1
Sensitivity= 0.83,
false-positive= .385

Criteria
- - - iCochin change
—— Invert iMKI change

3-2b. Using NCSS summary table output (truncated due to space) along with the ROC plot,

ROC for iCochin

iCochin change score in the furthest upper left corner of the plot = 1 point. A change of 1 iCochin point has sensitivity = 0.83, false-positive rate = 0.385, and specificity = 0.62.

Condition Variable (Criterion Standard) = Satisfaction

ROC Data

iCochin_change Cutoff Value	Count+|P A	Count+|A B	Count −|P C	Count −|A D	Sensitivity A/(A + C)	C/(A + C)	False+ B/(B+D)	Specificity D/(B + D)
−3.00	21	15	3	11	0.87500	0.12500	0.57692	0.42308
−2.00	20	14	4	12	0.83333	0.16667	0.53846	0.46154
−1.00	20	13	4	13	0.83333	0.16667	0.50000	0.50000
0.00	20	12	4	14	0.83333	0.16667	0.46154	0.53846
1.00	20	10	4	16	0.83333	0.16667	0.38462	0.61538
2.00	18	9	6	17	0.75000	0.25000	0.34615	0.65385
3.00	17	9	7	17	0.70833	0.29167	0.34615	0.65385

ROC for iMKI

Inverted_iMKI change score in the furthest upper left corner of the plot = 1 point. A change of 1 iMKI point has sensitivity = 0.96, a false-positive rate of 0.385, and specificity = 0.62.

Condition Variable (Criterion Standard) = Satisfaction

ROC Data

Invert_iMKI_ change Cutoff Value	Count+|P A	Count+|A B	Count −|P C	Count −|A D	Sensitivity A/(A + C)	C/(A + C)	False+ B/(B+D)	Specificity D/(B + D)
−9.00	23	14	1	12	0.95833	0.04167	0.53846	0.46154
−8.00	23	13	1	13	0.95833	0.04167	0.50000	0.50000
−7.00	23	12	1	14	0.95833	0.04167	0.46154	0.53846
−6.00	23	11	1	15	0.95833	0.04167	0.42308	0.57692
1.00	23	10	1	16	0.95833	0.04167	0.38462	0.61538
2.00	20	10	4	16	0.83333	0.16667	0.38462	0.61538
3.00	18	10	6	16	0.75000	0.25000	0.38462	0.61538
4.00	17	10	7	16	0.70833	0.29167	0.38462	0.61538
5.00	14	10	10	16	0.58333	0.41667	0.38462	0.61538

3-2c. The optimal points on the ROC curves for each hand function tool represent the MCID for that tool. Imaginary patients would need to change at least *one point* on each scale in order to have meaningful clinical change.

3-2d. Yes. Adding the counts for cells A + D, the inverted iMKI MCID identifies 39 true results; iCochin identifies 36 true results.

3-2e. Note that rounding sensitivity and specificity can produce results that are slightly different from the calculators created in Excel.

Applying eq 3-3 and eq3-5 Manually

iCochin change score ≥ 1

$$+LR = \text{Sensitivity}/1 - \text{Specificity} = 0.83/$$
$$(1 - 0.62) = 2.18$$
$$-LR = (1 - \text{Sensitivity})/\text{Specificity} =$$
$$(1 - 0.83)/0.62 = 0.27$$

Inverted iMKI change score ≥ 1

$$+LR = \text{Sensitivity}/1 - \text{Specificity} =$$
$$0.96/(1 - 0.62) = 2.53$$
$$-LR = (1 - \text{Sensitivity})/\text{Specificity} = (1 - 0.96)/0.62$$
$$= 0.07$$

3-2f. For *meaningful clinical change, the +Likelihood Ratio* is the likelihood that a person identified as "improved" by the change score on the clinical assessment will actually be classified as improved by the criterion standard.

For *meaningful clinical change, the −Likelihood Ratio* is the likelihood that a person identified as "not improved" by the change score on the clinical assessment will actually be classified as improved by the criterion standard. All +LRs and −LRs have 95% CIs that do not include the number 1 and therefore all are statistically significant. However, the magnitude of the +LRs never exceeds 5, so clinical impact for these imaginary data is minimal. The negative LR for the inverted iMKI is less than 0.20, so this value has clinical meaning with respect to the definition for −LR. Using the P_calculator from Chapter 3:

• For iCochin change score:

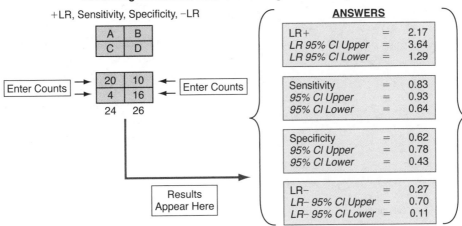

Estimating Confidence Intervals for Diagnostic Validity Statistics

+LR, Sensitivity, Specificity, −LR

A	B
C	D

Enter Counts → | 20 | 10 | ← Enter Counts
| 4 | 16 |
24 26

Results Appear Here

ANSWERS

LR+	=	2.17
LR 95% CI Upper	=	3.64
LR 95% CI Lower	=	1.29
Sensitivity	=	0.83
95% CI Upper	=	0.93
95% CI Lower	=	0.64
Specificity	=	0.62
95% CI Upper	=	0.78
95% CI Lower	=	0.43
LR−	=	0.27
LR− 95% CI Upper	=	0.70
LR− 95% CI Lower	=	0.11

• For inverted iMKI change score:

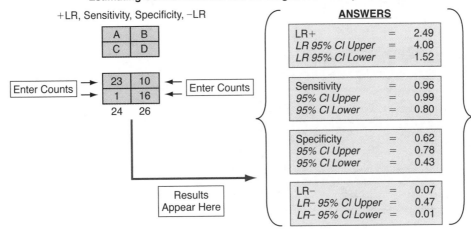

Estimating Confidence Intervals for Diagnostic Validity Statistics

+LR, Sensitivity, Specificity, −LR

A	B
C	D

Enter Counts → | 23 | 10 | ← Enter Counts
| 1 | 16 |
24 26

Results Appear Here

ANSWERS

LR+	=	2.49
LR 95% CI Upper	=	4.08
LR 95% CI Lower	=	1.52
Sensitivity	=	0.96
95% CI Upper	=	0.99
95% CI Lower	=	0.80
Specificity	=	0.62
95% CI Upper	=	0.78
95% CI Lower	=	0.43
LR−	=	0.07
LR− 95% CI Upper	=	0.47
LR− 95% CI Lower	=	0.01

3-2g. Statistical comparison of AUCs (edited from NCSS).

3-2g(i). The 95% CIs for AUC between each hand function *overlap* (highlighted), so there is no statistically significant difference in AUC, and therefore no responsiveness difference, between the tools based on AUC.

3-2g(ii). The 95% CI for AUC in each tool does not hold the meaningless value of AUC = 0.50. Therefore, each tool is more responsive than "meaningless."

NCSS						
Criterion	**Empirical Estimate of AUC**	**AUC's Standard Error**	**Lower 95.0% Confidence Limit**	**Upper 95.0% Confidence Limit**	**Prevalence of Satisfaction**	**Count**
iCochin_change	0.75881	0.06877	0.58869	0.86457	0.48000	50
Invert_iMKI_change	0.69631	0.08057	0.50320	0.82319	0.48000	50

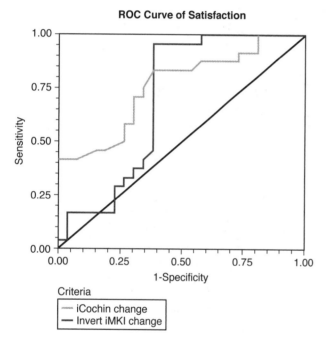

ROC Curve of Satisfaction

Criteria
— iCochin change
— Invert iMKI change

Hypothetical Study #4: Shoulder Sick Leave

4-1a. Statistically significant predictors of hypothetical sick leave use (highlighted). The hypothetical potential predictors of sick leave use due to shoulder dysfunction are *sick leave prior to initial evaluation, psychological complaints, and the shoulder pain score*. These variables were selected because they are statistically significant predictors using either the Wald z value (NCSS) or the forward Wald stepwise logistic regression in SPSS.

Alternatively in PSPP, this setup will yield the same result as NCSS.

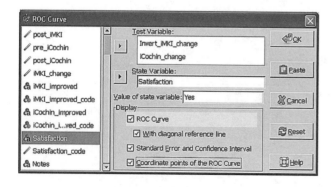

In NCSS:

Parameter	Regression Coefficient (B or Beta)	Standard Error	Wald Z Value (Beta = 0)	Wald Prob. Level	Odds Ratio Exp(B)
B0: Intercept	−9.82512	1.66550	−5.899	0.00000	0.00005
B1: Age_yrs	0.01286	0.01867	0.689	0.49093	1.01295
B2: BL_Sick_days_num	0.18180	0.05578	3.259	0.00112	1.19937
B4: (Neck_coded = 1)	−0.66705	0.40946	−1.629	0.10330	0.51322
B5: (Psych_coded = 1)	4.62143	1.10178	4.195	0.00003	101.63954
B6: Shoulder_Pain_score	0.94804	0.13069	7.254	0.00000	2.58064
B3: (Cause_Coded = 1)	0.11672	0.42021	0.278	0.78120	1.12380

Parameter Significance Tests Section (Reference Group: Dichotomous_sick_days = ZNO)

Alternatively, in SPSS (Forward Wald Logistic regression p <0.50 to enter, p >0.10 to leave model). Output edited.

Variables in the Equation

	B	S.E.	Wald*	df	Sig.	Exp(B)
BL_Sick_days_num	.178	.055	10.379	1	.001	1.195
Shoulder_Pain_score	.926	.127	53.082	1	.000	2.525
Psych_coded	4.465	1.085	16.944	1	.000	86.937
Constant	−9.283	1.373	45.704	1	.000	.000

*Wald score calculated differently in SPSS vs. NCSS.

4-1b. Estimated logistic regression model(s):

Model for Dichotomous_sick_days = YES

−9.28329386833599 + 4.46515850999457 * (Psych_coded = 1) + .926184603384217 * Shoulder_Pain_score + .177871588736232 * BL_Sick_days_num

4-1c.

Classification Table (Goodness-of-Fit = 91%)

Actual	Estimated YES	ZNO	Total
YES	82	22	104
ZNO	6	188	194
Total	88	210	298

Percent correctly classified = 90.6%

4-1d. Probability of sick leave use for the profile psychological symptoms present (code = 1), shoulder pain score = 8, and 10 days of sick leave prior to initial evaluation is 99%.

−9.28329386833599 + 4.46515850999457 * (**Psych_coded = 1**) + .926184603384217 * **Shoulder_Pain_score** + .177871588736232 * BL_Sick_days_num

−9.28329386833599 + 4.46515850999457 * **(1)** + .926184603384217 * **(8)** + .177871588736232 * **(10)**

logit	Odds	Probability of Sick Leave Use
4.370057	79.04817	0.987508 or 99%

4-2a. ROC analysis using Coded_Dichotomous_sick_days as the criterion standard found the optimal cut-points for the following continuous variables in the model (cells A + D were the highest value for the cut-point selected):

- "BL_Sick_days_num ≥ 1

BL_Sick_days_num Cutoff Value	Count A	Count B	Count C	Count D
0	104	194	0	0
1	**80**	9	24	**185**
2	68	9	36	185
3	58	9	46	185
4	48	9	56	185

- "Shoulder_Pain_score" ≥ 6

Shoulder_Pain_score Cutoff Value	Count A	Count B	Count C	Count D
0	104	194	0	0
1	104	167	0	27
2	104	138	0	56
3	101	101	3	93
4	97	66	7	128
5	90	30	14	164
6	**78**	7	26	**187**
7	58	7	46	187
8	44	5	60	189
9	32	1	72	193
10	21	1	83	193

The remaining variable in the model is already dichotomous:

- Psych_coded ≥ 1

4-3a. (Plot in SPSS.)

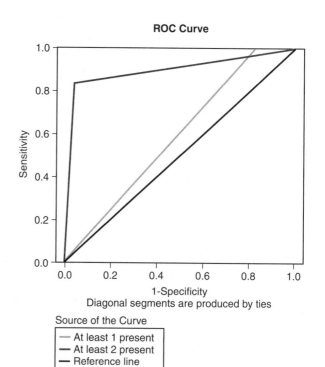

ROC Curve

Diagonal segments are produced by ties

Source of the Curve
- At least 1 present
- At least 2 present
- Reference line

4-3b.

Number of Clinical Variables Present at Initial Evaluation	Sensitivity	Specificity	+LR	95%CI
At_Least_2_present	0.83654	0.96392	23.18	11.15–48.22
At_Least_1_present	1.00000	0.18041	1.22	1.14–1.30

Analysis of LR 95% CIs for "**At least 2** clinical predictors present"

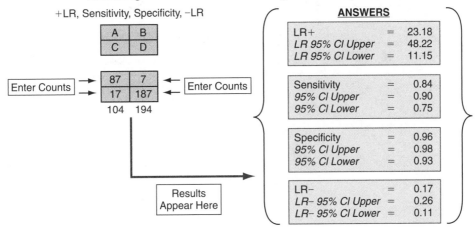

Analysis of LR 95% CIs for "**At least 1** clinical predictor present"

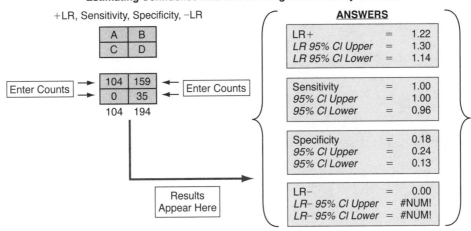

4-3c. Assuming 35% prevalence, if a patient has at least two clinical signs present, then the posttest probability is approximately 93%. For at least one clinical sign present, the posttest probability drops to the order of 38%.

4-3d. If these results were real and replicated in other studies, the clinician would be alerted to people at risk for future shoulder injuries and could implement preventative actions to reduce that risk.

Hypothetical Study #5: Pull Test

5-1a. $ICC_{inter\ rater\ fixed} = 0.70$; descriptive magnitude = "Good" (see **Table 6-3**). ICC calculations shown below.

Repeated Measures

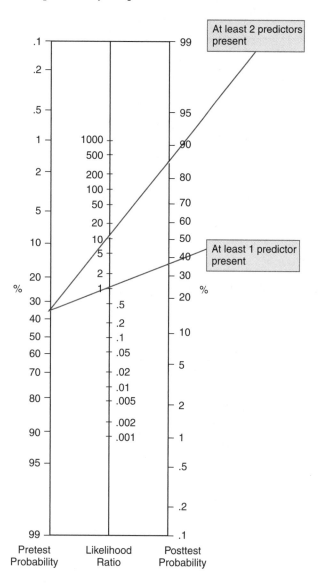

| Pretest Probability | Likelihood Ratio | Posttest Probability |

Analysis of Variance Table						
Source Term	**DF**	**Sum of Squares**	**Mean Square**	**F-Ratio**	**Prob Level**	**Power (Alpha=0.05)**
A: Patient_num	41	60.14286	1.466899			
B: Rater	1	5.761905	5.761905	28.68	0.000004*	0.999455
AB	41	8.238095	0.2009291			
S	0					
Total (Adjusted)	83	74.14286				
Total	84					

From the ANOVA Summary Table (Enter these values using the Chapter 6 P_Consensus calculator.xls in the section for ICC inter rater fixed):

PMS = 1.47
RMS = 5.76
EMS = 0.20   Enter
#raters = 2   (Section
#patients = 42

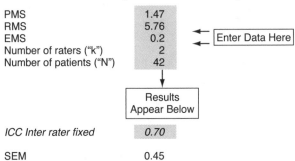

ICC Inter rater *fixed*
From the ANOVA Summary table enter the following values:

PMS	1.47
RMS	5.76
EMS	0.2
Number of raters ("k")	2
Number of patients ("N")	42

← ← Enter Data Here

Results Appear Below

ICC Inter rater fixed	0.70
SEM	0.45

5-1b. As calculated in the "Consensus Calculator" from Chapter 6 (or from eq 6-17), SEM = 0.45.

The 95% CI ("error interval") from **eq 6-18** is:

95% CI = patients mean score ± 1.96 * SEM/√m =
2 ± 1.96 * (0.45/1.41) =

Lower Boundary Patient's Mean Score Upper Boundary
1.37——————————2——————————2.63

Thus, the range of true scores could vary (when rounded) from 1 to 3.

5-2a. Weighted kappa = 0.65 (calculations below)

Step 1 (cross tabulation using statistical software)

Observed Counts

	Rater1_Nutt_score_trial1			
Rater2_Nutt_score_trial1	0	1	2	3
0	8	6	0	0
1	0	6	11	0
2	0	0	3	7
3	0	1	0	0

Counts Expected by Chance

	Rater1_Nutt_score_trial1			
Rater2_Nutt_score_trial1	0	1	2	3
0	2.7	4.3	4.7	2.3
1	3.2	5.3	5.7	2.8
2	1.9	3.1	3.3	1.7
3	0.2	0.3	0.3	0.2

Step 2 (create weights)

SQUARED Weights table created manually in Excel

	Clinician 1			
Clinician 2	0	1	2	3
0	0	1	0	9
1	1	0	1	4
2	4	1	0	1
3	9	4	1	0

WHERE disagreement of 1= 1 squared= 1
WHERE disagreement of 2= 2 squared= 4
WHERE disagreement of 2= 3 squared= 9

Step 3 (multiply counts by respective weights)

wfo

	Rater1_Nutt_score_trial1				
Rater2_Nutt_score_trial1	0	1	2	3	
0	0	6	0	0	6
1	0	0	11	0	11
2	0	0	0	7	7
3	0	4	0	0	4

28 Σ*wfo*

wfc

	Rater1_Nutt_score_trial1				
Rater2_Nutt_score_trial1	0	1	2	3	
0	0	4.3	18.8	20.7	43.8
1	3.2	0	5.7	11.2	20.1
2	7.6	3.1	0	1.7	12.4
3	1.8	1.2	0.3	0	3.3

79.6 Σ*wfc*

Step 4 (apply formula eq6_13)

$$kappa\ (w) = 1 - \frac{\Sigma wfo}{\Sigma wfc} = 1-(28/79.6)=0.65$$

5-2b. Weighted kappa (0.65) closely approximates $ICC_{inter\ rater}$ (0.70). There appears to be little bias in the weighting scheme for this demonstration example.

Hypothetical Study #6: Treatment Effect
6-1a.

Outcome Measure Initial Evaluation vs. 1-Month Re-assessment	Unbiased Effect Size
High Compliance	
• Oswestry scale (% disability)	0.70
• Fingertip-floor distance (cm)	0.71
• Maximum isometric lift (lb)	−0.62
Low Compliance	
• Oswestry scale (% disability)	0.18
• Fingertip-floor distance (cm)	0.65
• Maximum isometric lift (lb)	−0.60

6-1b. Maximum isometric lift ESs are negative because higher scores at the 1-month follow-up (improvement) create a negative effect size.

6-2a(i). Yes. Patients in the HIGH compliance group had a statistically significant improvement in Oswestry disability scores. The 95% CI for the high-compliance group is 3 to 17 Oswestry points and does not include the value "0."

Oswestry Scores			
HIGH compliance point estimate of mean change			10
n			28
Standard Error of Oswestry change scores		(Tab A_7)	3.43
critical t (df n−1, α2=0.05)	Tab B_2		2.05
		crit t*SE	7.03
Oswestry points	Upper boundary	point est+(crit t*SE)	17
Oswestry points	Lower boundary	point est−(crit t*SE)	3

6-2a(ii). No. Patients in the LOW compliance group *did not* show a statistically significant improvement in Oswestry disability scores. The 95% CI for the low-compliance group is −3 to 9 Oswestry points and *does* include the value "0."

Oswestry Scores			
LOW compliance point estimate of mean change			3
n			14
Standard Error of Oswestry change scores		(Tab A_7)	2.77
critical t (df n−1, α2=0.05)	Tab B_2		2.15
		crit t*SE	5.96
Oswestry points	Upper boundary	point est+(crit t*SE)	9
Oswestry points	Lower boundary	point est−(crit t*SE)	−3

6-2b. PLOT point estimates of the treatment effect and the 95% CIs (using eq 10-6). Data set up for stock plot in Excel 2007.

	HIGH Compliance			LOW Compliance		
	Oswestry (n=28)	FTFD (n=33)	MAX Lift (n=26)	Oswestry (n=14)	FTFD (n=13)	MAX Lift (n=10)
Upper CI	17.00	20.00	−28.00	9.00	17.00	−19.00
Lower CI	3.00	6.00	−72.00	−3.00	11.00	−61.00
Point est	10.00	13.00	−50.00	3.00	14.00	−40.00

Stock Plot

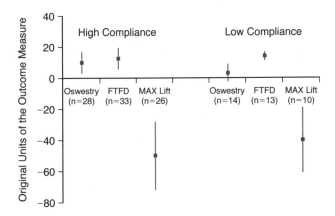

6-2b(i). Only the 95% CI for Oswestry outcome—low-compliance cohort includes the null value of 0.

6-2b(ii). Yes, all outcomes other than the low-compliance Oswestry score have both significant paired t-tests (Table A-5) as well as a 95% CI that does not include the null value of 0.

6-3. A nonrandomized pretest-posttest cohort study is II-B (see Fig. 11-1).

Index

Note: Page numbers followed by "f" and "t" indicate figures and tables, respectively.